D0429212

Women's Health Concerns

SOURCEBOOK

Fifth Edition

Health Reference Series

Fifth Edition

Women's Health Concerns

SOURCEBOOK

Basic Consumer Health Information about Breast and Gynecological Conditions, Menopause, Sexuality and Female Sexual Dysfunction, Birth Control, Infertility, Pregnancy, Common Cancers in Women, Cardiovascular Disease, Mental Health, and Chronic Disorders that Affect Women Disproportionally, Including Gastrointestinal Disorders, Thyroid Disease, Urinary Tract Disorders, Osteoporosis, Chronic Pain, and Migraines

Along with an Introduction to the Female Body, Information on Maintaining Wellness and Avoiding Risk Factors for Disease, a Glossary, and a Directory of Resources for Additional Help and Information

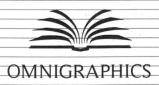

OMNIGRAPHICS
615 Griswold, Ste. 901, Detroit, MI 48226

Library of Congress Cataloging-in-Publication Data

Names: Omnigraphics, Inc., issuing body.

Title: Women's health concerns sourcebook: basic consumer health information
about breast and gynecological conditions, menopause, sexuality and female
sexual dysfunction, birth control, infertility, pregnancy, common cancers in
women, cardiovascular disease, mental health, and chronic disorders that affect
women disproportionally, including gastrointestinal disorders, thyroid disease,
urinary tract disorders, osteoporosis, chronic pain, and migraines; along with an
introduction to the female body, information on maintaining wellness and avoiding
risk factors for disease, a glossary, and a directory of resources for additional help
and information.

Description: Fifth edition. | Detroit, MI: Omnigraphics, [2017] | Series: Health
reference series | Includes bibliographical references and index.

Identifiers: LCCN 2017028219 (print) | LCCN 2017029245 (ebook) | ISBN
9780780815780 (eBook) | ISBN 9780780815773 (hardcover: alk. paper)

Subjects: LCSH: Women--Health and hygiene. | Women--Diseases.

Classification: LCC RA778 (ebook) | LCC RA778.W7543 2017 (print) | DDC
613/.04244--dc23

LC record available at https://lccn.loc.gov/2017028219

Table of Contents

Part III: Breast and Gynecological Concerns

Part V: Gynecological and High-Prevalence Cancers in Women

Part VI: Other Health Conditions with Issues of Significance to Women

Part VII: Additional Help and Information

Preface

About This Book

Statistics indicate that women—on average—live approximately five years longer than men, but this longevity is not linked to better overall health. According to the Health Resources and Services Administration (HRSA), part of the U.S. Department of Health and Human Services (HHS), women experience more physically and mentally unhealthy days than men. Part of this disparity is related to age. Because of their longer life expectancy, women are at greater risk for age-related conditions, like Alzheimer disease. Irrespective of their age, however, women experience gender-related healthcare needs and are more likely than men to have certain conditions, including asthma, arthritis, migraine headaches, osteoporosis, thyroid disorders, chronic pain, and activity limitations.

Women's Health Concerns Sourcebook, Fifth Edition provides updated information about the medical issues of most significance to women. It explains female anatomy and reports on women's health and wellness topics, including vaccination and screening recommendations, fitness and nutrition guidelines, and tips for healthy aging. It also discusses breast health, sexual and reproductive issues, conditions that disproportionately affect women, and the leading causes of death and disability in women, including heart disease, stroke, and diabetes. The book concludes with a glossary of terms related to women's health and a directory of resources for additional information.

How to Use This Book

This book is divided into parts and chapters. Parts focus on broad areas of interest. Chapters are devoted to single topics within a part.

Part I: Introduction to Women's Health provides basic information about female anatomy and physiology, including the reproductive system, menstruation, puberty, and menopause. Statistics related to women's health are included, and special concerns among specific female populations are addressed.

Part II: Maintaining Women's Health and Wellness provides guidelines for pursuing a healthy lifestyle. It includes nutrition and exercise recommendations, facts about obesity and weight management, and tips for handling sleep problems, stress, and common concerns associated with aging. It also discusses ways to prevent or mitigate risk factors for the leading causes of death among women. These tactics include following recommended health screenings, receiving appropriate immunizations, controlling high blood pressure and cholesterol, and avoiding the use of tobacco products.

Part III: Breast and Gynecological Concerns describes female-specific health matters, including breast disorders and changes, menstrual irregularities, and menopause. Disorders of the reproductive organs and pelvic floor are also explained, and the part concludes with information about common gynecological procedures.

Part IV: Sexual and Reproductive Concerns presents information about sexuality and sexual dysfunction from a female perspective. It also looks at topics related to fertility and pregnancy, including birth control methods, infertility treatments, abortion, prenatal and postnatal care, and labor and delivery. Other topics related to maternal health, such as breastfeeding, postpartum depression, and dealing with pregnancy loss, are also addressed.

Part V: Gynecological and High-Prevalence Cancers in Women takes a look at cancers that are of special significance to women. These include cervical, ovarian, uterine, and other cancers of the female reproductive system. Cancers that occur more often in women than in men—such as breast cancer and thyroid cancer—and other cancers that are among those most frequently diagnosed in women—including lung, colon, rectal, and skin cancers—are also discussed.

Part VI: Other Health Conditions with Issues of Significance to Women focuses on disorders with a high or disproportionate incidence among women, including Alzheimer disease, arthritis, autoimmune disorders, migraine headaches, osteoporosis, and thyroid disease. It also looks at the ways in which women experience some common disorders differently from men, and it describes special issues related to women's mental well-being.

Part VII: Additional Help and Information provides resources for readers seeking further assistance. It includes glossary of women's health terms and a directory of organizations related to women's healthcare needs.

Bibliographic Note

This volume contains documents and excerpts from publications issued by the following government agencies: Agency for Healthcare Research and Quality (AHRQ); Centers for Disease Control and Prevention (CDC); *Eunice Kennedy Shriver* National Institute of Child Health and Human Development (NICHD); National Cancer Institute (NCI); National Center for Complementary and Integrative Health (NCCIH); National Heart, Lung, and Blood Institute (NHLBI); National Institute of Arthritis and Musculoskeletal and Skin Diseases (NIAMS); National Institute of Diabetes and Digestive and Kidney Diseases (NIDDK); National Institute of Mental Health (NIMH); National Institute of Neurological Disorders and Stroke (NINDS); National Institute on Aging (NIA); National Institutes of Health (NIH); Office of Dietary Supplements (ODS); Office on Women's Health (OWH); U.S. Department of Agriculture (USDA); U.S. Department of Health and Human Services (HHS); and U.S. Food and Drug Administration (FDA).

It may also contain original material produced by Omnigraphics and reviewed by medical consultants.

About the Health Reference Series

The *Health Reference Series* is designed to provide basic medical information for patients, families, caregivers, and the general public. Each volume takes a particular topic and provides comprehensive coverage. This is especially important for people who may be dealing with a newly diagnosed disease or a chronic disorder in themselves or in a family member. People looking for preventive guidance, information about disease warning signs, medical statistics, and risk factors for health problems will also find answers to their questions in the *Health Reference Series*. The *Series*, however, is not intended to serve as a tool for diagnosing illness, in prescribing treatments, or as a substitute for the physician/patient relationship. All people concerned about medical symptoms or the possibility of disease are encouraged to seek professional care from an appropriate healthcare provider.

A Note about Spelling and Style

Health Reference Series editors use *Stedman's Medical Dictionary* as an authority for questions related to the spelling of medical terms and the *Chicago Manual of Style* for questions related to grammatical structures, punctuation, and other editorial concerns. Consistent adherence is not always possible, however, because the individual volumes within the *Series* include many documents from a wide variety of different producers, and the editor's primary goal is to present material from each source as accurately as is possible. This sometimes means that information in different chapters or sections may follow other guidelines and alternate spelling authorities. For example, occasionally a copyright holder may require that eponymous terms be shown in possessive forms (Crohn's disease vs. Crohn disease) or that British spelling norms be retained (leukaemia vs. leukemia).

Medical Review

Omnigraphics contracts with a team of qualified, senior medical professionals who serve as medical consultants for the *Health Reference Series*. As necessary, medical consultants review reprinted and originally written material for currency and accuracy. Citations including the phrase, "Reviewed (month, year)" indicate material reviewed by this team. Medical consultation services are provided to the *Health Reference Series* editors by:

Dr. Vijayalakshmi, MBBS, DGO, MD
Dr. Senthil Selvan, MBBS, DCH, MD
Dr. K. Sivanandham, MBBS, DCH, MS (Research), PhD

Our Advisory Board

We would like to thank the following board members for providing initial guidance on the development of this series:

- Dr. Lynda Baker, Associate Professor of Library and Information Science, Wayne State University, Detroit, MI

- Nancy Bulgarelli, William Beaumont Hospital Library, Royal Oak, MI

- Karen Imarisio, Bloomfield Township Public Library, Bloomfield Township, MI

- Karen Morgan, Mardigian Library, University of Michigan-Dearborn, Dearborn, MI

- Rosemary Orlando, St. Clair Shores Public Library, St. Clair Shores, MI

Health Reference Series *Update Policy*

The inaugural book in the *Health Reference Series* was the first edition of *Cancer Sourcebook* published in 1989. Since then, the *Series* has been enthusiastically received by librarians and in the medical community. In order to maintain the standard of providing high-quality health information for the layperson the editorial staff at Omnigraphics felt it was necessary to implement a policy of updating volumes when warranted.

Medical researchers have been making tremendous strides, and it is the purpose of the *Health Reference Series* to stay current with the most recent advances. Each decision to update a volume is made on an individual basis. Some of the considerations include how much new information is available and the feedback we receive from people who use the books. If there is a topic you would like to see added to the update list, or an area of medical concern you feel has not been adequately addressed, please write to:

Managing Editor
Health Reference Series
Omnigraphics
615 Griswold, Ste. 901
Detroit, MI 48226

Part One

Introduction to Women's Health

Chapter 1

The Female Body

Chapter Contents

Section 1.1

Breast Anatomy

This section includes text excerpted from "Site-Specific
Modules—Breast Cancer—Breast Anatomy," Surveillance,
Epidemiology and End Results Program (SEER), National
Cancer Institute (NCI), November 17, 2016.

The breasts of an adult woman are milk-producing, tear-shaped
glands. They are supported by and attached to the front of the chest
wall on either side of the breast bone or sternum by ligaments. They
rest on the major chest muscle, the pectoralis major.

The breast has no muscle tissue. A layer of fat surrounds the glands
and extends throughout the breast. The breast is responsive to a complex interplay of hormones that cause the tissue to develop, enlarge,
and produce milk.

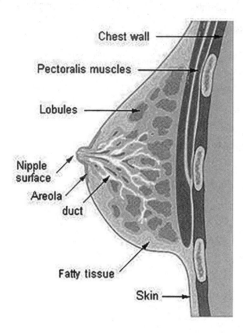

Figure 1.1. *Anatomy of the Breast*

The three major hormones affecting the breast are estrogen, progesterone and prolactin, which cause glandular tissue in the breast and the uterus to change during the menstrual cycle.

Each breast contains 15 to 20 lobes arranged in a circular fashion. The fat (subcutaneous adipose tissue) that covers the lobes gives the breast its size and shape. Each lobe is comprised of many lobules, at the end of which are tiny bulb like glands, or sacs, where milk is produced in response to hormonal signals.

Ducts connect the lobes, lobules, and glands in nursing mothers. These ducts deliver milk to openings in the nipple. The areola is the darker-pigmented area around the nipple.

Section 1.2

The Female Reproductive System

This section contains text excerpted from the following sources:
Text in this section begins with excerpts from "How the Female Reproductive System Works," girlshealth.gov, Office on Women's Health (OWH), May 23, 2014; Text under the heading "Common Reproductive Health Concerns for Women" is excerpted from "Common Reproductive Health Concerns for Women," Centers for Disease Control and Prevention (CDC), November 29, 2016.

The female reproductive system is all the parts of your body that help you reproduce, or have babies. And it is quite amazing! Consider these two fabulous facts:

- Your body likely has hundreds of thousands of eggs that could grow into a baby. And you have them from the time you're born.

- Right inside you, is a perfect place for those eggs to meet with sperm and grow a whole human being!

What's Inside the Female Reproductive System?

The **ovaries** are two small organs. Before puberty, it's as if the ovaries are asleep. During puberty, they "wake up." The ovaries start making more estrogen and other hormones, which cause body changes.

One important body change is that these hormones cause you to start getting your period, which is called menstruating.

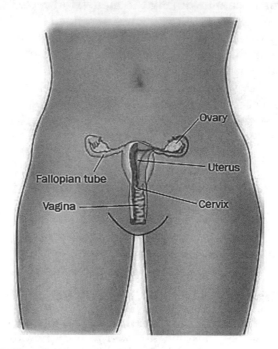

Figure 1.2. *The Female Reproductive System*

(Source: "The Healthy Woman: A Complete Guide for All Ages," Office on Women's Health (OWH), U.S. Department of Health and Human Services (HHS).)

Once a month, the ovaries release one egg (ovum). This is called ovulation.

The **fallopian tubes** connect the ovaries to the uterus. The released egg moves along a fallopian tube.

The **uterus**—or womb—is where a baby would grow. It takes several days for the egg to get to the uterus.

As the egg travels, estrogen makes the lining of the uterus (called the endometrium) thick with blood and fluid. This makes the uterus a good place for a baby to grow. You can get pregnant if you have sex with a male without birth control and his sperm joins the egg (called fertilization) on its way to your uterus.

If the egg doesn't get fertilized, it will be shed along with the lining of your uterus during your next period. But don't look for the egg—it's too small to see!

The blood and fluid that leave your body during your period passes through your cervix and vagina.

The **cervix** is the narrow entryway in between the vagina and uterus. The cervix is flexible so it can expand to let a baby pass through during childbirth.

The **vagina** is like a tube that can grow wider to deliver a baby that has finished growing inside the uterus.

The **hymen** covers the opening of the vagina. It is a thin piece of tissue that has one or more holes in it. Sometimes a hymen may be stretched or torn when you use a tampon or during a first sexual experience. If it does tear, it may bleed a little bit.

What's Outside the Vagina?

The **vulva** covers the entrance to the vagina. The vulva has five parts: mons pubis, labia, clitoris, urinary opening, and vaginal opening.

The **mons pubis** is the mound of tissue and skin above your legs, in the middle. This area becomes covered with hair when you go through puberty.

The **labia** are the two sets of skin folds (often called lips) on either side of the opening of the vagina.

The **labia majora** are the outer lips, and the **labia minora** are the inner lips. It is normal for the labia to look different from each other.

The **clitoris** is a small, sensitive bump at the bottom of the mons pubis that is covered by the labia minora.

The **urinary opening**, below the clitoris, is where your urine (pee) leaves the body.

The **vaginal opening** is the entry to the vagina and is found below the urinary opening.

These are the basics of the fabulous female.

Common Reproductive Health Concerns for Women

Endometriosis

Endometriosis is a problem affecting a woman's uterus—the place where a baby grows when a woman is pregnant. Endometriosis is when the kind of tissue that normally lines the uterus grows somewhere else. It can grow on the ovaries, behind the uterus, on the bowels, or on the bladder. Rarely, it grows in other parts of the body.

This "misplaced" tissue can cause pain, infertility, and very heavy periods. The pain is usually in the abdomen, lower back, or pelvic areas. Some women have no symptoms at all, and having trouble getting pregnant may be the first sign they have endometriosis.

Uterine Fibroids

Uterine fibroids are the most common noncancerous tumors in women of childbearing age. Fibroids are made of muscle cells and other tissues that grow in and around the wall of the uterus, or womb. The cause of fibroids is unknown. Risk factors include being African-American or being overweight. The symptoms of fibroids include:

- Heavy or painful periods or bleeding between periods.

- Feeling "full" in the lower abdomen.

- Urinating often.

- Pain during sex.

- Lower back pain.

- Reproductive problems, such as infertility, multiple miscarriages, or early labor.

But some women will have no symptoms. That is why it is important to see your healthcare provider for routine exams.

Gynecologic Cancer

Gynecologic cancer is any cancer that starts in a woman's reproductive organs. Gynecologic cancers begin in different places within a woman's pelvis, which is the area below the stomach and in between the hip bones.

- Cervical cancer begins in the cervix, which is the lower, narrow end of the uterus.

- Ovarian cancer begins in the ovaries, which are located on each side of the uterus.

- Uterine cancer begins in the uterus, the pear-shaped organ in a woman's pelvis where the baby grows when a woman is pregnant.

- Vaginal cancer begins in the vagina, which is the hollow, tube-like channel between the bottom of the uterus and the outside of the body.

- Vulvar cancer begins in the vulva, the outer part of the female genital organs.

Human Immunodeficiency Virus (HIV) / Acquired Immune Deficiency Syndrome (AIDS)

HIV is the human immunodeficiency virus. HIV affects specific cells of the immune system (called CD4 cells). Over time, HIV can destroy so many of these cells that the body can't fight off infection anymore. The human body cannot get rid of HIV—that means once a person has HIV, he or she has it for life. There is no cure at this time, but with proper medical care, the virus can be controlled. HIV is the virus that can lead to acquired immune deficiency syndrome, or AIDS. AIDS is the late stage of HIV infection, when a person's immune system is severely damaged.

HIV in Women

Women who are infected with HIV typically get it by having sex with a man who is infected or by sharing needles with an infected person. Women of minority races/ethnicities are especially affected, and black or African American women are the most affected group.

Pregnant Women

All pregnant women should know their HIV status. Pregnant women who are HIV-positive can work with their healthcare providers to ensure their babies do not contract HIV during pregnancy, delivery, or after delivery (through breast milk). It is possible for a mother to have HIV and not spread it to her baby, especially if she knows about her HIV status early and works with her healthcare provider to reduce the risk.

Interstitial Cystitis

Interstitial cystitis (IC) is a chronic bladder condition resulting in recurring discomfort or pain in the bladder or surrounding pelvic region. People with IC usually have inflamed or irritated bladder walls that can cause scarring and stiffening of the bladder. IC can affect anyone; however, it is more common in women than men. Some people have some or none of the following symptoms:

- Abdominal or pelvic mild discomfort.
- Frequent urination.
- A feeling of urgency to urinate.
- Feeling of abdominal or pelvic pressure.
- Tenderness.

- Intense pain in the bladder or pelvic region.

- Severe lower abdominal pain that intensifies as the urinary bladder fills or empties.

Polycystic Ovary Syndrome (PCOS)

Polycystic ovary syndrome (PCOS) happens when a woman's ovaries or adrenal glands produce more male hormones than normal. One result is that cysts (fluid-filled sacs) develop on the ovaries. Women who are obese are more likely to have PCOS. Women with PCOS are at increased risk of developing diabetes and heart disease. Symptoms may include:

- Infertility.

- Pelvic pain.

- Excess hair growth on the face, chest, stomach, thumbs, or toes.

- Baldness or thinning hair.

- Acne, oily skin, or dandruff.

- Patches of thickened dark brown or black skin.

Sexually Transmitted Diseases (STDs)

Sexually transmitted diseases (STDs) are infections that you can get from having sex with someone who has the infection. The causes of STDs are bacteria, parasites, and viruses. There are more than 20 types of STDs.

Most STDs affect both women and men, but in many cases the health problems they cause can be more severe for women. If a pregnant woman has an STD, it can cause serious health problems for the baby.

If you have an STD caused by bacteria or parasites, your healthcare provider can treat it with antibiotics or other medicines. If you have an STD caused by a virus, there is no cure, but antiviral medication can help control symptoms. Sometimes medicines can keep the disease under control. Correct usage of latex condoms greatly reduces, but does not completely eliminate, the risk of catching or spreading STDs.

Section 1.3

Menstruation and the Menstrual Cycle

This section includes text excerpted from "Menstruation and the Menstrual Cycle," Office on Women's Health (OWH), U.S. Department of Health and Human Services (HHS), February 6, 2017.

What Is Menstruation?

Menstruation is a woman's monthly bleeding. When you menstruate, your body sheds the lining of the uterus (womb). Menstrual blood flows from the uterus through the small opening in the cervix and passes out of the body through the vagina. Most menstrual periods last from 3 to 5 days.

What Is the Menstrual Cycle?

When periods (menstruations) come regularly, this is called the menstrual cycle. Having regular menstrual cycles is a sign that important parts of your body are working normally. The menstrual cycle provides important body chemicals, called hormones, to keep you healthy. It also prepares your body for pregnancy each month. A cycle is counted from the first day of 1 period to the first day of the next period. The average menstrual cycle is 28 days long. Cycles can range anywhere from 21 to 35 days in adults and from 21 to 45 days in young teens.

The rise and fall of levels of hormones during the month control the menstrual cycle.

What Happens during the Menstrual Cycle?

In the first half of the cycle, levels of estrogen (the "female hormone") start to rise. Estrogen plays an important role in keeping you healthy, especially by helping you to build strong bones and to help keep them strong as you get older. Estrogen also makes the lining of the uterus (womb) grow and thicken. This lining of the womb is a place that will nourish the embryo if a pregnancy occurs. At the same time, the lining of the womb is growing, an egg, or ovum, in one of the ovaries starts to mature. At about day 14 of an average 28-day cycle, the egg leaves the ovary. This is called ovulation.

After the egg has left the ovary, it travels through the fallopian tube to the uterus. Hormone levels rise and help prepare the uterine lining for pregnancy. A woman is most likely to get pregnant during the 3 days before or on the day of ovulation. Keep in mind, women with cycles that are shorter or longer than average may ovulate before or after day 14.

A woman becomes pregnant if the egg is fertilized by a man's sperm cell and attaches to the uterine wall. If the egg is not fertilized, it will break apart. Then, hormone levels drop, and the thickened lining of the uterus is shed during the menstrual period.

What Is a Typical Menstrual Period Like?

During your period, you shed the thickened uterine lining and extra blood through the vagina. Your period may not be the same every month. It may also be different than other women's periods. Periods can be light, moderate, or heavy in terms of how much blood comes out of the vagina. This is called menstrual flow. The length of the period also varies. Most periods last from 3 to 5 days. But, anywhere from 2 to 7 days is normal.

For the first few years after menstruation begins, longer cycles are common. A woman's cycle tends to shorten and become more regular with age. Most of the time, periods will be in the range of 21 to 35 days apart.

What Kinds of Problems Do Women Have with Their Periods?

Women can have a range of problems with their periods, including pain, heavy bleeding, and skipped periods.

- **Amenorrhea**—the lack of a menstrual period. This term is used to describe the absence of a period in:

  - Young women who haven't started menstruating by age 15
  - Women and girls who haven't had a period for 90 days, even if they haven't been menstruating for long

  Causes can include:

  - Pregnancy
  - Breastfeeding

- Extreme weight loss
- Eating disorders
- Excessive exercising
- Stress
- Serious medical conditions in need of treatment

As above, when your menstrual cycles come regularly, this means that important parts of your body are working normally. In some cases, not having menstrual periods can mean that your ovaries have stopped producing normal amounts of estrogen. Missing these hormones can have important effects on your overall health. Hormonal problems, such as those caused by polycystic ovary syndrome (PCOS) or serious problems with the reproductive organs, may be involved. It's important to talk to a doctor if you have this problem.

- **Dysmenorrhea**—painful periods, including severe cramps. Menstrual cramps in teens are caused by too much of a chemical called prostaglandin. Most teens with dysmenorrhea do not have a serious disease, even though the cramps can be severe. In older women, the pain is sometimes caused by a disease or condition such as uterine fibroids or endometriosis.

For some women, using a heating pad or taking a warm bath helps ease their cramps. Some over-the-counter pain medicines can also help with these symptoms.

They include:

- Ibuprofen (for instance, Advil, Motrin, Midol Cramp)
- Ketoprofen (for instance, Orudis KT)
- Naproxen (for instance, Aleve)

If these medicines don't relieve your pain or the pain interferes with work or school, you should see a doctor. Treatment depends on what's causing the problem and how severe it is.

- **Abnormal uterine bleeding**—vaginal bleeding that's different from normal menstrual periods. It includes:

- Bleeding between periods
- Bleeding after sex
- Spotting anytime in the menstrual cycle

13

- Bleeding heavier or for more days than normal
- Bleeding after menopause

Abnormal bleeding can have many causes. Your doctor may start by checking for problems that are most common in your age group. Some of them are not serious and are easy to treat. Others can be more serious. Treatment for abnormal bleeding depends on the cause.

In both teens and women nearing menopause, hormonal changes can cause long periods along with irregular cycles. Even if the cause is hormonal changes, you may be able to get treatment. You should keep in mind that these changes can occur with other serious health problems, such as uterine fibroids, polyps, or even cancer. See your doctor if you have any abnormal bleeding.

When Does a Girl Usually Get Her First Period?

In the United States, the average age for a girl to get her first period is 12. This does not mean that all girls start at the same age. A girl can start her period anytime between the ages of 8 and 15. Most of the time, the first period starts about 2 years after breasts first start to develop. If a girl has not had her first period by age 15, or if it has been more than 2 to 3 years since breast growth started, she should see a doctor.

How Long Does a Woman Have Periods?

Women usually have periods until menopause. Menopause occurs between the ages of 45 and 55, usually around age 50. Menopause means that a woman is no longer ovulating (producing eggs) or having periods and can no longer get pregnant. Like menstruation, menopause can vary from woman to woman and these changes may occur over several years.

The time when your body begins its move into menopause is called the menopausal transition. This can last anywhere from 2 to 8 years. Some women have early menopause because of surgery or other treatment, illness, or other reasons. If you don't have a period for 90 days, you should see your doctor. He or she will check for pregnancy, early menopause, or other health problems that can cause periods to stop or become irregular.

When Should I See a Doctor about My Period?

See your doctor about your period if:

- You have not started menstruating by the age of 15.

- You have not started menstruating within 3 years after breast growth began, or if breasts haven't started to grow by age 13.

- Your period suddenly stops for more than 90 days.

- Your periods become very irregular after having had regular, monthly cycles.

- Your period occurs more often than every 21 days or less often than every 35 days.

- You are bleeding for more than 7 days.

- You are bleeding more heavily than usual or using more than 1 pad or tampon every 1 to 2 hours.

- You bleed between periods.

- You have severe pain during your period.

- You suddenly get a fever and feel sick after using tampons.

How Often Should I Change My Pad and/or Tampon?

You should change a pad before it becomes soaked with blood. Each woman decides for herself what works best. You should change a tampon at least every 4 to 8 hours. Make sure to use the lowest absorbency tampon needed for your flow. For example, use junior or regular tampons on the lightest day of your period. Using a super absorbency tampon on your lightest days increases your risk for toxic shock syndrome (TSS).

TSS is a rare but sometimes deadly disease. TSS is caused by bacteria that can produce toxins. If your body can't fight the toxins, your immune (body defense) system reacts and causes the symptoms of TSS.

Young women may be more likely to get TSS. Using any kind of tampon puts you at greater risk for TSS than using pads. The U.S. Food and Drug Administration (FDA) recommends the following tips to help avoid tampon problems:

- Follow package directions for insertion.

- Choose the lowest absorbency for your flow.

- Change your tampon at least every 4 to 8 hours.

- Consider switching between pads and tampons.

- Know the warning signs of TSS.

- Don't use tampons between periods.

If you have any of these symptoms of TSS while using tampons, take the tampon out, and contact your doctor right away:

- Sudden high fever (over 102 degrees)

- Muscle aches

- Diarrhea

- Vomiting

- Dizziness and/or fainting

- Sunburn-like rash

- Sore throat

- Bloodshot eyes

Section 1.4

Puberty

This section includes text excerpted from "Body—Puberty,"
girlshealth.gov, Office on Women's Health (OWH), April 15, 2014.

Pimples. Growing breasts. Body hair. Moody moments. If any of this sounds familiar, you're likely on the path of puberty. It's a road everyone travels, and it certainly has its bumps. But it's also an amazing time.

Puberty is when you start making the change from being a child to being an adult. And it's when your body develops the ability to have a baby. It all happens thanks to changing hormones, or natural body chemicals.

With everything that's changing, life can feel a little overwhelming. But you can feel more in control if you take good care of your body. Knowing what to expect can help, too, so keep reading. (And don't forget that puberty also involves changes you can't see—like changes to your self-esteem and your feelings.

Timing and Stages of Puberty

Adolescence and puberty can be so confusing! Here's some info on what to expect and when:

- Puberty in girls usually starts between the ages of 8 and 13 and ends by around 14. For boys, puberty usually starts between 10 and 14, and ends by around 15 or 16.

- For girls, one of the first signs of puberty usually is their breasts starting to grow.

- Getting your period (menstruation) usually happens later, around two years after breast growth starts.

- In between, you'll probably start to see more hair in places like under your arms and in your pubic area.

- Puberty involves big changes to your shape, including getting taller (which stops when puberty ends).

Of course, it can be hard to have your body change at a slower or faster rate than your friends' bodies. If how fast or slow your body is changing is upsetting you, talk to an adult you trust.

If you're developing slower or faster than you think you should, your body may just be changing at its own natural rate. It's a good idea to let your doctor know if you start puberty before age 8. Also let your doctor know if you don't have any signs of puberty by the time you're 14. Your doctor can check whether a medical problem is involved.

Changes to Your Shape

How your body looks changes a lot during puberty. For one, usually between the ages of 9 and 13, girls grow much faster than they had been growing. This process, called a growth spurt, happens later for boys. That explains why you may be taller than the boys in your grade for a while.

You likely will also see lots of other changes in your body during puberty.

Changes in Your Body during Puberty

These are some of the changes you can expect during puberty:

- A curvier shape
- Wider hips, thighs, and bottom
- Normal weight gain as your body structure grows
- Stretch marks, or little scars, where your skin was pulled from growing fast (but that usually fade over time)

You'll also see more body hair, changes to your breasts, and possibly some acne.

Keep in mind that these changes all are common and normal! And make sure to take good care of your great, growing body. With everything that's going on, it's important to eat well, stay fit, and get enough sleep.

Your Feelings about Your Changing Body

During puberty your body may seem very different from what you're used to, and you might feel uncomfortable or shy about it. Remember that everyone goes through these changes—it's just part of life—and every girl grows at her own pace.

During puberty, it's common to struggle with body image, or how you feel about your body. This can be especially hard when models in magazines have bodies that seem "perfect." But a lot of what you see in magazines and online is either fake or unhealthy.

If you think you or a friend may have a problem with body image or an eating disorder, talk to a parent, a doctor, or another adult you trust. Help is available, and it's important to get treated. You can get better!

Remember, measure yourself by your great traits and loving heart—not by the size and shape of your body!

Changes to Your Breasts

It's natural for girls to wonder about their breasts: Are they too big? Too small? If your breasts are large, they may get you unwanted attention. If they're small, you may worry that they'll never grow. Remember that your breasts don't need to look like your friend's breasts or a magazine model's breasts. The world would be boring if everyone looked the same!

Here's some more info on your changing breasts.

What Happens to Breasts during Puberty?

Throughout puberty, you will experience changes in your breasts. The first change is developing a very small bump under the nipple. Early on, you may also notice that your breasts feel a little itchy or achy. Later on, they also may feel tender or sore during your period.

Keep in mind that it is very common for your two breasts to be different sizes, especially as they first start to grow. Other people can't tell that your breasts are different sizes. Give your body time to grow at its own rate and in its own way. Vitamins, herbal teas, and creams—even exercises—won't change the size of your breasts.

What about Lumps and Other Changes?

Most of the changes your breasts will go through are normal. Let your doctor know if you find a lump or have a pain that you are not sure about. Although lumps are common in young women, keep in mind that it is very rare for the lumps to be cancer.

Should I Wear a Bra?

Wearing a bra can help support and protect your breasts. If you find that exercise is not as comfortable when your breasts start to grow, try wearing a sports bra with a snug fit for support.

Are you having a hard time finding a bra that fits well? Often, you can get help in a department store or special bra store. There are certain steps people there can take for measuring your body to get a good fit.

Body Hair

Even before you get your first period, you will likely see new hair growing in your pubic area, under your arms, and on your legs. The hair may start out light and there won't be a lot of it, but then it will grow darker and thicker as you go through the stages of puberty. Hair in the pubic area starts near the opening and spreads up in a V shape over time.

Body hair is normal, and some people think it looks cool. Lots of women and girls remove body hair from places such as their legs and underarms, although there is no real health reason to do so.

If you are thinking about removing hair for the first time, it makes sense to talk to your parents or guardians. They may have an opinion about how old you should be to start removing hair or advice on ways to do it.

Removing body hair can cause skin irritation, cuts, and other problems. Some parts of your body, like areas around your eyes and vagina, can be especially sensitive. Also, if you have a lot of hair on your face, it could be a sign of a medical condition called PCOS.

Changes in Your Mind

During puberty, changes don't happen only to your body—changes happen in your mind, too.

- You are able to understand more complex matters.
- You are starting to make more of your own moral choices.
- You know more about who you are, and what your likes and dislikes are.
- You may have some new, strong emotions.

The teen years can seem like an emotional roller coaster, with worries about your changing looks, the demands of school, and pressure to fit in. You might feel alone on this ride, but everyone struggles with it. And some of your experiences have to do with the physical changes of this age, including shifts in your hormones and a brain that's developing just like your body is.

A New You

Even though this can be a stressful time, it's also a great chance to figure out who you are, what you care about, and how to value and respect the person you're becoming!

If you're feeling overwhelmed by some of the changes you're going through, talking can help. Don't be afraid to go to a parent, school counselor, or other adult you trust. They were young once, too!

Section 1.5

Perimenopause and Menopause

This section includes text excerpted from documents published by two public domain sources. Text under headings marked 1 are excerpted from "Menopause," National Institute on Aging (NIA), National Institutes of Health (NIH), July 23, 2017; Text under heading marked 2 is excerpted from "Menopause Basics," Office on Women's Health (OWH), U.S. Department of Health and Human Services (HHS), September 22, 2010. Reviewed August 2017.

What Is Menopause?[1]

Menopause is a normal part of life, just like puberty. It is the time of your last menstrual period. You may notice changes in your body before and after menopause. The transition usually has three parts: *perimenopause, menopause,* and *postmenopause.*

Changes usually begin with perimenopause. This can begin several years before your last menstrual period. Changing levels of estrogen and progesterone, which are two female hormones made in your ovaries, might lead to symptoms. Menopause comes next, the end of your menstrual periods. After a full year without a period, you can say you have been "through menopause," and perimenopause is over. Postmenopause follows perimenopause and lasts the rest of your life.

The average age of a woman having her last period, menopause, is 51. But, some women have their last period in their forties, and some have it later in their fifties.

Smoking can lead to early menopause. So, can some types of operations. For example, surgery to remove your uterus (called a hysterectomy) will make your periods stop, and that's menopause. But you might not have menopause symptoms like hot flashes right then because if your ovaries are untouched, they still make hormones. In time, when your ovaries start to make less estrogen, menopause symptoms could start. But, sometimes both ovaries are removed (called an oophorectomy), usually along with your uterus. In this case, menopause symptoms can start right away, no matter what age you are, because your body has lost its main supply of estrogen.

What Is Perimenopause?[2]

- Perimenopause, or the menopausal transition, is the time leading up to a woman's last period. Periods can stop and then start again, so you are in perimenopause until a year has passed since you've had a period. During perimenopause a woman will have changes in her levels of estrogen and progesterone, two female hormones made in the ovaries. These changes may lead to symptoms like hot flashes. Some symptoms can last for months or years after a woman's period stops.

- There is no way to tell in advance how long it will take you to go through the menopausal transition. It could take between two and eight years.

- Sometimes it's hard to tell if you are in the menopausal transition. Symptoms, a physical exam, and your medical history may provide clues to you and your doctor. Your doctor also could test the amount of hormones in your blood. But because hormones change during your menstrual cycle, these tests alone can't tell for sure that you have gone through menopause or are getting close to it. Unless there is a medical reason to test, doctors usually don't recommend it.

What Are the Signs of Menopause?[1]

Women may have different signs or symptoms at menopause. That's because estrogen is used by many parts of your body. As you have less estrogen, you could have various symptoms. Here are the most common changes you might notice at midlife. Some may be part of aging rather than directly related to menopause.

Change in your period. This might be what you notice first. Your periods may no longer be regular. They may be shorter or last longer. You might bleed less than usual or more. These are all normal changes, but to make sure there isn't a problem, see your doctor if:

- Your periods come very close together

- You have heavy bleeding

- You have spotting

- Your periods last more than a week

- Your periods resume after no bleeding for more than a year

Hot flashes. Many women have hot flashes, which can last a few years after menopause. They may be related to changing estrogen levels. A hot flash is a sudden feeling of heat in the upper part or all of your body. Your face and neck become flushed. Red blotches may appear on your chest, back, and arms. Heavy sweating and cold shivering can follow. Flashes can be very mild or strong enough to wake you from your sleep (called night sweats). Most hot flashes last between 30 seconds and 10 minutes.

Vaginal health and bladder control. Your vagina may get drier. This could make sexual intercourse uncomfortable. Or, you could have other health problems, such as vaginal or bladder infections. Some women also find it hard to hold their urine long enough to get to the bathroom. This loss of bladder control is called incontinence. You may have a sudden urge to urinate, or urine may leak during exercise, sneezing, or laughing.

Sleep. Around midlife, some women start having trouble getting a good night's sleep. Maybe you can't fall asleep easily, or you wake too early. Night sweats might wake you up. You might have trouble falling back to sleep if you wake up during the night.

Sex. You may find that your feelings about sex are changing. You could be less interested. Or, you could feel freer and sexier after menopause. After 1 full year without a period, you can no longer become pregnant. But remember, you could still be at risk for sexually transmitted diseases (STDs), such as gonorrhea or even human immunodeficiency virus (HIV) infection/acquired immune deficiency syndrome (AIDS). You increase your risk for an STD if you are having sex with more than one person or with someone who is having sex with others. If so, make sure your partner uses a condom each time you have sex.

Mood changes. You might find yourself more moody or irritable around the time of menopause. Scientists don't know why this happens. It's possible that stress, family changes such as growing children or aging parents, a history of depression, or feeling tired could be causing these mood changes.

Your body seems different. Your waist could get larger. You could lose muscle and gain fat. Your skin could get thinner. You might have memory problems, and your joints and muscles could feel stiff and achy. Are these a result of having less estrogen or just related to growing older? Experts don't know the answer.

23

In addition, in some women, symptoms may include aches and pains, headaches, and heart palpitations. Since menopausal symptoms may be caused by changing hormone levels, it is unpredictable how often women will have hot flashes and other symptoms and how severe they will be. Talk with your doctor if these symptoms are interfering with your everyday life. The severity of symptoms varies greatly around the world and by race and ethnicity.

How Can I Stay Healthy after Menopause?[1]

Staying healthy after menopause may mean making some changes in the way you live.

- **Don't smoke.** If you do use any type of tobacco, stop—it's never too late to benefit from quitting smoking.

- **Eat a healthy diet**, low in fat, high in fiber, with plenty of fruits, vegetables, and whole-grain foods, as well as all the important vitamins and minerals.

- **Make sure you get enough calcium and vitamin D**—in your diet or with vitamin/mineral supplements if recommended by your doctor.

- **Learn what your healthy weight is**, and try to stay there.

- **Do weight-bearing exercise**, such as walking, jogging, or dancing, at least 3 days each week for healthy bones. But try to be physically active in other ways for your general health.

Other things to remember:

- **Take medicine** if your doctor prescribes it for you, especially if it is for health problems you cannot see or feel—for example, high blood pressure, high cholesterol, or osteoporosis.

- **Use a water-based vaginal lubricant** (not petroleum jelly) or a vaginal estrogen cream or tablet to help with vaginal discomfort.

- **Get regular pelvic and breast exams, Pap tests, and mammograms.** You should also be checked for colon and rectal cancer and for skin cancer. Contact your doctor right away if you notice a lump in your breast or a mole that has changed.

Menopause is not a disease that has to be treated. But you might need help if symptoms like hot flashes bother you. Here are some ideas that have helped some women:

- Try to keep track of when hot flashes happen—a diary can help. You might be able to use this information to find out what triggers your flashes and then avoid those triggers.

- When a hot flash starts, try to go somewhere cool.

- If night sweats wake you, sleep in a cool room or with a fan on.

- Dress in layers that you can take off if you get too warm.

- Use sheets and clothing that let your skin "breathe."

- Have a cold drink (water or juice) when a flash is starting.

You could also talk to your doctor about whether there are any medicines to manage hot flashes. A few drugs that are approved for other uses (for example, certain antidepressants) seem to be helpful to some women.

Few Frequently Asked Questions on Menopause[1]

What's the Average Age of Menopause?

The average age of menopause is 51.

How Do I Know if I Am Starting Menopause?

The first thing many women notice, is a change in their periods.

Can I Get Pregnant after Menopause?

Even though your monthly periods are not regular anymore, you can get pregnant during the menopausal transition.

What Can I Do about Hot Flashes after Menopause?

There are some practical steps you can try to ease hot flashes and/or night sweats:

- Sleep in a cool room.

- Dress in layers, which can be removed at the start of a hot flash.

- Have a drink of cold water or juice when you feel a hot flash coming on.

- Use sheets and clothing that let your skin "breathe."

- Don't smoke.

- Talk to your doctor. Symptoms that might seem like menopause, even hot flashes, night sweats, and irregular periods, may have other causes.

Can I Have Periods after Menopause?

No, menopause is your final menstrual period.

Chapter 2

Women's Health Statistics

Heart Disease among Women

Heart disease is the leading cause of death for women in the United States, killing 289,758 women in 2013—that's about 1 in every 4 female deaths.

Although heart disease is sometimes thought of as a "man's disease," around the same number of women and men die each year of heart disease in the United States. Despite increases in awareness

This chapter contains text excerpted from the following sources: Text under the heading "Heart Disease among Women" is excerpted from "Women and Heart Disease Fact Sheet," Centers for Disease Control and Prevention (CDC), June 16, 2016; Text under the heading "Cancer among Women" is excerpted from "Cancer among Women," Centers for Disease Control and Prevention (CDC), June 5, 2017; Text under the heading "HIV among Women" is excerpted from "HIV among Women," Centers for Disease Control and Prevention (CDC), March 10, 2017; Text under the heading "Leading Causes of Death (LCOD) in Females" is excerpted from "Leading Causes of Death (LCOD) in Females United States, 2014," Centers for Disease Control and Prevention (CDC), January 11, 2017; Text under the heading "Pregnancy-Related Deaths" is excerpted from "Maternal Health," Centers for Disease Control and Prevention (CDC), June 18, 2016; Text under the heading "Drinking Levels among Women" is excerpted from "Excessive Alcohol Use and Risks to Women's Health," Centers for Disease Control and Prevention (CDC), March 7, 2016; Text under the heading "Health Statistics of Women" is excerpted from "Women's Health," Centers for Disease Control and Prevention (CDC), January 19, 2017.

over the past decade, only 54 percent of women recognize that heart disease is their number 1 killer.

Heart disease is the leading cause of death for African American and white women in the United States. Among Hispanic women, heart disease and cancer cause roughly the same number of deaths each year. For American Indian or Alaska Native and Asian or Pacific Islander women, heart disease is second only to cancer.

About 5.8 percent of all white women, 7.6 percent of black women, and 5.6 percent of Mexican American women have coronary heart disease.

Almost two-thirds (64%) of women who die suddenly of coronary heart disease have no previous symptoms. Even if you have no symptoms, you may still be at risk for heart disease.

Cancer among Women

Three Most Common Cancers among Women

1. **Breast cancer (123.9)**

   First among women of all races and Hispanic origin populations.

2. **Lung cancer (50.8)**

   - Second among white, black, Asian/Pacific Islander, and American Indian/Alaska Native women.

   - Third among Hispanic women.

3. **Colorectal cancer (32.8)**

   - Second among Hispanic women.

   - Third among white, black, Asian/Pacific Islander, and American Indian/Alaska Native women.

Leading Causes of Cancer Death among Women

1. **Lung cancer (34.7)**

   - First among white, black, Asian/Pacific Islander, and American Indian/Alaska Native women.

   - Second among Hispanic women.

2. **Breast cancer (20.5)**

   - First among Hispanic women.

- Second among white, black, Asian/Pacific Islander, and American Indian/Alaska Native women.

3. **Colorectal cancer (11.9)**

   Third among women of all races and Hispanic origin populations.

Note: The numbers in parentheses are the rates per 100,000 women of all races and Hispanic origins combined in the United States.

HIV among Women

Though HIV diagnoses among women have declined sharply in recent years, more than 7,000 women received an HIV diagnosis in 2015. Black/African American women are disproportionately affected by HIV, compared with women of other races/ethnicities. Of the total number of women living with diagnosed HIV at the end of 2014, 60 percent (139,058) were African American, 17 percent (39,343) were white, and 17 percent (40,252) were Hispanic/Latina.

The Numbers

HIV and AIDS Diagnoses

- Women made up 19 percent (7,402) of the 39,513 new HIV diagnoses in the United States in 2015.

- Overall, 86 percent (6,391) of HIV diagnoses among women were attributed to heterosexual sex, and 13 percent (980) were attributed to injection drug use. But among white women, 32 percent of HIV diagnoses were attributed to injection drug use.

- Among all women with HIV diagnosed in 2015, 61 percent (4,524) were African American, 19 percent (1,431) were white, and 15 percent (1,131) were Hispanic/Latina.

- Annual HIV diagnoses declined 20 percent among women from 2010 to 2014. They declined 24 percent among African American women, 16 percent among Hispanic/Latina women, and 9 percent among white women.

- Women accounted for 24 percent (4,459) of the 18,303 AIDS diagnoses in 2015 and represent 20 percent (248,270) of the 1,216,917 cumulative AIDS diagnoses in the United States from the beginning of the epidemic through the end of 2015.

Living with HIV and Deaths

- An estimated 287,400 women were living with HIV at the end of 2013, representing 23 percent of all Americans living with the virus. Of women living with HIV, around 11 percent do not know they are infected.

- Of women diagnosed with HIV in 2014, 76 percent were linked to HIV medical care within 1 month.

- Of women diagnosed with HIV in 2012 or earlier, 57 percent were retained in care (receiving continuous HIV medical care) at the end of 2013, and 52 percent had achieved viral suppression.

- In 2014, 1,783 women died from HIV or AIDS.

Leading Causes of Death (LCOD) in Females

Below are the leading causes of death in females for 2014.

Table 2.1. Leading Causes of Death (LCOD) in Females for 2014[*]

Rank	All Races	Hispanic	White	Black	American Indian/ Alaska Native	Asian/Pacific Islander
1	Heart disease (22.3%)	Cancer (22.6%)	Heart disease 22.3%)	Heart disease (23.2%)	Cancer (17.4%)	Cancer (27.3%)
2	Cancer (21.6%)	Heart disease (19.7%)	Cancer (21.4%)	Cancer (22.5%)	Heart disease (16.8%)	Heart disease (20.0%)
3	Chronic lower respiratory diseases (6.0%)	Stroke (6.0%)	Chronic lower respiratory diseases (6.5%)	Stroke (6.2%)	Unintentional injuries (8.1%)	Stroke (8.1%)
4	Stroke (6.0%)	Diabetes (4.7%)	Stroke (5.9%)	Diabetes (4.6%)	Chronic liver disease (5.7%)	Alzheimer disease (3.9%)
5	Alzheimer disease (5.0%)	Unintentional injuries (4.5%)	Alzheimer disease (5.3%)	Chronic lower respiratory diseases (3.2%)	Diabetes (5.4%)	Diabetes (3.8%)
6	Unintentional injuries (3.9%)	Alzheimer disease (4.3%)	Unintentional injuries (4.0%)	Alzheimer disease (3.1%)	Chronic lower respiratory diseases (5.2%)	Unintentional injuries (3.3%)
7	Diabetes (2.7%)	Chronic lower respiratory diseases (3.1%)	Diabetes (2.4%)	Unintentional injuries (3.0%)	Stroke (4.3%)	Influenza and pneumonia (3.0%)

Table 2.1. Continued

Rank	All Races	Hispanic	White	Black	American Indian/ Alaska Native	Asian/Pacific Islander
8	Influenza and pneumonia (2.2%)	Influenza and pneumonia (2.5%)	Influenza and pneumonia (2.2%)	Kidney disease (3.0%)	Alzheimer disease (2.7%)	Chronic lower respiratory diseases (2.6%)
9	Kidney disease (1.8%)	Chronic liver disease (2.3%)	Kidney disease (1.7%)	Septicemia (2.3%)	Influenza and pneumonia (2.7%)	Kidney disease (2.0%)
10	Septicemia (1.6%)	Kidney disease (2.0%)	Septicemia (1.5%)	Hypertension (1.9%)	Kidney disease (2.1%)	Hypertension (1.9%)

Percentages represent total deaths in the age group due to the cause indicated. Rankings are based on number of deaths. The white, black, American Indian/Alaska Native, and Asian/Pacific Islander race groups include persons of Hispanic and non-Hispanic origin. Persons of Hispanic origin may be of any race. Some terms have been shortened from those used in the National Vital Statistics Report.

Pregnancy-Related Deaths

Despite advances in medicine and medical technologies, the rate of pregnancy-related deaths in the United States has increased over the past 25 years. However, recent data show that this trend may be leveling off.

One in four pregnancy-related deaths are related to heart conditions. Women also die of infections (including flu), bleeding, blood clots, and high blood pressure. Although the risk of dying of pregnancy complications is low, some women are at higher risk than others.

- African American women are 3 to 4 times more likely to die of pregnancy complications than white women.

- Women aged 35 to 39 are almost twice as likely to die of pregnancy complications as women aged 20 to 24. The risk becomes even higher for women aged 40 or older

Drinking Levels among Women

- Approximately 46 percent of adult women report drinking alcohol in the last 30 days.

- Approximately 12 percent of adult women report binge drinking 3 times a month, averaging 5 drinks per binge.

- Most (90%) people who binge drink are not alcoholics or alcohol dependent.

- About 2.5 percent of women and 4.5 percent of men met the diagnostic criteria for alcohol dependence in the past year.

- About 10 percent of pregnant women drink alcohol.

- National surveys show that about 1 in 2 women of child-bearing age (i.e., aged 18–44 years) drink alcohol, and 18 percent of women who drink alcohol in this age group binge drink.

Health Statistics of Women

Health Status

Percent of women 18 years and over in fair or poor health: 13.3 percent

Alcohol Use

Percent of women 18 years and over who had four or more drinks in 1 day at least once in the past year: 18.9%

Physical Activity

Percent of women 18 years and over who met the 2008 federal physical activity guidelines for aerobic activity through leisure-time aerobic activity: 48.1%

Smoking

Percent of women 18 years and over who currently smoke cigarettes: 13.9%

Obesity

Percent of women 20 years and over who are obese: 38.5 percent (2011–2014)

Hypertension

Percent of women 20 years and over with hypertension (measured high blood pressure and/or taking antihypertensive medication): 33.4 percent (2011–2014)

Health Insurance Coverage

Percent of females under 65 years without health insurance coverage: 9.1%

Mortality

- Number of deaths (all ages): 1,298,177
- Deaths per 100,000 population: 892.9

Chapter 3

Health Concerns of Women with Disabilities

Women with Disabilities

About 27 million women in the United States have disabilities and the number is growing. More than 50 percent of women older than 65 are living with a disability. The most common cause of disability for women is arthritis or rheumatism.

Women with disabilities may need specialty care to address their individual needs. In addition, they need the same general healthcare as women without disabilities, and they may also need additional care to address their specific needs. However, research has shown that many women with disabilities may not receive regular health screenings within recommended guidelines.

Breast Cancer Screening: The Right to Know

Breast cancer is a major public health concern for all women, including women with disabilities. Women who have disabilities are just as likely as women without disabilities to have ever received a

This chapter contains text excerpted from the following sources: Text under the heading "Women with Disabilities" is excerpted from "Women with Disabilities," Centers for Disease Control and Prevention (CDC), March 8, 2016; Text beginning the heading "Healthy Living" is excerpted from "People with Disabilities," Centers for Disease Control and Prevention (CDC), March 17, 2016.

mammogram. However, they are significantly less likely to have been screened within the recommended guidelines.

Cervical Cancer Screening

Cervical cancer is the easiest female cancer to prevent, with regular screening tests and follow-up. It also is highly curable when found and treated early. All women are at risk for cervical cancer, including women with disabilities. It occurs most often in women over age 30. It is important to get tested for cervical cancer because 6 out of 10 cervical cancers occur in women who have never received a Pap test or have not been tested in the past five years.

Intimate Partner Violence (IPV)

Each year, women experience about 4.8 million intimate partner related physical assaults and rapes. Research has shown that women with a disability are more likely to experience IPV than those without a disability. In fact, researchers found that 37.3 percent of women with a disability were much more likely to report experiencing some form of IPV during their lifetime; this compared with 20.6 percent of women without a disability.

Healthy Living

Women with disabilities need healthcare and health programs for the same reasons anyone else does—to stay well, active, and a part of the community.

Having a disability does not mean a person is not healthy or that she cannot be healthy. Being healthy means the same thing for all of us—getting and staying well so we can lead full, active lives. That means having the tools and information to make healthy choices and knowing how to prevent illness.

Safety

Women with disabilities can be at higher risk for injuries and abuse. It is important for parents and other family members to teach their loved one how to stay safe and what to do if they feel threatened or have been hurt in any way.

Assistive Technology (AT)

Assistive technologies (ATs) are devices or equipment that can be used to help a person with a disability fully engage in life activities.

ATs can help enhance functional independence and make daily living tasks easier through the use of aids that help a person travel, communicate with others, learn, work, and participate in social and recreational activities. An example of an assistive technology can be anything from a low-tech device, such as a magnifying glass, to a high tech device, such as a special computer that talks and helps someone communicate. Other examples are wheelchairs, walkers, and scooters, which are mobility aids that can be used by persons with physical disabilities.

Independent Living

Independent living means that a person lives in her own apartment or house and needs limited or no help from outside agencies. The person may not need any assistance or might need help with only complex issues such as managing money, rather than day-to-day living skills. Whether an adult with disabilities continues to live at home or moves out into the community depends in large part on her ability to manage everyday tasks with little or no help. For example, can the person clean the house, cook, shop, and pay bills? Is she able to use public transportation? Many families prefer to start with some supported living arrangements and move towards increased independence.

Finding Support

For many women with disabilities and those who care for them, daily life may not be easy. Disabilities affect the entire family. Meeting the complex needs of a person with a disability can put families under a great deal of stress—emotional, financial, and sometimes even physical.

However, finding resources, knowing what to expect, and planning for the future can greatly improve overall quality of life. If you have a disability or care for someone who does, it might be helpful to talk with other people who can relate to your experience.

Find a Support Network

- By finding support within your community, you can learn more about resources available to meet the needs of families and people with disabilities. This can help increase confidence, enhance quality of life, and assist in meeting the needs of family members.

- A national organization that focuses on the disability, such as Spina Bifida Association, that has a state or local branch, such as Spina Bifida Association in your state, might exist. State or local area Centers for Independent Living could also be helpful. United Way offices may be able to point out resources. Look in the phone book or on the web for phone numbers and addresses.

- Other ways to connect with other people include camps, organized activities, and sports for people with disabilities. In addition, there are online support groups and networks for people with many different types of disabilities.

Talk with a Mental Health Professional

- Psychologists, social workers, and counselors can help you deal with the challenges of living with or caring for someone with a disability. Talk to your primary care physician for a referral.

Chapter 4

Lesbian and Bisexual Health Concerns

All women have specific health risks, and can take steps to improve their health through regular medical care and healthy living. Research tells us that lesbian and bisexual women are at a higher risk for certain problems than other women are, though. It is important for lesbian and bisexual women to talk to their doctors about their health concerns.

What Does It Mean to Be a Lesbian?

A lesbian is a woman who is sexually attracted to another woman or who has sex with another woman, even if it is only sometimes. A lesbian is currently only having sex with a woman, even if she has had sex with men in the past.

What Does It Mean to Be Bisexual?

A bisexual person is sexually attracted to, or sexually active with, both women and men.

This chapter includes text excerpted from "Lesbian and Bisexual Health," Office on Women's Health (OWH), U.S. Department of Health and Human Services (HHS), June 12, 2017.

What Are Important Health Issues That Lesbians and Bisexual Women Should Discuss with Their Healthcare Professionals?

All women have specific health risks, and can take steps to improve their health through regular medical care and healthy living. Research tells us that lesbian and bisexual women are at a higher risk for certain problems than other women are, though. It is important for lesbian and bisexual women to talk to their doctors about their health concerns, which include:

Heart disease. Heart disease is the No. 1 killer of all women. The more risk factors you have, the greater the chance that you will develop heart disease. There are some risk factors that you cannot control, such as age, family health history, and race. But you can protect yourself from heart disease by not smoking, controlling your blood pressure and cholesterol, exercising, and eating well. These things also help prevent type 2 diabetes, a leading cause of heart disease.

Lesbians and bisexual women have a higher rate of obesity, smoking, and stress. All of these are risk factors for heart disease. As such, lesbians and bisexual women should talk with their doctors about how to prevent heart disease.

Cancer. The most common cancers for all women are breast, lung, colon, uterine, and ovarian. Several factors put lesbian and bisexual women at higher risk for developing some cancers.

Remember:

- Lesbians are less likely than heterosexual women to have had a full-term pregnancy. Hormones released during pregnancy and breastfeeding are thought to protect women against breast, endometrial, and ovarian cancers.

- Lesbians and bisexual women are less likely to get routine screenings, such as a Pap test, which can prevent or detect cervical cancer. The viruses that cause most cervical cancer can be sexually transmitted between women. Bisexual women, who may be less likely than lesbians to have health insurance, are even more likely to skip these tests.

- Lesbians and bisexual women are less likely than other women to get routine mammograms and clinical breast exams. This may be due to lesbians' and bisexuals' lack of health insurance, fear of discrimination, or bad experiences with healthcare professionals. Failure to get these tests lowers women's chances of catching cancer early enough for treatments to work.

- Lesbians are more likely to smoke than heterosexual women are, and bisexual women are the most likely to smoke. This increases the risk for lung cancer in all women who have sex with women.

Depression and anxiety. Many factors cause depression and anxiety among all women. However, lesbian and bisexual women report higher rates of depression and anxiety than other women do. Bisexual women are even more likely than lesbians to have had a mood or anxiety disorder. Depression and anxiety in lesbian and bisexual women may be due to:

- Social stigma
- Rejection by family members
- Abuse and violence
- Unfair treatment in the legal system
- Stress from hiding some or all parts of one's life
- Lack of health insurance

Lesbians and bisexuals often feel they have to hide their sexual orientation from family, friends, and employers. Bisexual women may feel even more alone because they don't feel included in either the heterosexual community or the gay and lesbian community. Lesbians and bisexuals can also be victims of hate crimes and violence. Discrimination against these groups does exist, and can lead to depression and anxiety. Women can reach out to their doctors, mental health professionals, and area support groups for help dealing with depression or anxiety. These conditions are treatable, and with help, women can overcome them.

Polycystic ovary syndrome (PCOS). PCOS is the most common hormonal problem of the reproductive system in women of childbearing age. PCOS is a health problem that can affect a woman's:

- Menstrual cycle (monthly bleeding)
- Fertility (ability to get pregnant)
- Hormones
- Insulin production
- Heart

- Blood vessels

- Appearance

Five to 10 percent of women of childbearing age have PCOS. Lesbians may have a higher rate of PCOS than heterosexual women.

What Factors Put Lesbians' and Bisexual Women's Health at Risk?

There are a lot of things that can cause health problems for lesbians and bisexual women. Some of these may be outside of your control. Other things you can work to improve upon. These include:

Lack of fitness. Being obese and not exercising can raise your risk of heart disease, some cancers, and early death. Many studies show that lesbians and bisexual women have a higher body mass index (BMI) than other women. Studies suggest that lesbians may store more of their fat in the abdomen (stomach area). Belly fat increases the risk for heart disease and type 2 diabetes. Some studies also suggest that lesbians think less about weight issues than heterosexual women do.

Research shows that lesbian and bisexual women are more likely to have a higher BMI if they:

- Are African American or Latina

- Are older

- Have poor health

- Have a lower level of education

- Don't exercise often

- Live with a female partner

Smoking. Smoking can lead to heart disease and cancers of the lung, throat, stomach, colon, and cervix. The group of women most likely to smoke is bisexual women. Lesbians are also more likely to smoke than heterosexual women are. Researchers think that higher rates of smoking among lesbians and bisexual women are due to:

- Tobacco ads aimed at gays and lesbians

- Differences in community norms

- Low self-esteem

- Stress from bias

- Anxiety from hiding one's sexual orientation

Alcohol and drug abuse. Substance abuse is a serious health problem for all people in the United States. Recent data suggests that substance use among lesbians—mostly alcohol use—has gone down over the past two decades. Reasons for this may include:

- More general knowledge and concern about health

- More moderate drinking among women in general

- Some decrease in the social stigma and oppression of lesbians

- Changing norms around drinking in some lesbian groups

But, heavy drinking and drug abuse appear to be more common among lesbians (especially young women) than heterosexual women. Lesbian and bisexual women are also more likely to drink alcohol and smoke marijuana in moderation than other women are. Bisexual women are the most likely to have injected drugs, putting them at a higher risk for sexually transmitted infections (STIs).

Domestic violence. Also called intimate partner violence, this is when someone purposely causes either physical or mental harm to someone else. Domestic violence can occur in lesbian relationships (as it does in heterosexual ones). But, lesbian victims are more likely to stay silent about the violence. Some reasons include:

- Fewer services available to help lesbians and bisexual women

- Fear of discrimination

- Threats from the batterer to "out" the victim

- Fear of losing custody of children

There are many resources available to women who are victims of domestic violence. All women should seek help and safety from domestic violence.

Are Lesbian and Bisexual Women at Risk of Getting Sexually Transmitted Infections (STIs)?

Women who have sex with women are at risk for STIs. Lesbian and bisexual women can transmit STIs to each other through:

- Skin-to-skin contact

- Mucosa contact (e.g., mouth to vagina)
- Vaginal fluids
- Menstrual blood
- Sharing sex toys

Some STIs are more common among lesbians and bisexual women and may be passed easily from woman to woman (such as bacterial vaginosis). Other STIs are much less likely to be passed from woman to woman through sex (such as human immunodeficiency virus). When lesbians get these less common STIs, it may be because they also have had sex with men, especially when they were younger. It is also important to remember that some of the less common STIs may not be passed between women during sex, but through sharing needles used to inject drugs. Bisexual women may be more likely to get infected with STIs that are less common for lesbians, since bisexuals have typically had sex with men in the past or are presently having sex with a man.

Common STIs that can be passed between women include:

Bacterial vaginosis (BV). BV is more common in lesbian and bisexual women than in other women. The reason for this is unknown. BV often occurs in both members of lesbian couples.

The vagina normally has a balance of mostly "good" bacteria and fewer "harmful" bacteria. BV develops when the balance changes. With BV, there is an increase in harmful bacteria and a decrease in good bacteria.

Sometimes BV causes no symptoms. But over one-half of women with BV have vaginal itching or discharge with a fishy odor. BV can be treated with antibiotics.

Chlamydia. Chlamydia is caused by bacteria. It's spread through vaginal, oral, or anal sex. It can damage the reproductive organs, such as the uterus, ovaries, and fallopian tubes. The symptoms of chlamydia are often mild—in fact, it's known as a "silent infection." Because the symptoms are mild, you can pass it to someone else without even knowing you have it.

Chlamydia can be treated with antibiotics. Infections that are not treated, even if there are no symptoms, can lead to:

- Lower abdominal pain
- Lower back pain
- Nausea

- Fever

- Pain during sex

- Bleeding between periods

Genital herpes. Genital herpes is an STI caused by the herpes simplex viruses type 1 (HSV-1) or type 2 (HSV-2). Most genital herpes is caused by HSV-2. HSV-1 can cause genital herpes. But it more commonly causes infections of the mouth and lips, called "fever blisters or "cold sores." You can spread oral herpes to the genitals through oral sex.

Most people have few or no symptoms from a genital herpes infection. When symptoms do occur, they usually appear as one or more blisters on or around the genitals or rectum. The blisters break, leaving tender sores that may take up to four weeks to heal. Another outbreak can appear weeks or months later. But it almost always is less severe and shorter than the first outbreak.

Although the infection can stay in the body forever, the outbreaks tend to become less severe and occur less often over time. You can pass genital herpes to someone else even when you have no symptoms.

There is no cure for herpes. Drugs can be used to shorten and prevent outbreaks or reduce the spread of the virus to others.

Human papillomavirus (HPV). HPV can cause genital warts. If left untreated, HPV can cause abnormal changes on the cervix that can lead to cancer. Most people don't know they're infected with HPV because they don't have symptoms. Usually the virus goes away on its own without causing harm. But not always. The Pap test checks for abnormal cell growths caused by HPV that can lead to cancer in women. If you are age 30 or older, your doctor may also do an HPV test with your Pap test. This is a DNA test that detects most of the high-risk types of HPV. It helps with cervical cancer screening. If you're younger than 30 years old and have had an abnormal Pap test result, your doctor may give you an HPV test. This test will show if HPV caused the abnormal cells on your cervix.

Both women and men can spread the virus to others whether or not they have any symptoms. Lesbians and bisexual women can transmit HPV through direct genital skin-to-skin contact, touching, or sex toys used with other women. Lesbians who have had sex with men are also at risk of HPV infection. This is why regular Pap tests are just as important for lesbian and bisexual women as they are for heterosexual women.

45

There is no treatment for HPV, but a healthy immune (body defense) system can usually fight off HPV infection. Two vaccines (Cervarix and Gardasil) can protect girls and young women against the types of HPV that cause most cervical cancers. The vaccines work best when given before a person's first sexual contact, when she could be exposed to HPV. Both vaccines are recommended for 11 and 12-year-old-girls. But the vaccines also can be used in girls as young as 9 and in women through age 26 who did not get any or all of the shots when they were younger. These vaccines are given in a series of 3 shots. It is best to use the same vaccine brand for all 3 doses. Ask your doctor which brand vaccine is best for you. Gardasil also has benefits for men in preventing genital warts and anal cancer caused by HPV. It is approved for use in boys as young as 9 and for young men through age 26. The vaccine does not replace the need to wear condoms to lower your risk of getting other types of HPV and other sexually transmitted infections. If you do get HPV, there are treatments for diseases caused by it. Genital warts can be removed with medicine you apply yourself or treatments performed by your doctor. Cervical and other cancers caused by HPV are most treatable when found early. There are many options for cancer treatment.

Pubic lice. Also known as crabs, pubic lice are small parasites that live in the genital areas and other areas with coarse hair. Pubic lice are spread through direct contact with the genital area. They can also be spread through sheets, towels, or clothes. Pubic lice can be treated with creams or shampoos you can buy at the drug store.

Trichomoniasis or "Trich." Trichomoniasis is caused by a parasite that can be spread during sex. You can also get trichomoniasis from contact with damp, moist objects, such as towels or wet clothes. Symptoms include:

- Yellow, green, or gray vaginal discharge (often foamy) with a strong odor
- Discomfort during sex and when urinating
- Irritation and itching of the genital area
- Lower abdominal pain (in rare cases)

Trichomoniasis can be treated with antibiotics.

Less common STIs that may affect lesbians and bisexual women include:

Gonorrhea. Gonorrhea is a common STI but is not commonly passed during woman to woman sex. However, it could be since it does live in vaginal fluid. It is caused by a type of bacteria that can grow in warm, moist areas of the reproductive tract, like the cervix, uterus, and fallopian tubes in women. It can grow in the urethra in women and men. It can also grow in the mouth, throat, eyes, and anus. Even when women have symptoms, they are often mild and are sometimes thought to be from a bladder or other vaginal infection.

Symptoms include:

- Pain or burning when urinating
- Yellowish and sometimes bloody vaginal discharge
- Bleeding between menstrual periods

Gonorrhea can be treated with antibiotics.

Hepatitis B. Hepatitis B is a liver disease caused by a virus. It is spread through bodily fluids, including blood, semen, and vaginal fluid. People can get hepatitis B through sexual contact, by sharing needles with an infected person, or through mother-to-child transmission at birth. Some women have no symptoms if they get infected with the virus.

Women with symptoms may have:

- Mild fever
- Headache and muscle aches
- Tiredness
- Loss of appetite
- Nausea or vomiting
- Diarrhea
- Dark-colored urine and pale bowel movements
- Stomach pain
- Yellow skin and whites of eyes

There is a vaccine that can protect you from hepatitis B.

Human Immunodeficiency Virus (HIV)/ Acquired Immunodeficiency Syndrome (AIDS). The HIV is spread through body fluids, such as blood, vaginal fluid, semen, and breast milk. It is primarily spread through sex with men or by sharing needles. Women who have sex with women can spread HIV, but this is rare. Some women with HIV may have no symptoms for 10 years or more.

Women with HIV symptoms may have:

- Extreme fatigue (tiredness)
- Rapid weight loss
- Frequent low-grade fevers and night sweats
- Frequent yeast infections (in the mouth)
- Vaginal yeast infections
- Other STIs
- Pelvic inflammatory disease (an infection of the uterus, ovaries, or fallopian tubes)
- Menstrual cycle changes
- Red, brown, or purplish blotches on or under the skin or inside the mouth, nose, or eyelids

AIDS, or acquired immunodeficiency syndrome, is the final stage of HIV infection. HIV infection turns to AIDS when you have one or more opportunistic infections, certain cancers, or a very low CD4 cell count.

Syphilis. Syphilis is an STI caused by bacteria. It's passed through direct contact with a syphilis sore during vaginal, anal, or oral sex. Untreated syphilis can infect other parts of the body. It is easily treated with antibiotics. Syphilis is very rare among lesbians. But, you should talk to your doctor if you have any sores that don't heal.

What Challenges Do Lesbian and Bisexual Women Face in the Healthcare System?

Lesbians and bisexual women face unique problems within the healthcare system that can hurt their health. Many healthcare professionals have not had enough training to know the specific health issues that lesbians and bisexuals face. They may not ask about sexual orientation when taking personal health histories. Healthcare professionals may not think that a lesbian or bisexual woman, like any woman, can be a healthy, normal female.

Things that can stop lesbians and bisexual women from getting good healthcare include:

- Being scared to tell your doctor about your sexuality or your sexual history
- Having a doctor who does not know your disease risks or the issues that affect lesbians and bisexual women

- Not having health insurance. Many lesbians and bisexuals don't have domestic partner benefits. This means that one person does not qualify to get health insurance through the plan that the partner has (a benefit usually available to married couples).

- Not knowing that lesbians are at risk for STIs and cancer

For these reasons, lesbian and bisexual women often avoid routine health exams. They sometimes even delay seeking healthcare when feeling sick. It is important to be proactive about your health, even if you have to try different doctors before you find the right one. Early detection—such as finding cancer early before it spreads—gives you the best chance to do something about it. That's one example of why it's important to find a doctor who will work with you to identify your health concerns and make a plan to address them.

What Can Lesbian and Bisexual Women Do to Protect Their Health?

Find a doctor who is sensitive to your needs and will help you get regular check-ups. The Gay and Lesbian Medical Association provides online healthcare referrals. You can access its Provider Directory accessible on the Internet at www.glma.org or contact the Association at 202-600-8037.

Get a Pap test. The Pap test finds changes in your cervix early, so you can be treated before a problem becomes serious. Begin getting Pap tests at age 21. In your 20s, get a Pap test every two years. Women 30 and older should get a Pap test every three years. If you are HIV-positive, your doctor may recommend more frequent testing.

Get an HPV test. Combined with a Pap test, an HPV test helps prevent cervical cancer. It can detect the types of HPV that cause cervical cancer. Talk to your doctor about an HPV test if you've had an abnormal Pap or if you're 30 or older.

Talk to your doctor or nurse about other screening tests you may need. You need regular preventive screenings to stay healthy. Lesbian and bisexual women need all the same tests that heterosexual women do. Learn more about what tests you need, based on your age.

Practice safer sex. Get tested for STIs before starting a sexual relationship. If you are unsure about a partner's status, practice methods to reduce the chances of sharing vaginal fluid, semen, or blood. If you have sex with men, use a condom every time. You should also use condoms on sex toys. Oral sex with men or with women can also spread STIs, including, rarely, HIV. HIV can potentially be passed through a mucous membrane (such as the mouth) by vaginal fluids or blood, especially if the membrane is torn or cut.

Eat a balanced, healthy diet. Your diet should include a variety of whole grains, fruits, and vegetables. These foods give you energy, plus vitamins, minerals, and fiber. Reduce the amount of sodium you eat to less than 2,300 mg per day.

Drink moderately. If you drink alcohol, don't have more than one drink per day. Too much alcohol raises blood pressure and can increase your risk for stroke, heart disease, osteoporosis, many cancers, and other problems.

Get moving. An active lifestyle can help any woman. You will benefit most from about 2 hours and 30 minutes of moderate-intensity aerobic physical activity each week. More physical activity means additional health and fitness benefits. On two or more days every week, adults should engage in muscle-strengthening activities, such as lifting weights or doing squats or push-ups.

Don't smoke. If you do smoke, try to quit. Avoid secondhand smoke as much as you can.

Try different things to deal with your stress. Stress from discrimination and from loneliness is hard for every lesbian and bisexual woman. Relax using deep breathing, yoga, meditation, and massage therapy. You can also take a few minutes to sit and listen to soft music or read a book. Talk to your friends or get help from a mental health professional if you need it.

Get help for domestic violence. Call the police or leave if you or your children are in danger. Call a crisis hotline or the National Domestic Violence Hotline at 800-799-SAFE or TDD 800-787-3224, which is available 24 hours a day, 365 days a year, in English, Spanish, and other languages. The helpline can give you the phone numbers of local hotlines and other resources.

Build strong bones. Take the following steps to help build strong bones and prevent osteoporosis:

- Exercise

- Get a bone density test

- Get enough calcium and vitamin D each day

- Reduce your chances of falling by making your home safer. For example, use a rubber bath mat in the shower or tub and keep your floors free from clutter.

- Talk to your doctor about medicines to prevent or treat bone loss

Know the signs of a heart attack. Women are less likely than men to know when they are having a heart attack. So, they are more likely to delay in seeking treatment. For women, chest pain may not be the first sign your heart is in trouble. Before a heart attack, women have said that they have **unusual tiredness, trouble sleeping, problems breathing, indigestion, and anxiety.** These symptoms can happen a month or so before the heart attack. During a heart attack, women often have:

- Pain or discomfort in the center of the chest

- Pain or discomfort in the arms, back, neck, jaw, or stomach

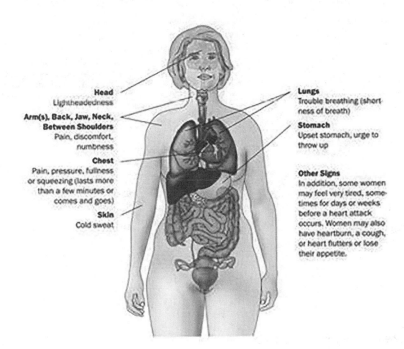

Figure 4.1. *Heart Attack: Warning Signs*

- Shortness of breath

- A cold sweat

- Nausea

- Light-headedness

Know the signs of a stroke. The signs of a stroke appear suddenly and are different from those of a heart attack. Signs you should look for include:

- Weakness or numbness on one side of your body

- Dizziness

- Loss of balance

- Confusion

- Trouble talking or understanding speech

- Headache

- Nausea

- Trouble walking or seeing

Remember: Even if you have a "mini-stroke," you may have some of these signs.

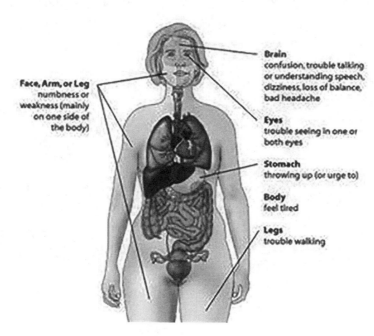

Figure 4.2. *Signs of a Stroke*

Chapter 5

Violence against Women and How to Get Help

Am I Being Abused?

It can be hard to know if you're being abused. You may think that your husband is allowed to make you have sex. That's not true. Forced sex is rape, no matter who does it. You may think that cruel or threatening words are not abuse. They are. And sometimes emotional abuse is a sign that a person will become physically violent.

Signs of Abuse

Below is a list of possible signs of abuse. Some of these are illegal. All of them are wrong. You may be abused if your partner:

* Monitors what you're doing all the time

This chapter contains text excerpted from the following sources: Text under the heading "Am I Being Abused?" is excerpted from "Am I Being Abused?" Office on Women's Health (OWH), U.S. Department of Health and Human Services (HHS), September 30, 2015; Text under the heading "Get Help for Violence" is excerpted from "Get Help for Violence," Office on Women's Health (OWH), U.S. Department of Health and Human Services (HHS), September 30, 2015; Text under the heading "How to Help a Friend Who is Being Abused" is excerpted from "How to Help a Friend Who is Being Abused," Office on Women's Health (OWH), U.S. Department of Health and Human Services (HHS), September 4, 2015; Text under the heading "Help End Violence against Women" is excerpted from "Help End Violence against Women," Office on Women's Health (OWH), U.S. Department of Health and Human Services (HHS), September 30, 2015.

- Unfairly accuses you of being unfaithful all the time
- Prevents or discourages you from seeing friends or family
- Prevents or discourages you from going to work or school
- Gets very angry during and after drinking alcohol or using drugs
- Controls how you spend your money
- Controls your use of needed medicines
- Decides things for you that you should be allowed to decide (like what to wear or eat)
- Humiliates you in front of others
- Destroys your property or things that you care about
- Threatens to hurt you, the children, or pets
- Hurts you (by hitting, beating, pushing, shoving, punching, slapping, kicking, or biting)
- Uses (or threatens to use) a weapon against you
- Forces you to have sex against your will
- Controls your birth control or insists that you get pregnant
- Blames you for his or her violent outbursts
- Threatens to harm himself or herself when upset with you
- Says things like, "If I can't have you then no one can."

If you think someone is abusing you, get help. Abuse can have serious physical and emotional effects. No one has the right to hurt you.

Healthy versus Unhealthy Relationships

Sometimes a relationship might not be abusive, but it might have some serious problems that make it unhealthy. If you think you might be in an unhealthy relationship, you should be able to talk to your partner about your concerns. If you feel like you can't talk to your partner, try talking to a trusted friend, family member, or counselor. Consider calling a confidential hotline to get the support you need and to explore next steps. If you're afraid to end the relationship, call a hotline for help.

Signs of an unhealthy relationship include:

- Focusing all your energy on your partner

- Dropping friends and family or activities you enjoy

- Feeling pressured or controlled a lot

- Having more bad times in the relationship than good

- Feeling sad or scared when with your partner

Signs of a healthy relationship include:

- Having more good times in the relationship than bad

- Having a life outside the relationship, with your own friends and activities

- Making decisions together, with each partner compromising at times

- Dealing with conflicts by talking honestly

- Feeling comfortable and able to be yourself

- Feeling able to take care of yourself

- Feeling like your partner supports you

Get Help for Violence

If you have experienced violence, you may feel shock, fear, sadness, and confusion. You may even feel numb, or think that what happens to you doesn't matter. But no one has the right to hurt you or make you feel afraid. Many groups and people want to help you live a healthier, happier life.

Ways to get help include:

- **Calling the police.** If you are in immediate danger, call 911.

- **Calling hotlines.** Learn more about different help hotlines. Hotlines provide support and resources. They also can help you create a safety plan for leaving an abuser.

- **Reaching out to people you trust.** People who care want to help. You can start with family, friends, or community organizations.

- **Talking to a healthcare professional.** Doctors, nurses, and counselors can offer physical aid, emotional support, and resources. Go to a hospital emergency room if you need immediate help for injuries.

- **Contacting a shelter or rape crisis center.** Shelters provide food, housing, and other types of help. You can find shelters and services by contacting a hotline or through state resources.

- **Contacting an advocate.** Advocates are people who are trained to help someone who has lived through domestic violence, dating violence, or sexual assault. You can talk to an advocate on the phone or in person, confidentially and for free. Advocates can explain options and programs in your community that may include legal support, counseling, emergency services, and other resources. Advocates work in shelters and in community-based programs. You can learn more by calling help hotlines.

How to Help a Friend Who Is Being Abused

Here are some ways to help a friend who is being abused:

- **Set up a time to talk.** Try to make sure you have privacy and won't be distracted or interrupted.

- **Let your friend know you're concerned about her safety.** Be honest. Tell her about times when you were worried about her. Help her see that what she's going through is not right. Let her know you want to help.

- **Be supportive.** Listen to your friend. Keep in mind that it may be very hard for her to talk about the abuse. Tell her that she is not alone, and that people want to help.

- **Offer specific help.** You might say you are willing to just listen, to help her with child care, or to provide transportation, for example.

- **Don't place shame, blame, or guilt on your friend.** Don't say, "You just need to leave." Instead, say something like, "I get scared thinking about what might happen to you." Tell her you understand that her situation is very difficult.

- **Help her make a safety plan.** Safety planning includes picking a place to go and packing important items.

- **Encourage your friend to talk to someone who can help.** Offer to help her find a local domestic violence agency. Offer to go with her to the agency, the police, or court.

- **If your friend decides to stay, continue to be supportive.** Your friend may decide to stay in the relationship, or she may leave and then go back many times. It may be hard for you to understand, but people stay in abusive relationships for many reasons. Be supportive, no matter what your friend decides to do.

- **Encourage your friend to do things outside of the relationship.** It's important for her to see friends and family.

- **If your friend decides to leave, continue to offer support.** Even though the relationship was abusive, she may feel sad and lonely once it is over. She also may need help getting services from agencies or community groups.

- **Keep in mind that you can't "rescue" your friend.** She has to be the one to decide it's time to get help. Support her no matter what her decision.

- **Let your friend know that you will always be there no matter what.**

Help End Violence Against Women

Violence does not hurt only the person who has experienced it. It hurts the whole community. Learn ways you can work to help end violence against women. Here are some suggestions:

- **Call the police** if you see or hear evidence of domestic violence.

- **Support a friend or family member** who may be in an abusive relationship. Learn more about how to help.

- **Volunteer** at a local domestic violence shelter or other organization that helps survivors or works to prevent violence.

- **Raise children to respect others.** Teach children to treat others as they would like to be treated.

- **Lead by example.** Work to create a culture that rejects violence as a way to deal with problems. Speak up against messages that say violence or mistreating women is okay.

- **Become an activist.** Participate in an anti-violence event like a local Take Back the Night march. Tell your congressional representatives that you want them to support domestic violence services and violence prevention programs.

- **Volunteer in youth programs.** Become a mentor. Get involved in programs that teach young people to solve problems without violence. Get involved with programs that teach teens about healthy relationships.

- **Ask about anti-violence policies and programs at work and school.** At work, ask about policies that deal with sexual harassment, for example. On campus, ask about services to escort students to dorms safely at night and other safety measures.

Part Two

Maintaining Women's Health and Wellness

Chapter 6

Nutrition and Exercise Recommendations

Chapter Contents

Section 6.1

Nutrition and Vitamins for Women

This section includes text excerpted from "Nutrition Basics,"
Office on Women's Health (OWH), U.S. Department of Health and
Human Services (HHS), February 28, 2017.

The basics of good nutrition are the same for women and men:
Choose healthy foods most of the time and limit the amount of
unhealthy foods you eat. Healthy eating means choosing the right
amount of foods from all the food groups and getting the nutrients
your body needs.

What Is a Nutrient?

A nutrient is any substance in food that:

- Provides energy

- Helps your body "burn" another nutrient to provide energy

- Helps build or repair tissue

The different types of nutrients include:

- Proteins
- Carbohydrates
- Fats

- Vitamins
- Minerals
- Water

Proteins

Proteins are an important part of your bones, muscles, and skin. In
fact, proteins are in every living cell in your body. Inside cells, proteins
perform many functions, including:

- Helping to break down food for energy

- Building structures

- Breaking down toxins

Proteins are made up of building blocks called amino acids. Your body can make some amino acids but not others. Proteins that you get from meat and other animal products contain all the amino acids you need. These include both those your body can make and those it can't. Proteins from meat and other animal products are known as complete protein.

Proteins from plant products are incomplete proteins. That means that the proteins from one plant product don't contain all the amino acids your body needs. But another plant product may have the amino acids that the first one is missing. To get complete protein from plants, you need to eat a variety of plant foods. For instance, eating rice with beans or peanut butter with bread will give you complete protein.

You may have seen ads for protein powders and shakes that say their products contain amino acids that your body can't make. Although this is true, most people can get all the protein they need from food and don't need protein supplements.

Good Sources of Protein

Good sources of protein include:

- Fish and shellfish
- Poultry
- Red meat (beef, pork, lamb)
- Eggs
- Nuts
- Peanut butter
- Nut butters
- Seeds
- Beans
- Peas
- Lentils
- Soy products (tofu, tempeh, vegetarian burgers)
- Milk
- Milk products (cheese, cottage cheese, yogurt)

63

Carbohydrates

The foods you eat contain different types of carbohydrates. Some kinds are better for you than others. The different types of carbohydrates are:

- **Sugars** are found naturally in fruits, vegetables, milk, and milk products. Foods such as cakes and cookies have had sugars added. Table sugar also is an added sugar. All of these sugars can be converted in your body to glucose, or blood sugar. Your cells "burn" glucose for energy.

- **Starches** are broken down in your body into sugars. Starches are found in certain vegetables, such as potatoes, beans, peas, and corn. They are also found in breads, cereals, and grains.

- **Dietary fibers** are carbohydrates that your body cannot digest. They pass through your body without being broken down into sugars. Even though your body does not get energy from fiber, you still need fiber to stay healthy. Fiber helps get rid of excess fats in the intestine, which helps prevent heart disease. Fiber also helps push food through the intestines, which helps prevent constipation. Foods high in fiber include fruits, vegetables, beans, peas, nuts, seeds, and whole-grain foods (such as whole-wheat bread, oatmeal, and brown rice).

Healthy and Unhealthy Carbohydrates

In general, you want to limit carbohydrates that increase your blood glucose levels. If your blood glucose stays high for too long, you can develop type 2 diabetes. To keep your blood glucose in check, limit the amount of table sugar you eat. Also, limit foods with added sugars. You can tell if a food has added sugars by looking at the ingredients list on the package. Look for terms such as:

- Corn sweetener
- Corn syrup
- High-fructose corn syrup
- Dextrose
- Fructose
- Glucose
- Lactose
- Maltose
- Sucrose
- Honey
- Sugar
- Brown sugar
- Invert sugar
- Molasses
- Malt syrup
- Syrup

You also should limit the amount of white potatoes you eat. Eating white potatoes occasionally is fine because they contain important vitamins and minerals. But your body rapidly digests the starch in white potatoes. This can raise your blood glucose level.

Healthy carbohydrates include:

- Natural sugars in fruits, vegetables, milk, and milk products

- Dietary fiber

- Starches in whole-grain foods, beans, peas, and corn

Fats

Your body needs some fat to function properly.
Fat:

- Is a source of energy

- Is used by your body to make substances it needs

- Helps your body absorb certain vitamins from food

But not all fats are the same. Some are better for your health than others. To help prevent heart disease and stroke, most of the fats you eat should be monounsaturated and polyunsaturated fats.

Foods high in monounsaturated fats include:

- Olive oil

- Peanut oil

- Canola oil

- Avocados

- Most nuts

Foods high in polyunsaturated fats include:

- Safflower oil

- Corn oil

- Sunflower oil

- Soybean oil

- Cottonseed oil

Healthy and Unhealthy Fats

Omega-3 fatty acids are a type of polyunsaturated fat that appear to reduce your risk of heart disease. Good sources of omega-3s are fatty fish. These include salmon, trout, herring, mackerel, anchovies, and sardines. You can also get omega-3s from plant sources. These include ground flaxseed (linseed), flaxseed oil, and walnuts. Small amounts are also found in soybean and canola oils.

Less healthy kinds of fats are saturated and *trans* fats. They can increase your risk of heart disease by causing the buildup of a fatty substance in the arteries carrying oxygen-rich blood to your heart. When this happens, your heart does not get all the blood it needs to work properly. The result can be chest pain or a heart attack. These fats can also increase your risk of stroke by causing the buildup of the same fatty substance in arteries carrying blood to your brain. Research also suggests that eating lots of *trans* fats may increase your risk of breast cancer.

Foods high in saturated fats include:

- Red meat (beef, pork, lamb)

- Poultry

- Butter

- Whole milk and whole milk products

- Coconut oil

- Palm oil

Trans fats are found in foods made with hydrogenated and partially hydrogenated oils. Look on the ingredients list on the food package to see if the food contains these oils. You are likely to find them in commercial baked goods, such as crackers, cookies, and cakes. *Trans* fats are also found in fried foods, such as doughnuts and french fries. Stick or hard margarine and shortening are also high in *trans* fats.

As with saturated and *trans* fats, eating too much cholesterol can raise your risk of heart disease and stroke. Cholesterol is a fat-like substance found in animal products, such as:

- Red meat

- Poultry

- Seafood

- Egg yolks

- Milk and milk products
- Lard
- Butter

Although monounsaturated and polyunsaturated fats are better for your health than saturated and *trans* fats, eating large amounts of any fat can cause weight gain. You should eat fats in moderation. And make sure that fatty foods don't replace more nutritious foods, such as fruits, vegetables, and whole grains.

Vitamins

Vitamins are substances found in foods that your body needs for growth and health. There are 13 vitamins your body needs. Each vitamin has specific jobs. Below is a list of the vitamins, some of their actions, and good food sources.

Table 6.1. Vitamins, Some of Their Actions, and Good Food Sources

Vitamin	Actions	Sources
A	Needed for vision Helps your body fight infections Helps keep your skin healthy	Kale, broccoli, spinach, carrots, squash, sweet potatoes, liver, eggs, whole milk, cream, and cheese.
B1	Helps your body use carbohydrates for energy Good for your nervous system	Yeasts, ham and other types of pork, liver, peanuts, whole-grain and fortified cereals and breads, and milk.
B2	Helps your body use proteins, carbohydrates, and fats Helps keep your skin healthy	Liver, eggs, cheese, milk, leafy green vegetables, peas, navy beans, lima beans, and whole-grain breads.
B3	Helps your body use proteins, carbohydrates, and fats Good for your nervous system and skin	Liver, yeast, bran, peanuts, lean red meats, fish, and poultry.
B5	Helps your body use carbohydrates and fats Helps your body make red blood cells	Beef, chicken, lobster, milk, eggs, peanuts, peas, beans, lentils, broccoli, yeast, and whole grains.
B6	Helps your body use proteins and fats Good for your nervous system Helps your blood carry oxygen	Liver, whole grains, egg yolk, peanuts, bananas, carrots, and yeast.

Table 6.1. Continued

Vitamin	Actions	Sources
B9 (folic acid or folate)	Helps your body make and maintain new cells Prevents some birth defects	Green leafy vegetables, liver, yeast, beans, peas, oranges, and fortified cereals and grain products.
B12	Helps your body make red blood cells Good for your nervous system	Milk, eggs, liver, poultry, clams, sardines, flounder, herring, eggs, blue cheese, cereals, nutritional yeast, and foods fortified with vitamin B12, including cereals, soy-based beverages, and veggie burgers.
C	Needed for healthy bones, blood vessels, and skin	Broccoli, green and red peppers, spinach, brussels sprouts, oranges, grapefruits, tomatoes, potatoes, papayas, strawberries, and cabbage.
D	Needed for healthy bones	Fish liver oil, milk and cereals fortified with vitamin D. Your body may make enough vitamin D if you are exposed to sunlight for about 5 to 30 minutes at least twice a week.
E	Helps prevent cell damage Helps blood flow Helps repair body tissues	Wheat germ oil, fortified cereals, egg yolk, beef liver, fish, milk, vegetable oils, nuts, fruits, peas, beans, broccoli, and spinach.
H (biotin)	Helps your body use carbohydrates and fats Needed for growth of many cells	Liver, egg yolk, soy flour, cereals, yeast, peas, beans, nuts, tomatoes, nuts, green leafy vegetables, and milk.
K	Helps in blood clotting Helps form bones	Alfalfa, spinach, cabbage, cheese, spinach, broccoli, brussels sprouts, kale, cabbage, tomatoes, and plant oils. Your body usually makes all the vitamin K you need.

Minerals

Like vitamins, minerals are substances found in food that your body needs for growth and health. There are two kinds of minerals: macrominerals and trace minerals. Macrominerals are minerals your body needs in larger amounts. They include calcium, phosphorus, magnesium, sodium, potassium, and chloride. Your body needs just small amounts of trace minerals. These include iron, copper, iodine, zinc, fluoride, and selenium.

Table 6.2. Minerals, Some of Their Actions, and Good Food Sources

Mineral	Actions	Sources
Calcium	Needed for forming bones and teeth Helps nerves and muscles function	Canned salmon with bones, sardines, milk, cheese, yogurt, Chinese cabbage, bok choy, kale, collard greens, turnip greens, mustard greens, broccoli, and calcium-fortified orange juice.
Chloride	Needed for keeping the right amounts of water in the different parts of your body	Salt, seaweed, rye, tomatoes, lettuce, celery, olives, sardines, beef, pork, and cheese.
Copper	Helps protect cells from damage Needed for forming bone and red blood cells	Organ meats, shellfish (especially oysters), chocolate, mushrooms, nuts, beans, and whole-grain cereals.
Fluoride	Needed for forming bones and teeth	Saltwater fish, tea, coffee, and fluoridated water.
Iodine	Needed for thyroid gland function	Seafood, iodized salt, and drinking water (in regions with iodine-rich soil, which are usually regions near an ocean).
Iron	Helps red blood cells deliver oxygen to body tissues Helps muscles function	Red meats, poultry, fish, liver, soybean flour, eggs, beans, lentils, peas, molasses, spinach, turnip greens, clams, dried fruit (apricots, prunes, and raisins), whole grains, and fortified breakfast cereals.
Magnesium	Needed for forming bones and teeth Needed for normal nerve and muscle function	Green leafy vegetables, nuts, bran cereal, seafood, milk, cheese, and yogurt.
Phosphorus	Needed for forming bones and teeth Needed for storing energy from food	Milk, yogurt, cheese, red meat, poultry, fish, eggs, nuts, peas, and some cereals and breads.
Potassium	Needed for normal nerve and muscle function Needed for keeping the right amounts of water in the different parts of your body	Milk, bananas, tomatoes, oranges, melons, potatoes, sweet potatoes, prunes, raisins, spinach, turnip greens, collard greens, kale, most peas and beans, and salt substitutes (potassium chloride).
Selenium	Helps protect cells from damage Needed for thyroid gland function	Vegetables, fish, shellfish, red meat, grains, eggs, chicken, liver, garlic, brewer's yeast, wheat germ, and enriched breads.

Table 6.2. Continued

Mineral	Actions	Sources
Sodium	Needed for normal nerve and muscle function Needed for keeping the right amounts of water in the different parts of your body	Salt, milk, cheese, beets, celery, beef, pork, sardines, and green olives.
Zinc	Needed for healthy skin Needed for wound healing Helps your body fight off illnesses and infections	Liver, eggs, seafood, red meats, oysters, certain seafood, milk products, eggs, beans, peas, lentils, peanuts, nuts, whole grains, fortified cereals, wheat germ, and pumpkin seeds.

Water

Water is an important part of your body. In fact, it makes up more than 60 percent of your body weight. Among other functions, water:

- Moistens tissues, such as those around your mouth, eyes, and nose
- Regulates your body temperature
- Cushions your joints
- Helps your body get nutrients
- Flushes out waste products

How Much Water Should I Drink?

Without water, you would die in a few days. So it's important that you get enough water. But how much water is enough? Experts generally recommend that you drink six to eight 8-ounce glasses of fluid every day. But it doesn't have to be all water. You could satisfy some of your fluid needs by drinking milk, tea, soda, coffee, or juice, which are composed mostly of water. Just remember that juice and sodas are high in sugar. Many fruits and vegetables, such as watermelon and tomatoes, are also mostly water.

If you're being physically active and sweating a lot, you'll need more fluid. You'll also need more if the weather is hot. Women who are pregnant should drink about 10 cups of fluids daily. And women who breastfeed should drink about 13 cups of fluids daily.

It's generally not a good idea to use thirst alone as a guide for when to drink. By the time you're thirsty, you may already be a bit dehydrated. On the other hand, you don't need to be constantly carrying around water bottles and drinking lots of water. You are probably getting all the fluid you need if you are rarely thirsty and you produce a little more than six cups of colorless or slightly yellow urine a day. Dark urine can be a signal that you need more fluid.

Section 6.2

Heart-Healthy Eating

This section includes text excerpted from "Heart-Healthy Eating,"
Office on Women's Health (OWH), U.S. Department of Health
and Human Services (HHS), June 23, 2017.

Heart-healthy eating is an important way to lower your risk for heart disease and stroke. Heart disease is the number one cause of death for American women. Stroke is the number three cause of death. To get the most benefit for your heart, you should choose more fruits, vegetables, and foods with whole grains and healthy protein. You also should eat less food with added sugar, calories, and unhealthy fats.

Why Is Heart-Healthy Eating Important?

Heart-healthy eating, along with regular exercise or physical activity, can lower your risk for heart disease and stroke. Heart disease is the number one cause of death for American women. Stroke is the number three cause of death for American women.

What Foods Should I Eat to Help Lower My Risk for Heart Disease and Stroke?

You should choose these foods most of the time:

- **Fruits and vegetables.** At least half of your plate should be fruits and vegetables.

- **Whole grains.** At least half of your grains should be whole grains. Whole grains include:

  - whole wheat
  - whole oats
  - Oatmeal
  - whole-grain corn
  - brown rice
  - wild rice

  - whole rye
  - whole-grain barley
  - Buckwheat
  - Bulgur
  - Millet
  - Sorghum

- **Fat-free or low-fat dairy products.** These include milk, calcium-fortified soy drinks (soy milk), cheese, yogurt, and other milk products.

- **Seafood, skinless poultry, lean meats, beans, eggs, and unsalted nuts.**

What Foods Should I Limit to Lower My Risk of Heart Disease and Stroke?

You should limit:

- **Saturated fats.** Saturated fat is usually in pizza, ice cream, fried chicken, many cakes and cookies, bacon, and hamburgers. Check the Nutrition Facts label for saturated fat. Less than 10% of your daily calories should be from saturated fats.

- ***Trans* fats.** These are found mainly in commercially prepared baked goods, snack foods, fried foods, and margarine. The U.S. Food and Drug Administration (FDA) is taking action to remove artificial *trans* fats from our food supply because of their risk to heart health. Check the Nutrition Facts label on packaged food products and choose foods with no *trans* fats as much as possible.

- **Cholesterol.** Cholesterol is found in foods made from animals, such as bacon, whole milk, cheese made from whole milk, ice cream, full-fat frozen yogurt, and eggs. Fruits and vegetables do not contain cholesterol. Eggs are a major source of dietary cholesterol for Americans, but studies show that eating one egg a day does not increase the risk for heart disease in healthy people. You should eat less than 300 milligrams of cholesterol per day. Check the Nutrition Facts label for cholesterol. Foods with

20 percent or more of the "Daily Value" of cholesterol are high in cholesterol.

- **Sodium.** Sodium is found in salt, but most of the sodium we eat does not come from salt that we add while cooking or at the table. Most of our sodium comes from breads and rolls, cold cuts, pizza, hot dogs, cheese, pasta dishes, and condiments (like ketchup and mustard). Limit your daily sodium to less than 2,300 milligrams (equal to a teaspoon), unless your doctor says something else. Check the Nutrition Facts label for sodium. Foods with 20 percent or more of the "Daily Value" of sodium are high in sodium.

- **Added sugars.** Foods like fruit and dairy products naturally contain sugar. But you should limit foods that contain added sugars. These include sodas, sports drinks, cake, candy, and ice cream. Check the Nutrition Facts label for added sugars and limit the how much food you eat with added sugars. Look for these other names for sugar in the list of ingredients:

  - Corn syrup
  - Corn sweetener
  - Fructose
  - Glucose
  - Sucrose
  - Dextrose
  - Lactose
  - Maltose
  - Honey
  - Molasses
  - Raw sugar
  - Invert sugar
  - Syrup
  - Caramel
  - Fruit juice concentrates

How Can I Tell What Is in the Foods I Eat?

Most packaged foods have a Nutrition Facts label. This label has information about how many calories, saturated fat, *trans* fat, cholesterol, sodium, and added sugars are in each serving. It also lists the amounts of certain vitamins and minerals. Learn to read the Nutrition Facts label to know what is in the packaged food you buy.

For food that does not have a Nutrition Facts label, such as fresh salmon or a raw apple, you can use the MyPlate SuperTracker "Food-a-pedia" tool accessible on the Internet at www.supertracker.usda.gov/foodapedia.aspx. The "Food-a-pedia" tool shows whether a food is high or low in cholesterol, saturated fat, or sodium.

How Many Calories Should I Eat?

The number of calories you should eat each day depends on your age, sex, body size, physical activity, and other factors.

For instance, a woman between 31 and 50 years old who is of normal weight and is moderately active (gets 30 minutes of exercise on most days of the week) should eat and drink about 2,000 calories each day to maintain her weight. To find your personalized daily calorie limit, use the SuperTracker tool accessible on the Internet at www.supertracker. usda.gov/MyWeightManager.aspx.

How Does Sodium in Food Affect My Heart?

Eating foods high in sodium may cause high blood pressure, also called hypertension. Hypertension is a risk factor for heart disease and stroke. You should limit the amount of sodium you eat each day to less than 2,300 milligrams (about 1 teaspoon of salt), including the sodium found in packaged foods that you cannot see.

You should limit your sodium intake to less than 1,500 milligrams (about two-thirds of a teaspoon of salt) if you:

- Have high blood pressure

- Are African-American

- Are 51 years or older

- Have diabetes

- Have chronic kidney disease

You can lower the amount of sodium you eat each day by:

- **Eating fewer processed foods.** Most of the salt we eat comes from processed foods rather than salt we add to foods we cook.

- **Checking the sodium content on the Nutrition Facts label.** The sodium content in similar foods can vary a lot. For instance, the sodium content in regular tomato soup may be 700 milligrams (about a third of a teaspoon) per cup in one brand and 1,100 milligrams (about a half a teaspoon) per cup in another brand.

- **Seasoning your food with herbs and spices instead of salt.** Look for salt-free seasoning combinations in your grocery store.

How Does Potassium in Food Affect My Heart?

Potassium lessens the harmful effects of sodium on blood pressure. Try to eat or drink at least 4,700 milligrams of potassium a day. Good sources of potassium include:

- Bananas (442 milligrams for a medium banana)
- Milk, nonfat and low fat (up to 370 milligrams per cup)
- Orange juice (496 milligrams per 8-ounce glass of 100% orange juice)
- Plain yogurt, nonfat or low fat (up to 579 milligrams per 8-ounce carton)
- Prunes and prune juice (707 milligrams per 8-ounce glass)
- Spinach (up to 419 milligrams per half cup)
- Sweet potatoes (542 milligrams for a medium-sized sweet potato)
- Tomatoes and tomato products (664 milligrams for one-half cup of tomato paste; 405 milligrams for one-half cup of tomato sauce)
- White potatoes (738 milligrams per small potato)

How Does Cholesterol in Food Affect My Heart?

Cholesterol is a waxy, fat-like substance made by your body. It also is found in foods made from animals, like meat and dairy. Fruits and vegetables do not contain cholesterol.

There are two types of cholesterol:

1. High-Density Lipoprotein (HDL), or "good" cholesterol
2. Low-Density Lipoprotein (LDL), or "bad" cholesterol.

Higher levels of total cholesterol and LDL or "bad" cholesterol raise your risk for heart disease. Almost half of American women have high or borderline high cholesterol.

You can lower your cholesterol and LDL or "bad" cholesterol by:

- **Limiting foods that are high in saturated fats, *trans* fats, and cholesterol.**
- **Limiting cholesterol.** Try to eat or drink less than 300 milligrams of cholesterol each day. For comparison, a fast food double-patty plain cheeseburger has about 100 milligrams of cholesterol.

Is Eating Seafood Good for My Heart?

Yes. Seafood contains a type of fat called omega-3 fatty acids. Research suggests that eating about 8 ounces of seafood with omega-3 fatty acids per week can lower your risk of dying from heart disease.

Seafood that naturally contain more oil and are better sources of omega-3 fatty acids include:

- Salmon

- Trout

- Mackerel

- Anchovies

- Sardines

Lean fish (such as cod, haddock, and catfish) have less omega-3 fatty acids.

Is Drinking Alcohol Good for My Heart?

Maybe. Research suggests that moderate drinkers are less likely to develop heart disease than people who do not drink any alcohol or who drink too much. For women, moderate drinking means up to one drink per day. For men, it means up to two drinks per day. One drink is:

- One glass of wine (5 ounces)

- One can of beer (12 ounces)

- One shot of 80-proof hard liquor (1.5 ounces)

The reasons behind the benefit of moderate drinking on heart disease are not clear. But, moderate drinking is also linked to breast cancer, violence, and injuries. So, if you do not already drink, you should not start for the potential benefits to your heart.

You should also not drink alcohol if you are pregnant or may be pregnant, as there is no amount of alcohol that is known to be safe during pregnancy. You should not drink alcohol if you have another health condition that makes alcohol harmful.

Who Can Help Me Work Out an Eating Plan That Is Best for Me?

You may want to talk with a registered dietitian. A dietitian is a nutrition expert who can give you advice about what foods to eat and how much of each type. Ask your doctor to recommend a dietitian. You can also contact the Academy of Nutrition and Dietetics on the Internet at www.eatright.org.

How Can I Get Free or Low-Cost Nutrition Counseling?

Nutrition counseling for adults at higher risk of chronic disease must be covered by most insurers under the Affordable Care Act (the healthcare law). If you are at risk for heart disease or another chronic disease that is affected by what you eat, most insurance plans now cover nutrition counseling at no cost to you.

- If you have insurance, check with your insurance provider before you visit a health professional for diet counseling to find out what types of services are covered.

- If you have Medicare, find out how Medicare covers nutrition counseling.

- If you have Medicaid, the benefits covered are different in each state, but certain benefits must be covered by every Medicaid program. Check with your state's Medicaid program to find out what is covered.

Section 6.3

Folic Acid

This section includes text excerpted from "Folic Acid,"
Office on Women's Health (OWH), U.S. Department of
Health and Human Services (HHS), February 23, 2017.

Folic acid is a form of folate (a B vitamin) that everyone needs. If you can get pregnant or are pregnant, folic acid is especially important. Folic acid protects unborn babies against serious birth defects. You can get folic acid from vitamins and fortified foods, such as breads, pastas, and cereals. Folate is found naturally in foods such as leafy green vegetables, oranges, and beans.

What Are Folic Acid and Folate?

Folic acid is the man-made form of folate, a B vitamin. Folate is found naturally in certain fruits, vegetables, and nuts. Folic acid is found in vitamins and fortified foods.

Folic acid and folate help the body make healthy new red blood cells. Red blood cells carry oxygen to all the parts of your body. If your body does not make enough red blood cells, you can develop anemia. Anemia happens when your blood cannot carry enough oxygen to your body, which makes you pale, tired, or weak. Also, if you do not get enough folic acid, you could develop a type of anemia called folate-deficiency anemia.

Why Do Women Need Folic Acid?

Everyone needs folic acid to be healthy. But it is especially important for women:

- **Before and during pregnancy.** Folic acid protects unborn children against serious birth defects called neural tube defects. These birth defects happen in the first few weeks of pregnancy, often before a woman knows she is pregnant. Folic acid might also help prevent other types of birth defects and early pregnancy loss (miscarriage). Since about half of all pregnancies in the United States are unplanned, experts recommend all women get enough folic acid even if you are not trying to get pregnant.

- **To keep the blood healthy by helping red blood cells form and grow.** Not getting enough folic acid can lead to a type of anemia called folate-deficiency anemia. Folate-deficiency anemia is more common in women of childbearing age than in men.

How Do I Get Folic Acid?

You can get folic acid in two ways.

- **Through the foods you eat.** Folate is found naturally in some foods, including spinach, nuts, and beans. Folic acid is found in fortified foods (called "enriched foods"), such as breads, pastas, and cereals. Look for the term "enriched" on the ingredients list to find out whether the food has added folic acid.

- **As a vitamin.** Most multivitamins sold in the United States contain 400 micrograms, or 100% of the daily value, of folic acid. Check the label to make sure.

How Much Folic Acid do Women Need?

All women need 400 micrograms of folic acid every day. Women who can get pregnant should get 400 to 800 micrograms of folic acid from a vitamin or from food that has added folic acid, such as breakfast cereal. This is in addition to the folate you get naturally from food.

Some women may need more folic acid each day. See the below table to find out how much folic acid you need.

Table 6.3. Folic Acid Requirement

If You:	Amount of Folic Acid You May Need Daily
Could get pregnant or are pregnant	400–800 micrograms. Your doctor may prescribe a prenatal vitamin with more.
Had a baby with a neural tube defect (such as spina bifida) and want to get pregnant again	4,000 micrograms. Your doctor may prescribe this amount. Research shows taking this amount may lower the risk of having another baby with spina bifida.
Have a family member with spina bifida and could get pregnant	4,000 micrograms. Your doctor may prescribe this amount.
Have spina bifida and want to get pregnant	4,000 micrograms. Your doctor may prescribe this amount. Women with spina bifida have a higher risk of having children with the condition.
Take medicines to treat epilepsy, type 2 diabetes, rheumatoid arthritis, or lupus	Talk to your doctor or nurse. Folic acid supplements can interact with these medicines.
Are on dialysis for kidney disease	Talk to your doctor or nurse.
Have a health condition, such as inflammatory bowel disease or celiac disease, that affects how your body absorbs folic acid	Talk to your doctor or nurse.

Are Some Women at Risk for Not Getting Enough Folic Acid?

Yes, certain groups of women do not get enough folic acid each day.

- Women who can get pregnant need more folic acid (400 to 800 micrograms).

- Nearly one in three African-American women does not get enough folic acid each day.

- Spanish-speaking Mexican-American women often do not get enough folic acid. However, Mexican-Americans who speak English usually get enough folic acid.

Not getting enough folic acid can cause health problems, including folate-deficiency anemia, and problems during pregnancy for you and your unborn baby.

What Can Happen If I Do Not Get Enough Folic Acid during Pregnancy?

If you do not get enough folic acid before and during pregnancy, your baby is at higher risk for neural tube defects.

Neural tube defects are serious birth defects that affect the spine, spinal cord, or brain and may cause death. These include:

- **Spina bifida.** This condition happens when an unborn baby's spinal column does not fully close during development in the womb, leaving the spinal cord exposed. As a result, the nerves that control the legs and other organs do not work. Children with spina bifida often have lifelong disabilities. They may also need many surgeries.

- **Anencephaly**. This means that most or all of the brain and skull does not develop in the womb. Almost all babies with this condition die before or soon after birth.

Do I Need to Take Folic Acid Every Day Even If I'm Not Planning to Get Pregnant?

Yes. All women who can get pregnant need to take 400 to 800 micrograms of folic acid every day, even if you're not planning to get pregnant. There are several reasons why:

- Your birth control may not work or you may not use birth control correctly every time you have sex. In a survey by the Centers for Disease Control and Prevention (CDC), almost 40 percent of women with unplanned pregnancies were using birth control.

- Birth defects of the brain and spine can happen in the first few weeks of pregnancy, often before you know you are pregnant. By the time you find out you are pregnant, it might be too late to prevent the birth defects.

- You need to take folic acid every day because it is a water soluble B-vitamin. Water soluble means that it does not stay in the body for a long time. Your body metabolizes (uses) folic acid quickly, so your body needs folic acid each day to work properly.

What Foods Contain Folate?

Folate is found naturally in some foods. Foods that are naturally high in folate include:

- Spinach and other dark green, leafy vegetables
- Oranges and orange juice
- Nuts
- Beans
- Poultry (chicken, turkey, etc.) and meat
- Whole grains

What Foods Contain Folic Acid?

Folic acid is added to foods that are refined or processed (not whole grain):

- Breakfast cereals (Some have 100% of the recommended daily value—or 400 micrograms—of folic acid in each serving.)
- Breads and pasta
- Flours
- Cornmeal
- White rice

Since 1998, the U.S. Food and Drug Administration (FDA) has required food manufacturers to add folic acid to processed breads, cereals, flours, cornmeal, pastas, rice, and other grains.

For other foods, check the Nutrition Facts label on the package to see if it has folic acid. The label will also tell you how much folic acid is in each serving. Sometimes, the label will say "folate" instead of folic acid.

How Can I Be Sure I Get Enough Folic Acid?

You can get enough folic acid from food alone. Many breakfast cereals have 100% of your recommended daily value (400 micrograms) of folic acid.

If you are at risk for not getting enough folic acid, your doctor or nurse may recommend that you take a vitamin with folic acid every day. Most U.S. multivitamins have at least 400 micrograms of folic acid. Check the label on the bottle to be sure. You can also take a pill that contains only folic acid. If swallowing pills is hard for you, try a chewable or liquid product with folic acid.

What Should I Look for When Buying Vitamins with Folic Acid?

Look for "USP" or "NSF" on the label when choosing vitamins. These "seals of approval" mean the pills are made properly and have the amounts of vitamins it says on the label. Also, make sure the pills have not expired. If the bottle has no expiration date, do not buy it.

Ask your pharmacist for help with selecting a vitamin or folic acid-only pill. If you are pregnant and already take a daily prenatal vitamin, you probably get all the folic acid you need. Check the label to be sure.

Vitamin Label

Check the "Supplement Facts" label to be sure you are getting 400 to 800 micrograms (mcg) of folic acid.

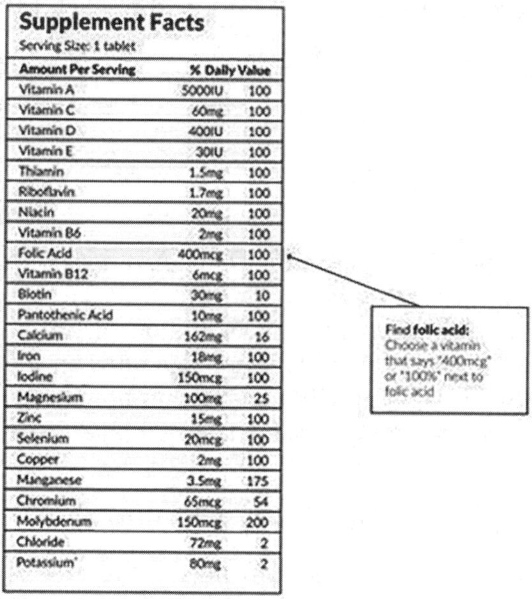

Supplement Facts
Serving Size: 1 tablet

Amount Per Serving		% Daily Value
Vitamin A	5000IU	100
Vitamin C	60mg	100
Vitamin D	400IU	100
Vitamin E	30IU	100
Thiamin	1.5mg	100
Riboflavin	1.7mg	100
Niacin	20mg	100
Vitamin B6	2mg	100
Folic Acid	400mcg	100
Vitamin B12	6mcg	100
Biotin	30mg	10
Pantothenic Acid	10mg	100
Calcium	162mg	16
Iron	18mg	100
Iodine	150mcg	100
Magnesium	100mg	25
Zinc	15mg	100
Selenium	20mcg	100
Copper	2mg	100
Manganese	3.5mg	175
Chromium	65mcg	54
Molybdenum	150mcg	200
Chloride	72mg	2
Potassium'	80mg	2

Find folic acid:
Choose a vitamin that says "400mcg" or "100%" next to folic acid

Figure 6.1. *Supplement Facts Label*

Can I Get Enough Folic Acid from Food Alone?

Yes, many people get enough folic acid from food alone. Some foods have high amounts of folic acid. For example, many breakfast cereals have 100% of the recommended daily value (400 micrograms) of folic acid in each serving. Check the label to be sure.

Some women, especially women who could get pregnant, may not get enough folic acid from food. African-American women and Mexican Americans are also at higher risk for not getting enough folic acid each day. Talk to your doctor or nurse about whether you should take a vitamin to get the 400 micrograms of folic acid you need each day.

What Is Folate-Deficiency Anemia?

Folate-deficiency anemia is a type of anemia that happens when you do not get enough folate. Folate-deficiency anemia is most common during pregnancy. Other causes of folate-deficiency anemia include alcoholism and certain medicines to treat seizures, anxiety, or arthritis.

The symptoms of folate-deficiency anemia include:

- Fatigue
- Headache
- Pale skin
- Sore mouth and tongue

If you have folate-deficiency anemia, your doctor may recommend taking folic acid vitamins and eating more foods with folate.

Can I Get Too Much Folic Acid?

Yes, you can get too much folic acid, but only from man-made products such as multivitamins and fortified foods, such as breakfast cereals. You can't get too much from foods that naturally contain folate.

You should not get more than 1,000 micrograms of folic acid a day, unless your doctor prescribes a higher amount. Too much folic acid can hide signs that you lack vitamin B12, which can cause nerve damage.

Do I Need Folic Acid after Menopause?

Yes. Women who have gone through menopause still need 400 micrograms of folic acid every day for good health. Talk to your doctor or nurse about how much folic acid you need.

Are Folic Acid Pills Covered under Insurance?

Yes. Under the Affordable Care Act (the healthcare law), all Health Insurance Marketplace plans and most other insurance plans cover folic acid pills for women who could get pregnant at no cost to you. Check with your insurance provider to find out what's included in your plan.

Section 6.4

Physical Activity Guidelines for Women

This section includes text excerpted from "Physical Activity,"
Office on Women's Health (OWH), U.S. Department of
Health and Human Services (HHS), June 12, 2017.

Studies show that an active lifestyle can lower your risk of early death from a variety of causes. For older adults, activity can improve mental function.

How Can Physical Activity Improve My Health?

The *Physical Activity Guidelines for Americans* state that an active lifestyle can lower your risk of early death from a variety of causes. There is strong evidence that regular physical activity can also lower your risk of:

- Heart disease
- Stroke
- High blood pressure
- Unhealthy cholesterol levels
- Type 2 diabetes
- Metabolic syndrome
- Colon cancer

- Breast cancer

- Falls

- Depression

Regular activity can help prevent unhealthy weight gain and also help with weight loss, when combined with lower calorie intake. If you are overweight or obese, losing weight can lower your risk for many diseases. Being overweight or obese increases your risk of heart disease, high blood pressure, stroke, type 2 diabetes, breathing problems, osteoarthritis, gallbladder disease, sleep apnea (breathing problems while sleeping), and some cancers.

Regular physical activity can also improve your cardiorespiratory (heart, lungs, and blood vessels) and muscular fitness. For older adults, activity can improve mental function.

Physical activity may also help:

- Improve functional health for older adults

- Reduce waistline size

- Lower risk of hip fracture

- Lower risk of lung cancer

- Lower risk of endometrial cancer

- Maintain weight after weight loss

- Increase bone density

- Improve sleep quality

What Is Body Mass Index?

You can get an idea of whether you are obese, overweight, or of normal weight by figuring out your body mass index (BMI). BMI is a number calculated from your weight and height. Women with a BMI of 25 to 29.9 are considered overweight. Women with a BMI of 30 or more are considered obese. All adults (aged 18 years or older) with a BMI of 25 or higher are considered at risk for serious health problems. These health risks increase as your BMI rises. Your doctor or nurse can help you figure out your BMI, or you can use this online BMI calculator (www.cdc.gov/healthyweight/assessing/bmi/adult_bmi/english_bmi_calculator/bmi_calculator.html) from the Centers for Disease Control and Prevention (CDC).

85

How Much Physical Activity Should I Do?

Health benefits are gained by doing the following each week:

- 2 hours and 30 minutes of moderate-intensity aerobic physical activity or
- 1 hour and 15 minutes of vigorous-intensity aerobic physical activity or
- A combination of moderate and vigorous-intensity aerobic physical activity and
- Muscle-strengthening activities on 2 or more days

This physical activity should be in addition to your routine activities of daily living, such as cleaning or spending a few minutes walking from the parking lot to your office.

Moderate Activity

During moderate-intensity activities you should notice an increase in your heart rate, but you should still be able to talk comfortably. An example of a moderate-intensity activity is walking on a level surface at a brisk pace (about 3 to 4 miles per hour). Other examples include ballroom dancing, leisurely bicycling, moderate housework, and waiting tables.

Vigorous Activity

If your heart rate increases a lot and you are breathing so hard that it is difficult to carry on a conversation, you are probably doing vigorous-intensity activity. Examples of vigorous-intensity activities include jogging, bicycling fast or uphill, singles tennis, and pushing a hand mower.

How Much Physical Activity Do I Need to Do to Lose Weight?

If you want to lose a substantial (more than 5 percent of body weight) amount of weight, you need a high amount of physical activity unless you also lower calorie intake. This is also the case if you are trying to keep the weight off. Many people need to do more than 300 minutes of moderate-intensity activity a week to meet weight-control goals.

Does the Type of Physical Activity I Choose Matter?

Yes! Engaging in different types of physical activity is important to overall physical fitness. Your fitness routine should include aerobic and strength-training activities, and may also include stretching activities.

Aerobic Activities

These activities move large muscles in your arms, legs, and hips over and over again. Examples include walking, jogging, bicycling, swimming, and tennis.

Strength-Training Activities

These activities increase the strength and endurance of your muscles. Examples of strength-training activities include working out with weight machines, free weights, and resistance bands. (A resistance band looks like a giant rubber band. You can buy one at a sporting goods store.) Push-ups and sit-ups are examples of strength-training activities you can do without any equipment. You also can use soup cans to work out your arms.

Aim to do strength-training activities at least twice a week. In each strength-training session, you should do 8 to 10 different activities using the different muscle groups throughout your body, such as the muscles in your abdomen, chest, arms, and legs. Repeat each activity 8 to 12 times, using a weight or resistance that will make you feel tired. When you do strength-training activities, slowly increase the amount of weight or resistance that you use. Also, allow one day in between sessions to avoid excess strain on your muscles and joints.

Stretching

Stretching improves flexibility, allowing you to move more easily. This will make it easier for you to reach down to tie your shoes or look over your shoulder when you back the car out of your driveway. You should do stretching activities after your muscles are warmed up—for example, after strength training. Stretching your muscles before they are warmed up may cause injury.

How Can I Prevent Injuries When I Work Out?

Being physically active is safe if you are careful. Take these steps to prevent injury:

- If you're not active at all or have a health problem, start your program with short sessions (5 to 10 minutes) of physical activity and build up to your goal. (Be sure to ask a doctor before you start if you have a health problem.)

- Use safety equipment such as a helmet for bike riding or supportive shoes for walking or jogging.

- Start every workout with a warm-up. If you plan to walk at a brisk pace, start by walking at an easy pace for 5 to 10 minutes. When you're done working out, do the same thing until your heart rate returns to normal.

- Drink plenty of fluids when you are physically active, even if you are not thirsty.

- Use sunscreen when you are outside.

- Always bend forward from the hips, not the waist. If you keep your back straight, you're probably bending the right way. If your back "humps," that's probably wrong.

- Stop your activity if you feel very out of breath, dizzy, nauseous, or have pain. If you feel tightness or pain in your chest, or you feel faint or have trouble breathing, stop the activity right away and talk to your doctor.

Exercise should not hurt or make you feel really tired. You might feel some soreness, a little discomfort, or a bit weary. But you should not feel pain. In fact, in many ways, being active will probably make you feel better.

Can I Stay Active If I Have a Disability?

A disability may make it harder to stay active, but it shouldn't stop you. In most cases, people with disabilities can improve their flexibility, mobility, and coordination by becoming physically active. Getting regular physical activity can also help you stay independent by preventing illnesses, such as heart disease, that can make caring for yourself more difficult.

Even though you have a disability, you should still aim to meet the physical activity goals. Work with a doctor to develop a physical activity plan that works for you.

What Are Some Tips to Help Me Get Moving?

Fit it into a busy schedule

- If you can't set aside one block of time, do short activities throughout the day, such as three 10-minute walks.

- Create opportunities for activity. Try parking your car farther away from where you are headed. If you ride the bus or train, get off one or two stops early and walk.

- Walk or bike to work or to the store.

- Use stairs instead of the elevator or escalator.

- Take breaks at work to stretch or take quick walks, or do something active with coworkers at lunch.

- Walk while you talk, if you're using a cellphone or cordless phone.

- Doing yard work or household chores counts as physical activity. Turn on some upbeat music to help you do chores faster and speed up your heart rate.

Make it fun

- Choose activities that you enjoy.

- Vary your activities, so you don't get bored. For instance, use different jogging, walking, or biking paths. Or bike one day, and jog the next.

- Reward yourself when you achieve your weekly goals. For instance, reward yourself by going to a movie.

- If you have children, make time to play with them outside. Set a good example!

- Plan active vacations that will keep you moving, such as taking tours and sightseeing on foot.

Make it social

- Join a hiking or running club.

- Go dancing with your partner or friends.

- Turn activities into social occasions—for example, go to a movie after you and a friend work out.

Overcome challenges

- Don't let cold weather keep you on the couch. You can find activities to do in the winter, such as indoor fitness classes or exercising to a workout video.

- If you live in a neighborhood where it is unsafe to be active outdoors, contact your local recreational center or church to see if they have indoor activity programs that you can join. You can also find ways to be active at home. For instance, you can do push-ups or lift hand weights. If you don't have hand weights, you can use canned foods or bottles filled with water or sand.

Don't expect to notice body changes right away. It can take weeks or months before you notice some of the changes from being physically active, such as weight loss. And keep in mind, many benefits of physical activity are happening inside you and you cannot see them.

Do I Need to Talk to My Doctor before I Start?

You should talk to your doctor before you begin any physical activity program if you:

- Have heart disease, had a stroke, or are at high risk for these diseases
- Have diabetes or are at high risk for diabetes
- Are obese (BMI of 30 or greater)
- Have an injury or disability
- Are pregnant
- Have a bleeding or detached retina, eye surgery, or laser treatment on your eye
- Have had recent hip surgery

Chapter 7

Obesity and Weight Loss

Over 60 percent of U.S. adult women are overweight, according to estimates from the National Center for Health Statistics (NCHS) of the Center for Disease Control and Prevention (CDC). Just over one-third of overweight adult women are obese.

How Do I know If I'm Overweight or Obese?

Find out your body mass index (BMI). BMI is a measure of body fat based on height and weight. People with a BMI of 25 to 29.9 are considered overweight. People with a BMI of 30 or more are considered obese.

What Causes Someone to Become Overweight or Obese?

You can become overweight or obese when you eat more calories than you use. A calorie is a unit of energy in the food you eat. Your body needs this energy to function and to be active. But if you take in more energy than your body uses, you will gain weight.

Many factors can play a role in becoming overweight or obese. These factors include:

- Behaviors, such as eating too many calories or not getting enough physical activity

---

This chapter includes text excerpted from "Overweight, Obesity, and Weight Loss," Office on Women's Health (OWH), U.S. Department of Health and Human Services (HHS), June 12, 2017.

- Environment and culture
- Genes

Overweight and obesity problems keep getting worse in the United States. Some cultural reasons for this include:

- Bigger portion sizes
- Little time to exercise or cook healthy meals
- Using cars to get places instead of walking

What Are the Health Effects of Being Overweight or Obese?

Being overweight or obese can increase your risk of:

- Heart disease
- Stroke
- Type 2 diabetes
- High blood pressure
- Breathing problems
- Arthritis
- Gallbladder disease
- Some kinds of cancer

But excess body weight isn't the only health risk. The places where you store your body fat also affect your health. Women with a "pear" shape tend to store fat in their hips and buttocks. Women with an "apple" shape store fat around their waists. If your waist is more than 35 inches, you may have a higher risk of weight-related health problems.

What Is the Best Way for Me to Lose Weight?

The best way to lose weight is to use more calories than you take in. You can do this by following a healthy eating plan and being more active. Before you start a weight-loss program, talk to your doctor.

Safe weight-loss programs that work well:

- Set a goal of slow and steady weight loss—1 to 2 pounds per week

- Offer low-calorie eating plans with a wide range of healthy foods
- Encourage you to be more physically active
- Teach you about healthy eating and physical activity
- Adapt to your likes and dislikes and cultural background
- Help you keep weight off after you lose it

How Can I Make Healthier Food Choices?

The U.S. Department of Health and Human Services (HHS) and Department of Agriculture (USDA) offer tips for healthy eating in *Dietary Guidelines for Americans.*

- **Focus on fruits.** Eat a variety of fruits—fresh, frozen, canned, or dried—rather than fruit juice for most of your fruit choices. For a 2,000-calorie diet, you will need 2 cups of fruit each day. An example of 2 cups is 1 small banana, 1 large orange, and 1/4 cup of dried apricots or peaches.

- **Vary your veggies.** Eat more:
  - dark green veggies, such as broccoli, kale, and other dark leafy greens
  - orange veggies, such as carrots, sweet potatoes, pumpkin, and winter squash
  - beans and peas, such as pinto beans, kidney beans, black beans, garbanzo beans, split peas, and lentils

- **Get your calcium-rich foods.** Each day, drink 3 cups of low-fat or fat-free milk. Or, you can get an equivalent amount of low-fat yogurt and/or low-fat cheese each day. 1.5 ounces of cheese equals 1 cup of milk. If you don't or can't consume milk, choose lactose-free milk products and/or calcium-fortified foods and drinks.

- **Make half your grains whole.** Eat at least 3 ounces of whole-grain cereals, breads, crackers, rice, or pasta each day. One ounce is about 1 slice of bread, 1 cup of breakfast cereal, or 1/2 cup of cooked rice or pasta. Look to see that grains such as wheat, rice, oats, or corn are referred to as "whole" in the list of ingredients.

- **Go lean with protein.** Choose lean meats and poultry. Bake it, broil it, or grill it. Vary your protein choices with more fish, beans, peas, nuts, and seeds.

- **Limit saturated fats.** Get less than 10 percent of your calories from saturated fatty acids. Most fats should come from sources of polyunsaturated and monounsaturated fatty acids, such as fish, nuts, and vegetable oils. When choosing and preparing meat, poultry, dry beans, and milk or milk products, make choices that are lean, low-fat, or fat-free.

- **Limit salt.** Get less than 2,300 mg of sodium (about 1 teaspoon of salt) each day.

How Can Physical Activity Help?

The *Physical Activity Guidelines for Americans* state that an active lifestyle can lower your risk of early death from a variety of causes. There is strong evidence that regular physical activity can also lower your risk of:

- Heart disease

- Stroke

- High blood pressure

- Unhealthy cholesterol levels

- Type 2 diabetes

- Metabolic syndrome

- Colon cancer

- Breast cancer

- Falls

- Depression

Regular activity can help prevent unhealthy weight gain and also help with weight loss, when combined with lower calorie intake. If you are overweight or obese, losing weight can lower your risk for many diseases. Being overweight or obese increases your risk of heart disease, high blood pressure, stroke, type 2 diabetes, breathing problems, osteoarthritis, gallbladder disease, sleep apnea (breathing problems while sleeping), and some cancers.

Regular physical activity can also improve your cardiorespiratory (heart, lungs, and blood vessels) and muscular fitness. For older adults, activity can improve mental function.

Physical activity may also help:

- Improve functional health for older adults
- Reduce waistline size
- Lower risk of hip fracture
- Lower risk of lung cancer
- Lower risk of endometrial cancer
- Maintain weight after weight loss
- Increase bone density
- Improve sleep quality

Health benefits are gained by doing the following each week:

- 2 hours and 30 minutes of moderate-intensity aerobic physical activity, or
- 1 hour and 15 minutes of vigorous-intensity aerobic physical activity, or
- A combination of moderate and vigorous-intensity aerobic physical activity and
- Muscle-strengthening activities on 2 or more days

This physical activity should be in addition to your routine activities of daily living, such as cleaning or spending a few minutes walking from the parking lot to your office.

If you want to lose a substantial (more than 5 percent of body weight) amount of weight, you need a high amount of physical activity unless you also lower calorie intake. This is also the case if you are trying to keep the weight off. Many people need to do more than 300 minutes of moderate-intensity activity a week to meet weight-control goals.

Moderate Activity

During moderate-intensity activities you should notice an increase in your heart rate, but you should still be able to talk comfortably. An example of a moderate-intensity activity is walking on a level surface at a brisk pace (about 3 to 4 miles per hour). Other examples include ballroom dancing, leisurely bicycling, moderate housework, and waiting tables.

Vigorous Activity

If your heart rate increases a lot and you are breathing so hard that it is difficult to carry on a conversation, you are probably doing vigorous-intensity activity. Examples of vigorous-intensity activities include jogging, bicycling fast or uphill, singles tennis, and pushing a hand mower.

How Can You Increase Your Physical Activity?

Table 7.1. Increasing Physical Activity

If You Normally...	Try This Instead!
Park as close as possible to the store	Park farther away
Let the dog out back	Take the dog for a walk
Take the elevator	Take the stairs
Have lunch delivered	Walk to pick up lunch
Relax while the kids play	Get involved in their activity

What Are the Medicines Approved for Long-Term Treatment of Obesity?

The U.S. Food and Drug Administration (FDA) has approved two medicines for long-term treatment of obesity:

- Sibutramine suppresses your appetite.

- Orlistat keeps your body from absorbing fat from the food you eat.

These medicines are for people who:

- Have a BMI of 30 or higher

- Have a BMI of 27 or higher and weight-related health problems or health risks

If you take these medicines, you will need to follow a healthy eating and physical activity plan at the same time.

Before taking these medicines, talk with your doctor about the benefits and the side effects.

- Sibutramine can raise your blood pressure and heart rate. You should not take this medicine if you have a history of high blood pressure, heart problems, or strokes. Other side effects include dry mouth, headache, constipation, anxiety, and trouble sleeping.

- Orlistat may cause diarrhea, cramping, gas, and leakage of oily stool. Eating a low-fat diet can help prevent these side effects. This medicine may also prevent your body from absorbing some vitamins. Talk with your doctor about whether you should take a vitamin supplement.

What Surgical Options Are Used to Treat Obesity?

Weight loss surgeries—also called bariatric surgeries—can help treat obesity. You should only consider surgical treatment for weight loss if you:

- Have a BMI of 40 or higher

- Have a BMI of 35 or higher and weight-related health problems

- Have not had success with other weight-loss methods
Common types of weight loss surgeries are:

- **Roux-en-Y gastric bypass.** The surgeon uses surgical staples to create a small stomach pouch. This limits the amount of food you can eat. The pouch is attached to the middle part of the small intestine. Food bypasses the upper part of the small intestine and stomach, reducing the amount of calories and nutrients your body absorbs.

- **Laparoscopic gastric banding.** A band is placed around the upper stomach to create a small pouch and narrow passage into the rest of the stomach. This limits the amount of food you can eat. The size of the band can be adjusted. A surgeon can remove the band if needed.

- **Biliopancreatic diversion (BPD) or BPD with duodenal switch (BPD/DS).** In BPD, a large part of the stomach is removed, leaving a small pouch. The pouch is connected to the last part of the small intestine, bypassing other parts of the small intestine. In BPD/DS, less of the stomach and small intestine are removed. This surgery reduces the amount of food you can eat and the amount of calories and nutrients your body absorbs from food. This surgery is used less often than other types of surgery because of the high risk of malnutrition.

If you are thinking about weight-loss surgery, talk with your doctor about changes you will need to make after the surgery. You will need to:

- Follow your doctor's directions as you heal

- Make lasting changes in the way you eat
- Follow a healthy eating plan and be physically active
- Take vitamins and minerals if needed

You should also talk to your doctor about risks and side effects of weight loss surgery. Side effects may include:

- Infection
- Leaking from staples
- Hernia
- Blood clots in the leg veins that travel to your lungs (pulmonary embolism)
- Dumping syndrome, in which food moves from your stomach to your intestines too quickly
- Not getting enough vitamins and minerals from food

Is Liposuction a Treatment for Obesity?

Liposuction is not a treatment for obesity. In this procedure, a surgeon removes fat from under the skin. Liposuction can be used to reshape parts of your body. But this surgery does not promise lasting weight loss.

Chapter 8

Dealing with Sleep Disorders and Tips for Getting Better Sleep

How Much Sleep Is Enough?[1]

Experts say most teens need a little more than nine hours of sleep each night. Only a tiny number get that much, though. Here are some ways to see if you are getting enough sleep:

- Do you have trouble getting up in the morning?

- Do you have trouble focusing?

- Do you sometimes fall asleep during class?

If you answered yes to these questions, try using the tips above for getting better sleep.

This chapter includes text excerpted from documents published by four public domain sources. Text under the heading marked 1 is excerpted from "Getting Enough Sleep," girlshealth.gov, Office on Women's Health (OWH), April 15, 2014; Text under the heading marked 2 is excerpted from "Key Sleep Disorders," Centers for Disease Control and Prevention (CDC), December 10, 2014; Text under the headings marked 3 are excerpted from "For Women—Sleep Problems," U.S. Food and Drug Administration (FDA), April 24, 2017; Text under the heading marked 4 is excerpted from "Sleep Problems and Menopause: What Can I Do?" National Institute on Aging (NIA), National Institutes of Health (NIH), August 1, 2017.

Also keep in mind that good sleep isn't just about the number of hours you're in bed. If you wake up a lot in the night, snore, or have headaches, you may not be getting enough quality sleep to keep you fresh and healthy.

Major Sleep Disorders[2]

Sleep-related difficulties affect many people. The following is a description of some of the major sleep disorders. If you, or someone you know, is experiencing any of the following, it is important to receive an evaluation by a healthcare provider or, if necessary, a provider specializing in sleep medicine.

Insomnia

Insomnia is characterized by an inability to initiate or maintain sleep. It may also take the form of early morning awakening in which the individual awakens several hours early and is unable to resume sleeping. Difficulty initiating or maintaining sleep may often manifest itself as excessive daytime sleepiness, which characteristically results in functional impairment throughout the day. Before arriving at a diagnosis of primary insomnia, the healthcare provider will rule out other potential causes, such as other sleep disorders, side effects of medications, substance abuse, depression, or other previously unde-tected illness. Chronic psychophysiological insomnia (or "learned" or "conditioned" insomnia) may result from a stressor combined with fear of being unable to sleep. Individuals with this condition may sleep better when not in their own beds. Healthcare providers may treat chronic insomnia with a combination of use of sedative-hypnotic or sedating antidepressant medications, along with behavioral techniques to promote regular sleep.

Narcolepsy

Excessive daytime sleepiness (including episodes of irresistible sleepiness) combined with sudden muscle weakness are the hallmark signs of narcolepsy. The sudden muscle weakness seen in narcolepsy may be elicited by strong emotion or surprise. Episodes of narcolepsy have been described as "sleep attacks" and may occur in unusual cir-cumstances, such as walking and other forms of physical activity. The healthcare provider may treat narcolepsy with stimulant medications combined with behavioral interventions, such as regularly scheduled naps, to minimize the potential disruptiveness of narcolepsy on the individual's life.

Restless Legs Syndrome (RLS)

Restless legs syndrome (RLS) is characterized by an unpleasant "creeping" sensation, often feeling like it is originating in the lower legs, but often associated with aches and pains throughout the legs. This often causes difficulty initiating sleep and is relieved by movement of the leg, such as walking or kicking. Abnormalities in the neurotransmitter dopamine have often been associated with RLS. Healthcare providers often combine a medication to help correct the underlying dopamine abnormality along with a medicine to promote sleep continuity in the treatment of RLS.

Sleep Apnea

Snoring may be more than just an annoying habit–it may be a sign of sleep apnea. Persons with sleep apnea characteristically make periodic gasping or "snorting" noises, during which their sleep is momentarily interrupted. Those with sleep apnea may also experience excessive daytime sleepiness, as their sleep is commonly interrupted and may not feel restorative. Treatment of sleep apnea is dependent on its cause. If other medical problems are present, such as congestive heart failure or nasal obstruction, sleep apnea may resolve with treatment of these conditions. Gentle air pressure administered during sleep (typically in the form of a nasal continuous positive airway pressure device) may also be effective in the treatment of sleep apnea. As interruption of regular breathing or obstruction of the airway during sleep can pose serious health complications, symptoms of sleep apnea should be taken seriously. Treatment should be sought from a healthcare provider.

Getting Enough Sleep[1]

What's up with sleep? It may seem like a waste of time when you've got so much going on. But sleep can help you do better in school, stress less, and generally be more pleasant to have around. Sound good? Now consider some possible effects of not getting enough sleep:

- Feeling angry or depressed

- Having trouble learning, remembering, and thinking clearly

- Having more accidents, including when driving or using machines

- Getting sick more often
- Feeling less motivated
- Possibly gaining weight
- Having lower self-esteem

Medicines to Help You Sleep[3]

There are medicines that may help you fall asleep or stay asleep. You need a doctor's prescription for some sleep drugs. You can get other over-the-counter (OTC) medicines without a prescription.

Prescription

Prescription sleep medicines work well for many people but they can cause serious side effects.

- Talk to your doctor about all of the risks and benefits of using prescription sleep medicines.
- Sleep drugs taken for insomnia can affect your driving the morning after use.
- Sleep drugs can cause rare side effects like:
  - Severe allergic reactions
  - Severe face swelling
  - Behaviors like making phone calls, eating, having sex or driving while you are not fully awake

Over-the-Counter (OTC)

OTC sleep drugs have side effects too. Read the 'Drug Facts Label' to learn more about the side effects of your OTC sleep medicine.

Tips for Better Sleep[3]

Making some changes to your night time habits may help you get the sleep you need.

- Go to bed and get up at the same times each day.
- Sleep in a dark, quiet room.
- Limit caffeine.

- Don't drink alcohol before bedtime.

- Do something to help you relax before bedtime.

- Don't exercise before bedtime.

- Don't take a nap after 3 p.m.

- Don't eat a large meal before you go to sleep.

Talk to your healthcare provider if you have trouble sleeping almost every night for more than 2 weeks.

Sleep Problems and Menopause[4]

The years of the menopausal transition are often a time when there are other changes in a woman's life. You may be caring for aging parents, supporting children as they move into adulthood, and reflecting on your own life journey. Add hot flashes on top of all this, and you may find yourself having trouble sleeping at night.

Not getting enough sleep can affect all areas of life. Lack of sleep can make you feel irritable or depressed, might cause you to be more forgetful than normal, and could lead to more falls or accidents.

Some women who have trouble sleeping may use over-the-counter sleep aids like melatonin. Others use prescription medicines to help them sleep, which may help when used for a short time. But, medicines are not a cure for insomnia. Developing healthy habits at bedtime can help you get a good night's sleep.

Getting a Good Night's Sleep during the Menopausal Transition

To improve your sleep through the menopausal transition and beyond:

- Follow a regular sleep schedule. Go to sleep and get up at the same time each day.

- Avoid napping in the late afternoon or evening if you can. It may keep you awake at night.

- Develop a bedtime routine. Some people read a book, listen to soothing music, or soak in a warm bath.

- Try not to watch television or use your computer or mobile device in the bedroom. The light from these devices may make it difficult for you to fall asleep.

- Keep your bedroom at a comfortable temperature, not too hot or too cold, and as quiet as possible.

- Exercise at regular times each day but not close to bedtime.

- Avoid eating large meals close to bedtime.

- Stay away from caffeine (found in some coffees, teas, or chocolate) late in the day.

- Remember, alcohol won't help you sleep. Even small amounts make it harder to stay asleep.

If these changes to your bedtime routine don't help as much as you'd like, you may want to consider cognitive behavioral therapy. This problem-solving approach to therapy has recently been shown to help sleep disturbances in women with menopausal symptoms. Cognitive behavioral therapy can be found through a class or in one-on-one sessions. Be sure that your therapy is guided by a trained professional with experience working with women during their menopausal transition. Your doctor may be able to recommend a therapist in your area.

Chapter 9

Managing Stress

Stress is a feeling you get when faced with a challenge. Feeling stressed for a long time can take a toll on your mental and physical health. Even though it may seem hard to find ways to de-stress with all the things you have to do, it's important to find those ways. Your health depends on it.

What Is Stress?

Stress is a feeling you get when faced with a challenge. In small doses, stress can be good for you because it makes you more alert and gives you a burst of energy. For instance, if you start to cross the street and see a car about to run you over, that jolt you feel helps you to jump out of the way before you get hit. But feeling stressed for a long time can take a toll on your mental and physical health. Even though it may seem hard to find ways to de-stress with all the things you have to do, it's important to find those ways. Your health depends on it.

What Are the Most Common Causes of Stress?

Stress happens when people feel like they don't have the tools to manage all of the demands in their lives. Stress can be short term or long term. Missing the bus or arguing with your spouse or partner can cause short-term stress. Money problems or trouble at work can

This chapter includes text excerpted from "Stress and Your Health," Office on Women's Health (OWH), U.S. Department of Health and Human Services (HHS), June 12, 2017.

cause long-term stress. Even happy events, like having a baby or getting married can cause stress. Some of the most common stressful life events include:

- Death of a spouse
- Death of a close family member
- Divorce
- Losing your job
- Major personal illness or injury
- Marital separation
- Marriage
- Pregnancy
- Retirement
- Spending time in jail

What Are Some Common Signs of Stress?

Everyone responds to stress a little differently. Your symptoms may be different from someone else's. Here are some of the signs to look for:

- Not eating or eating too much
- Feeling like you have no control
- Needing to have too much control
- Forgetfulness
- Headaches
- Lack of energy
- Lack of focus
- Trouble getting things done
- Poor self-esteem
- Short temper
- Trouble sleeping
- Upset stomach
- Back pain
- General aches and pains

These symptoms may also be signs of depression or anxiety, which can be caused by long-term stress.

Do Women React to Stress Differently than Men?

One recent survey found that women were more likely to experience physical symptoms of stress than men. But we don't have enough proof to say that this applies to all women. We do know that women often cope with stress in different ways than men. Women "tend and befriend," taking care of those closest to them, but also drawing support from friends and family. Men are more likely to have the "fight or flight" response. They cope by "escaping" into a relaxing activity or other distraction.

Can Stress Affect My Health?

The body responds to stress by releasing stress hormones. These hormones make blood pressure, heart rate, and blood sugar levels go up. Long-term stress can help cause a variety of health problems, including:

- Mental health disorders, like depression and anxiety
- Obesity
- Heart disease
- High blood pressure
- Abnormal heart beats
- Menstrual problems
- Acne and other skin problems

Does Stress Cause Ulcers?

No, stress doesn't cause ulcers, but it can make them worse. Most ulcers are caused by a germ called *Helicobacter pylori*. Researchers think people might get it through food or water. Most ulcers can be cured by taking a combination of antibiotics and other drugs.

What Is Posttraumatic Stress Disorder (PTSD)?

Posttraumatic stress disorder (PTSD) is a type of anxiety disorder that can occur after living through or seeing a dangerous event. It can also occur after a sudden traumatic event. This can include:

- Being a victim of or seeing violence

- Being a victim of sexual or physical abuse or assault
- The death or serious illness of a loved one
- Fighting in a war
- A severe car crash or a plane crash
- Hurricanes, tornadoes, and fires

You can start having PTSD symptoms right after the event. Or symptoms can develop months or even years later. Symptoms may include:

- Nightmares
- Flashbacks, or feeling like the event is happening again
- Staying away from places and things that remind you of what happened
- Being irritable, angry, or jumpy
- Feeling strong guilt, depression, or worry
- Trouble sleeping
- Feeling "numb"
- Having trouble remembering the event

Women are 2 to 3 times more likely to develop PTSD than men. Also, people with ongoing stress in their lives are more likely to develop PTSD after a dangerous event.

How Can I Help Handle My Stress?

Everyone has to deal with stress. There are steps you can take to help you handle stress in a positive way and keep it from making you sick. Try these tips to keep stress in check:

Develop a New Attitude

- **Become a problem solver.** Make a list of the things that cause you stress. From your list, figure out which problems you can solve now and which are beyond your control for the moment. From your list of problems that you can solve now, start with the little ones. Learn how to calmly look at a problem, think of possible solutions, and take action to solve the problem. Being able to solve small problems will give you confidence to tackle the big ones. And feeling confident that you can solve problems will go a long way to helping you feel less stressed.

- **Be flexible.** Sometimes, it's not worth the stress to argue. Give in once in awhile or meet people halfway.

- **Get organized.** Think ahead about how you're going to spend your time. Write a to-do list. Figure out what's most important to do and do those things first.

- **Set limits.** When it comes to things like work and family, figure out what you can really do. There are only so many hours in the day. Set limits for yourself and others. Don't be afraid to say NO to requests for your time and energy.

Relax

- **Take deep breaths.** If you're feeling stressed, taking a few deep breaths makes you breathe slower and helps your muscles relax.

- **Stretch.** Stretching can also help relax your muscles and make you feel less tense.

- **Massage tense muscles.** Having someone massage the muscles in the back of your neck and upper back can help you feel less tense.

- **Take time to do something you want to do.** We all have lots of things that we have to do. But often we don't take the time to do the things that we really want to do. It could be listening to music, reading a good book, or going to a movie. Think of this as an order from your doctor, so you won't feel guilty!

Take Care of Your Body

- **Get enough sleep.** Getting enough sleep helps you recover from the stresses of the day. Also, being well-rested helps you think better so that you are prepared to handle problems as they come up. Most adults need 7 to 9 hours of sleep a night to feel rested.

- **Eat right.** Try to fuel up with fruits, vegetables, beans, and whole grains. Don't be fooled by the jolt you get from caffeine or high-sugar snack foods. Your energy will wear off, and you could wind up feeling more tired than you did before.

- **Get moving.** Getting physical activity can not only help relax your tense muscles but improve your mood. Research shows that physical activity can help relieve symptoms of depression and anxiety.

- **Don't deal with stress in unhealthy ways.** This includes drinking too much alcohol, using drugs, smoking, or overeating.

Connect with Others

- **Share your stress.** Talking about your problems with friends or family members can sometimes help you feel better. They might also help you see your problems in a new way and suggest solutions that you hadn't thought of.

- **Get help from a professional if you need it.** If you feel that you can no longer cope, talk to your doctor. She or he may suggest counseling to help you learn better ways to deal with stress. Your doctor may also prescribe medicines, such as antidepressants or sleep aids.

- **Help others.** Volunteering in your community can help you make new friends and feel better about yourself.

Chapter 10

Preventing Vision and Hearing Problems

Vision and hearing losses can happen as you age. Other problems with your eyes and ears can happen as you work and play. Prevention, early detection, and proper treatment for injury or disease to your eyes and ears will help you enjoy independence and a better quality of life.

Steps you can take:

- Get your eyes examined according to this schedule:
  - If you are between the ages of 18 and 39, discuss with your doctor when you should have a comprehensive dilated eye exam.
  - Get a baseline exam at age 40, then every 2 to 4 years (or as your doctor advises) until age 49.
  - Have an exam every 2 to 4 years until age 55, then every 1 to 3 years until age 65, or as your doctor advises.
  - At ages 65 and older, get an exam every 1 to 2 years.

People at higher risk for eye diseases need to be examined more often. For example, adults with diabetes should have a dilated eye

This chapter includes text excerpted from "A Lifetime of Good Health: Your Guide to Staying Healthy," Office on Women's Health (OWH), U.S. Department of Health and Human Services (HHS), April 9, 2011. Reviewed August 2017.

exam at least once a year. African-Americans over age 40, people with a family history, and everyone over age 60 are at higher risk for glaucoma and should have a dilated eye exam every 1 to 2 years. Eye diseases often have no warning signs in their early stage and can only be detected by an eye care professional.

- Have regular dilated eye exams. This is the best thing you can do to make sure your eyes are healthy and you are seeing your best. Your eye care professional will tell you how often you need to have one.

- Wear sunglasses to protect your eyes from harmful ultraviolet (UV) rays when outdoors. Choose sunglasses with 99 to 100 percent UVA and UVB protection, to block both forms of ultraviolet rays.

- Wear protective eyewear, such as polycarbonate safety glasses, safety goggles, or face shields, when working outdoors or with materials that can harm eyes and when playing sports.

- Eating a diet rich in fruits and vegetables, particularly dark leafy greens such as spinach, kale, or collard greens is important to keep your eyes healthy.

- Reduce eyestrain by adjusting your computer monitor appropriately, taking rest breaks when working on a computer, and sitting upright with your feet flat on the floor when working on a computer.

- Prevent hearing loss from noise. Pay attention to sounds around you that are at or above 85 decibels, such as concerts, fireworks, or lawn mowers. If you are around loud sounds for too long, wear earplugs or move away from the sound.

- Get a hearing exam every 10 years between the ages of 18 and 49 and every 3 years after that.

- Prevent ear infections. You can help prevent upper respiratory infections—and a resulting ear infection—by washing your hands often. Also, get a flu vaccine every year to help prevent flu-related ear infections.

- Ask your doctor if your medicines may hurt your ears. Some medicine (like certain antibiotics) can damage hearing.

- Be careful when listening to music through headphones. Many devices that people use today have noise levels much higher than 85 decibels. For example, an MP3 player at maximum level is roughly 105 decibels. Scientists recommend no more than 15 minutes of unprotected exposure to sounds that are 100 decibels. In addition, regular exposure to sounds at 110 decibels for more than 1 minute risks permanent hearing loss.

Chapter 11

Healthy Aging Tips for Women

Chapter Contents

Section 11.1

Food Choices for Healthy Aging

This section includes text excerpted from "Make Better Food
Choices—10 Tips for Women's Health," ChooseMyPlate.gov,
U.S. Department of Agriculture (USDA), January 2014.

Make yourself a priority and take time to care for yourself. Choose-
MyPlate.gov helps you choose the types and amounts of food and beverages you need. And, make time to be physically active, so you can
do the things you want to do.

Find out What You Need

Get personalized nutrition information based on your age, gender,
height, weight, and physical activity level. SuperTracker provides your
calorie level, shows foods and beverages you need, and tracks progress
toward your goals. Learn more at www.SuperTracker.usda.gov.

Enjoy Your Food but Eat Less

Use a smaller plate at meals to help control the amount of food and
calories you eat. Take time to enjoy smaller amounts of food.

Strengthen Your Bones

Choose foods like fat-free and low-fat milk, cheese, yogurt, and fortified soymilk to help strengthen bones. Be sure your morning coffee
includes fat-free or low-fat milk.

Make Half Your Plate Fruits and Vegetables

Add fruit to meals as part of main or side dishes. Choose red, orange,
or dark-green vegetables like tomatoes, sweet potatoes, and broccoli,
along with other vegetables for meals.

Drink Water

Sip water or other drinks with few or no calories to help maintain a healthy weight. Keep a water bottle in your bag or at your desk to satisfy your thirst throughout the day.

Eat Whole Grains More Often

Choose whole grains like brown rice and whole-grain pastas and breads more often. Foods with a high-fiber content can help give you a feeling of fullness and also provide key nutrients.

Learn What Is in Foods

Use both ingredient and Nutrition Facts labels to discover what various foods contain. SuperTracker's Food-A-Pedia (www.supertracker. usda.gov/foodapedia.aspx) makes it easy to compare nutrition information for more than 8,000 foods.

Cut Back on Some Foods

Cut calories by cutting out foods high in solid fats and added sugar. Limit fatty meats like ribs, bacon, and hot dogs. Choose cakes, cookies, candies, and ice cream as just occasional treats.

Be a Better Cook

Try out healthier recipes that use less solid fat, salt, and sugar. Eat at home more often so you can control what you are eating. If you eat out, check and compare nutrition information. Choose healthier options such as baked chicken instead of fried chicken.

Be Active Whenever You Can

Set a goal to fit in at least 2½ hours of moderate physical activity in your week. Being active 10 minutes at a time also adds to your weekly total. Ask your friends or family to keep you company as you bike, jog, walk, or dance. Don't forget to do some muscle strengthening activities twice a week.

Section 11.2

How to Be Active for Health

This section contains text excerpted from the following sources: Text beginning with the heading "Start out Slowly" is excerpted from "Exercise: How to Get Started: Safety First," NIHSeniorHealth, National Institute on Aging (NIA), October 2015; Text under the heading "Endurance Exercises: Endurance Exercises" is excerpted from "Exercise: Exercises to Try," NIHSeniorHealth, National Institute on Aging (NIA), January 2015.

Start out Slowly

Most older adults, regardless of age or condition, will do just fine increasing their physical activity to a moderate level. However, if you haven't been active for a long time, it's important to start out at a low level of effort and work your way up slowly.

When to Check with Your Doctor

If you are at high risk for any chronic diseases such as heart disease or diabetes, or if you smoke or are obese, you should check first with your doctor before becoming more physically active.

Other reasons to check with your doctor before you exercise include:

- any new, undiagnosed symptom
- chest pain
- irregular, rapid, or fluttery heartbeat
- severe shortness of breath

Check with your doctor if you have:

- ongoing, significant, and undiagnosed weight loss
- infections, like pneumonia, accompanied by fever which can cause rapid heart beat and dehydration
- an acute blood clot
- a hernia that is causing symptoms such as pain and discomfort.

- foot or ankle sores that won't heal
- persistent pain or problems walking after a fall—you might have a fracture and not know it
- eye conditions such as bleeding in the retina or a detached retina. Also consult your doctor after a cataract removal or lens implant, or after laser treatment or other eye surgery
- a weakening in the wall of the heart's major outgoing blood vessel called an abdominal aortic aneurysm
- a narrowing of one of the heart's valves called critical aortic stenosis
- joint swelling

If You've Had Hip Replacement

If you have had hip repair or replacement:

- check with your doctor before doing lower-body exercises
- don't cross your legs
- don't bend your hips farther than a 90-degree angle
- avoid locking the joints in your legs into a strained position

Discuss Your Activity Level

Your activity level is an important topic to discuss with your doctor as part of your ongoing preventive healthcare. Talk about exercise at least once a year if your health is stable, and more often if your health is getting better or worse over time so that you can adjust your exercise program. Your doctor can help you choose activities that are best for you and reduce any risks.

When to Stop Exercising

Stop exercising if you:

- have pain or pressure in your chest, neck, shoulder, or arm
- feel dizzy or sick to your stomach
- break out in a cold sweat
- have muscle cramps
- feel severe pain in joints, feet, ankles, or legs

117

Endurance Exercises

To get all of the benefits of physical activity, try all four types of exercise—endurance, strength, balance, and flexibility. This section addresses endurance activities.

Increasing Your Breathing and Heart Rate

Endurance exercises are activities that increase your breathing and heart rate for an extended period of time. Examples are walking, jogging, swimming, raking, sweeping, dancing, and playing tennis. Endurance exercises will make it easier for you to walk farther, faster, or uphill. They also should make everyday activities such as gardening, shopping, or playing a sport easier.

How Much, How Often?

Refer to your starting goals, and build up your endurance gradually. If you haven't been active for a long time, it's especially important to work your way up over time. It may take a while to go from a long-standing inactive lifestyle to doing some of the activities listed below.

For example, start out with 5 or 10 minutes at a time, and then build up to at least 30 minutes of moderate-intensity endurance activity. Doing less than 10 minutes at a time won't give you the desired heart and lung benefits. Try to build up to at least 150 minutes (2 1/2 hours) of moderate endurance activity a week. Being active at least 3 days a week is best.

Going Further

When you're ready to do more, build up the amount of time you spend doing endurance activities first, then build up the difficulty of your activities. For example, gradually increase your time to 30 minutes over several days to weeks (or even months, depending on your condition) by walking longer distances. Then walk more briskly or up steeper hills.

Safety Tips

- Do a little light activity, such as easy walking, before and after your endurance activities to warm up and cool down.
- Drink liquids when doing any activity that makes you sweat.
- Dress appropriately for the heat and cold. Dress in layers if you're outdoors so you can add or remove clothes as needed.

- Wear proper shoes.

- When you're out walking, watch out for low-hanging branches and uneven sidewalks.

- Walk during the day or in well-lit areas at night, and be aware of your surroundings.

- To prevent injuries, use safety equipment such as helmets for biking.

- Endurance activities should not make you breathe so hard that you can't talk and should not cause dizziness, or chest pain or pressure, or a feeling like heartburn.

Indoor Endurance Activities

Don't let bad weather stop you from exercising. Here are some options for exercising indoors.

- going to a gym or fitness center and using the treadmill, elliptical machine, stationary bike, or rowing machine

- swimming laps

- joining a water aerobics class

- dancing

- performing martial arts

- bowling

Outdoor Endurance Activities

Use your exercise program as a chance to get outside and enjoy nature. Here are some ideas for being active outdoors.

- biking, hand-crank bicycling, or tandem biking

- horseback riding

- sailing

- jogging or running

- skating

- snorkeling

Endurance Activities around the House

You don't need to leave your house to be active. Check out these ways to exercise at home.

- gardening
- heavy housework
- sweeping
- raking
- shoveling snow

Walking or Rolling

Walking or wheelchair rolling are simple ways to be active. You can do it alone, with friends, even with your dog! Try one of these types of walking or rolling to get active today.

- nordic walking
- hiking
- walking the dog
- mall walking
- wheelchair rolling
- race walking

Section 11.3

Medication for Older Women

This section includes text excerpted from "Medicines and You: A Guide for Older Adults," U.S. Food and Drug Administration (FDA), October 7, 2015.

Aging and Health: You and Your Medicines

As you age, it is important to know about your medicines to avoid possible problems. As you get older you may be faced with more health conditions that you need to treat on a regular basis. It is important to be aware that more use of medicines and normal body changes caused by aging can increase the chance of unwanted or maybe even harmful drug interactions.

The more you know about your medicines and the more you talk with your healthcare professionals, the easier it is to avoid problems with medicines.

As you age, body changes can affect the way medicines are absorbed and used. For example, changes in the digestive system can affect how fast medicines enter the bloodstream. Changes in body weight can influence the amount of medicine you need to take and how long it stays in your body. The circulation system may slow down, which can affect how fast drugs get to the liver and kidneys. The liver and kidneys also may work more slowly affecting the way a drug breaks down and is removed from the body.

Because of these body changes, there is also a bigger risk of drug interactions for older adults. Drug-drug interactions happen when two or more medicines react with each other to cause unwanted effects. This kind of interaction can also cause one medicine to not work as well or even make one medicine stronger than it should be. For example, you should not take aspirin if you are taking a prescription blood thinner, such as Warfarin, unless your healthcare professional tells you to.

Drug-condition interactions happen when a medical condition you already have makes certain drugs potentially harmful. For example, if you have high blood pressure or asthma, you could have an unwanted reaction if you take a nasal decongestant.

Drug-food interactions result from drugs reacting with foods or drinks. In some cases, food in the digestive tract can affect how a drug is absorbed. Some medicines also may affect the way nutrients are absorbed or used in the body.

Drug-alcohol interactions can happen when the medicine you take reacts with an alcoholic drink. For instance, mixing alcohol with some medicines may cause you to feel tired and slow your reactions.

It is important to know that many medicines do not mix well with alcohol. As you grow older, your body may react differently to alcohol, as well as to the mix of alcohol and medicines. Keep in mind that some problems you might think are medicine-related, such as loss of coordination, memory loss, or irritability, could be the result of a mix between your medicine and alcohol.

What Are Side Effects?

Some medicines can interact with other medicines, foods, drinks, or health conditions. Side effects are unplanned symptoms or feelings you have when taking a medicine. Most side effects are not serious and go away on their own; others can be more bothersome and even serious. To help prevent possible problems with medicines, seniors must know about the medicine they take and how it makes them feel.

Keep track of side effects to help your doctor know how your body is responding to a medicine. New symptoms or mood changes may not be a result of getting older but could be from the medicine you're taking or another factor, such as a change in diet or routine. If you have an unwanted side effect, call your doctor right away.

Tips for Seniors on Safe Medicine Use

- Learn about your medicines. Read medicine labels and package inserts and follow the directions. If you have questions, ask your doctor or other healthcare professionals.

- Talk to your team of healthcare professionals about your medical conditions, health concerns, and all the medicines you take (prescription and OTC medicines), as well as dietary supplements, vitamins, and herbals. The more they know, the more they can help. Don't be afraid to ask questions.

- Keep track of side effects or possible drug interactions and let your doctor know right away about any unexpected symptoms or changes in the way you feel.

- Make sure to go to all doctor appointments and to any appointments for monitoring tests done by your doctor or at a laboratory.

- Use a calendar, pill box or other things, to help you remember what you need to take and when. Write down information your doctor gives you about your medicines or your health condition.

- Take along a friend or relative to your doctor's appointments if you think you might need help to understand or to remember what the doctor tells you.

- Have a "Medicine Check-Up" at least once a year. Go through your medicine cabinet to get rid of old or expired medicines and also ask your doctor or pharmacist to go over all of the medicines you now take. Don't forget to tell them about all the OTC medicines or any vitamins, dietary supplements, and herbals you take.

- Keep all medicines out of the sight and reach of children.

Section 11.4

Talking with Your Healthcare Provider

This section includes text excerpted from "Talking with Your Doctor," NIHSeniorHealth, National Institute on Aging (NIA), June 2015.

How well you and your doctor talk to each other is one of the most important parts of getting good healthcare. Unfortunately, talking with your doctor isn't always easy. In the past, the doctor typically took the lead and the patient followed. Today, a good patient-doctor relationship is a partnership. You and your doctor can work as a team.

Creating a basic plan before you go to the doctor can help you make the most of your visit. The tips in this chapter will make it easier for you and your doctor to cover everything you need to talk about.

Make a List of Your Symptoms

Talking about your health means sharing information about how you feel. Sometimes it can be hard to remember everything that is bothering you during your doctor visit. Making a list of your symptoms before your visit will help you not forget to tell the doctor anything.

Symptoms can be physical, such as pain, fever, a lump or bump, unexplained weight gain or loss, change in energy level, or having a hard time sleeping. Symptoms can also involve your thoughts and your feelings. For example, you would want to tell your doctor if you are often confused, or if you feel sad a lot.

What to Include

When you list your symptoms, be specific. Your list should include:

- what the symptom is
- when it started
- what time of day it happens and how long it lasts
- how often it happens
- anything that makes it worse or better
- anything it prevents you from doing

List Your Medications

Your doctor needs to know about ALL the medications you take. Medications include:

- prescription drugs
- over-the-counter (non-prescription) drugs
- vitamins, herbal remedies or supplements
- laxatives
- eye drops

Sometimes doctors may ask you to bring all your medications in a bag to your visit. Other doctors suggest making a list of all your medications to bring to your visit.

Note Dosages, Frequency, Side Effects

If you do make a list of the medications you take, do not forget to write down how much you take and how often you take it. Make sure to tell the doctor if a dose has changed or if you are taking a new medicine since your last visit.

Write down or bring all your medications even if you think that one or some of them are not important. The doctor needs to know everything you take because sometimes medicines cause problems when taken together. Also, sometimes a medicine you take for one health problem, like a headache, can cause another health problem to get worse. Write down any medication allergies you have and any bad side effects you have had with the medicines you take. Also, write down which medications work best for you.

To provide the best care, your doctor must understand you as a person and know what your life is like.

Do You Use Assistive Devices?

Be sure to let your doctor know if you use any assistive devices to help you in your daily activities. Assistive devices can help you see, hear, stand, reach, balance, grasp items, go up or down stairs, and move around. Devices used by older adults may include canes, walkers, scooters, hearing aids, reachers, grab bars, and stair lifts.

What Are Your Everyday Habits?

Be prepared to tell your doctor about where you live, if you drive or how you get around, what you eat, how you sleep, what you do each day, what activities you enjoy, what your sex life is like, and if you smoke or drink alcohol.

Be open and honest. It will help your doctor to better understand your medical conditions and figure out the best treatment choices for you.

Any Life Changes?

Sometimes things happen in life that are sad or stressful. Your doctor needs to know about any life changes that have occurred since your last visit because they can affect your health. Examples of life changes are divorce, death of a loved one, or changing where you live.

Your list should include all your life changes but does not need to go into detail. It can be short like "had to sell home and move in with daughter."

Any Other Medical Encounters?

Also, write down and tell your doctor if you had to go to the emergency room, stay in the hospital or see a different doctor, such as a specialist, since your last visit. It may be helpful to bring that doctor's contact information.

What Else to Bring

Bring your insurance cards, names and phone numbers of your other doctors, and the phone number of the pharmacy you use. Also, bring your medical records if your doctor does not have them.

Chapter 12

Women-Related Health Conditions and CAM

About Complementary and Alternative Medicine

Complementary and alternative medicine (CAM) is a group of diverse medical and healthcare systems, practices, and products that are not generally considered part of conventional medicine. Complementary medicine is used together with conventional medicine, and alternative medicine is used in place of conventional medicine. Integrative medicine combines conventional and CAM treatments for which there is evidence of safety and effectiveness. While scientific evidence

This chapter contains text excerpted from the following sources: Text under the heading "About Complementary and Alternative Medicine" is excerpted from "The Use of Complementary and Alternative Medicine in the United States," National Center for Complementary and Integrative Health (NCCIH), March 22, 2016; Text under the heading "What Is Natural Childbirth?" is excerpted from "What Is Natural Childbirth?" *Eunice Kennedy Shriver* National Institute of Child Health and Human Development (NICHD), December 17, 2014; Text under the heading "Menopausal Symptoms and Complementary Health Practices" is excerpted from "Menopausal Symptoms and Complementary Health Practices," National Center for Complementary and Integrative Health (NCCIH), February 24, 2016; Text under the heading "Four Things to Know About Menopausal Symptoms and Complementary Health Practices" is excerpted from "4 Things to Know About Menopausal Symptoms and Complementary Health Practices," National Center for Complementary and Integrative Health (NCCIH), August 11, 2016.

exists regarding some CAM therapies, for most there are key questions that are yet to be answered through well-designed scientific studies— questions such as whether these therapies are safe and whether they work for the purposes for which they are used.

What Is Natural Childbirth?

Natural childbirth can refer to many different ways of giving birth without using pain medication, either in the home or at the hospital or birthing center.

Natural Forms of Pain Relief

Women who choose natural childbirth can use a number of natural ways to ease pain. These include:

• Emotional support

• Relaxation techniques

• A soothing atmosphere

• Moving and changing positions frequently

• Using a birthing ball

• Using soothing phrases and mental images

• Placing a heating pad or ice pack on the back or stomach

• Massage

• Taking a bath or shower

• Hypnosis

• Using soothing scents (aromatherapy)

• Acupuncture or acupressure

• Applying small doses of electrical stimulation to nerve fibers to activate the body's own pain-relieving substances (called transcutaneous electrical nerve stimulation, or TENS)

• Injecting sterile water into the lower back, which can relieve the intense discomfort and pain in the lower back known as back labor

A woman should discuss the many aspects of labor with her healthcare provider well before labor begins to ensure that she understands all of the options, risks, and benefits of pain relief during labor and delivery. It might also be helpful to put all the decisions in writing to clarify the options chosen.

Menopausal Symptoms and Complementary Health Practices

- A number of studies and systematic reviews on complementary health practices for menopausal symptoms have been published. There is limited evidence on the effects of mind and body practices for menopausal symptoms, but a few approaches hold promise. Scientists have found little evidence that natural products, such as herbs and other dietary supplements, are helpful. The long-term safety of phytoestrogens has not been established.

- This issue of the digest provides highlights from current evidence on several frequently used complementary health approaches for menopausal symptoms, including phytoestrogens, black cohosh, dehydroepiandrosterone (DHEA), hypnotherapy and mindfulness meditation, acupuncture, and yoga.

Natural Products

Phytoestrogens (Red Clover, Soy)

Studies of phytoestrogens such as the isoflavones found in soy and red clover have had inconsistent results on relieving menopausal symptoms. Clinical practice guidelines issued by the American Association of Clinical Endocrinologists (AACE) for the diagnosis and management of menopause state that phytoestrogens, including soy-derived isoflavonoids, result in inconsistent relief of symptoms. The guidelines advise that women with a personal or strong family history of hormone-dependent cancers, thromboembolic events, or cardiovascular events should not use soy-based therapies. Likewise, guidelines from the American College of Obstetricians and Gynecologists (ACOG) state that phytoestrogens and herbal supplements have not been shown to be useful for treating hot flashes.

Black Cohosh

Research suggests that there is overall insufficient evidence to support the use of black cohosh for menopausal symptoms.

DHEA (Dehydroepiandrosterone)

DHEA is a naturally occurring substance that is changed in the body to the hormones estrogen and testosterone. DHEA is manufactured and sold as a dietary supplement. A few small studies have suggested that DHEA might possibly have some benefit for hot flashes and decreased sexual arousal, although small randomized controlled trials have shown no benefit.

Four Things to Know about Menopausal Symptoms and Complementary Health Practices

Menopause is the permanent end of a woman's menstrual periods. Menopause can occur naturally or be caused by surgery, chemotherapy, or radiation. During the years around menopause, some women have hot flashes, night sweats, difficulty sleeping, or other bothersome symptoms. Natural products or mind and body practices are sometimes used in an effort to relieve menopausal symptoms such as hot flashes and night sweats. Here are 4 things to know if you are considering a complementary health approach for managing menopausal symptoms:

1. **Mind and body practices such as hypnosis, mindfulness meditation, and tai chi may help improve some menopausal symptoms.** Researchers looked at mind and body therapies for menopausal symptoms and found that tai chi and meditation-based programs may be helpful in reducing common menopausal symptoms including the frequency and intensity of hot flashes, sleep and mood disturbances, stress, and muscle and joint pain. There is also some evidence that hypnotherapy may help women manage hot flashes.

2. **Many natural products, such as black cohosh, soy isoflavone supplements, and DHEA, have been studied for their effects on menopausal symptoms, but scientists have found little evidence that they are helpful.** There is also no conclusive evidence that the herbs red clover, kava, or dong quai reduce hot flashes.

3. **Natural products used for menopausal symptoms can have side effects and can interact with other botanicals or supplements or with medications.** For example, rare cases of liver damage—some of them very serious—have been reported in people taking commercial black cohosh products. Also, concerns have been raised about the safety of DHEA because it is converted in the body to hormones, which are known to carry risks.

4. **Tell all your healthcare providers about any complementary health practices you use.** Give them a full picture of what you do to manage your health. This will help ensure coordinated and safe care.

Chapter 13

Avoiding Risk Factors for Common Health Concerns

Chapter Contents

Section 13.1

Women and High Cholesterol Prevention

This section includes text excerpted from "The Healthy Heart Handbook for Women," National Heart, Lung, and Blood Institute (NHLBI), February 29, 2012. Reviewed August 2017.

High blood cholesterol is another major risk factor for heart disease that you can do something about. The higher your blood cholesterol level, the greater your risk for developing heart disease or having a heart attack. To prevent these disorders, all women should make a serious effort to keep their cholesterol at healthy levels.

If you already have heart disease, it is particularly important to lower an elevated blood cholesterol level to reduce your high risk for a heart attack. Women with diabetes also are at especially high risk for a heart attack. If you have diabetes, you will need to take steps to keep both your cholesterol and your diabetes under control.

Although young women tend to have lower cholesterol levels than young men, between the ages of 45 and 55, women's levels begin to rise higher than men's. After age 55, this "cholesterol gap" between women and men becomes still wider. Although women's overall risk of heart disease at older ages continues to be somewhat lower than that of men, the higher a woman's blood cholesterol level, the greater her chances of developing heart disease.

Cholesterol and Your Heart

The body needs cholesterol to function normally. However, your body makes all the cholesterol it needs. Over a period of years, extra cholesterol and fat circulating in the blood buildup in the walls of the arteries that supply blood to the heart. This buildup, called plaque, makes the arteries narrower and narrower. As a result, less blood gets to the heart. Blood carries oxygen to the heart. If not enough oxygen-rich blood can reach your heart, you may suffer chest pain. If the blood supply to a portion of the heart is completely cut off, the result is a heart attack.

Cholesterol travels in the blood in packages called lipoproteins. Low-density lipoprotein (LDL) carries most of the cholesterol in the blood. Cholesterol packaged in LDL is often called "bad" cholesterol, because too much LDL in the blood can lead to cholesterol buildup and blockage in the arteries.

Another type of cholesterol is high density lipoprotein (HDL), known as "good" cholesterol. That's because HDL helps remove cholesterol from the body, preventing it from building up in the arteries.

Getting Tested

High blood cholesterol itself does not cause symptoms, so if your cholesterol level is too high, you may not be aware of it. That's why it's important to get your cholesterol levels checked regularly. Starting at age 20, all women should have their cholesterol levels checked by means of a blood test called a "fasting lipoprotein profile." Be sure to ask for the test results, so you will know whether you need to lower your cholesterol. Ask your doctor how soon you should be retested.

Total cholesterol is a measure of the cholesterol in all of your lipoproteins, including the "bad" cholesterol in LDL and the "good" cholesterol in HDL. An LDL level below 100 mg/dL* is considered "optimal," or ideal. However, not every woman needs to aim for so low a level. As you can see on the next page, there are four other categories of LDL level. The higher your LDL number, the higher your risk of heart disease. Knowing your LDL number is especially important because it will determine the kind of treatment you may need.

Your HDL number tells a different story. The lower your HDL level, the higher your heart disease risk.

Your lipoprotein profile test will also measure levels of triglycerides, another fatty substance in the blood.

* Cholesterol levels are measured in milligrams (mg) of cholesterol per deciliter (dL) of blood.

What's Your Number?

Table 13.1. Blood Cholesterol Levels and Heart Disease Risk

Total Cholesterol Level	Category
Less than 200 mg/dL	Desirable
200-239 mg/dL	Borderline high
240 mg/dL and above	High

Table 13.1. Continued

LDL Cholesterol Level	Category
Less than 100mg/dL	Optimal (ideal)
100-129 mg/dL	Near optimal/above optimal
130-159 mg/dL	Borderline high
160-189 mg/dL	High
190 mg/dL and above	Very high

Heart Disease Risk and Your Low-Density Lipoprotein (LDL) Goal

In general, the higher your LDL level and the more other risk factors you have, the greater your chances of developing heart disease or having a heart attack. The higher your risk, the lower your LDL goal level will be. Here is how to determine your LDL goal:

Step One: Count your risk factors. Below are risk factors for heart disease that will affect your LDL goal. Check to see how many of the following risk factors you have:

- Cigarette smoking
- High blood pressure (140/90 mmHg or higher, or if you are on blood pressure medication)
- Low HDL cholesterol (less than 40 mg/dL)
- Family history of early heart disease (your father or brother before age 55, or your mother or sister before age 65)
- Age (55 or older)

Step Two: Find Out Your Risk Score. If you have two or more risk factors in Step One, you will need to figure out your "risk score." This score will show your chances of having a heart attack in the next 10 years.

Step Three: Find Out Your Risk Category. Use your number of risk factors, risk score, and medical history to find out your history to find out your category of risk for heart disease or heart attack.

What Are Triglycerides?

Triglycerides are another type of fat found in the blood and in food. Triglycerides are produced in the liver. When you drink alcohol or take in more calories than your body needs, your liver produces more

Table 13.2. Blood Cholesterol Levels and Risk Category

If You Have	Your Category Is
Heart disease, diabetes, or a risk score of more than 20 percent	High Risk
2 or more risk factors and a risk score of 10 to 20 percent	Next Highest Risk
2 or more risk factors and a risk score of less than 10 percent	Moderate Risk
0 to 1 risk factor	Low-to-Moderate Risk

triglycerides. Triglyceride levels that are borderline high (150–199 mg/dL) or high (200–499 mg/dL) are signals of an increased risk for heart disease. To reduce blood triglyceride levels, it is important to control your weight, get more physical activity, quit smoking, and avoid alcohol. You should also follow an eating plan that is not too high in carbohydrates (less than 60 percent of calories) and is low in saturated fat, trans fat, and cholesterol. Sometimes, medication is also needed.

A Special Type of Risk

Some women have a group of risk factors known as "metabolic syndrome," which is usually caused by overweight or obesity and by not getting enough physical activity. This cluster of risk factors increases your risk of heart disease and diabetes, regardless of your LDL cholesterol level. Women have metabolic syndrome if they have three or more of the following conditions:

- A waist measurement of 35 inches or more
- Triglycerides of 150 mg/dL or more
- An HDL level of less than 50 mg/dL
- Blood pressure of 130/85 mmHg or more (either number counts)
- Blood sugar of 100 mg/dL or more

If you have metabolic syndrome, you should calculate your risk score and risk category as indicated in Steps 2 and 3 on the previous page. You should make a particularly strong effort to reach and maintain your LDL goal. You should emphasize weight control and physical activity to correct the risk factors of the metabolic syndrome.

135

Your LDL Goal

The main goal of cholesterol-lowering treatment is to lower your LDL level enough to reduce your risk of heart disease or heart attack. The higher your risk category, the lower your LDL goal will be. To find your personal LDL goal, see the below table:

Table 13.3. LDL Risk Category and Your Goal

If You Are in This Risk Category	Your LDL Goal Is
High Risk	Less than 100 mg/dL
Next Highest Risk or Moderate Risk	Less than 130 mg/dL
Low-to-Moderate Risk	Less than 160 mg/dL

If you have heart disease, work with your doctor to lower your LDL cholesterol as much as possible. But even if you can't lower your LDL cholesterol to less than 70 mg/dL because of a high starting level, lowering your LDL cholesterol to less than 100 mg/dL will still greatly reduce your risk.

How to Lower Your LDL

There are two main ways to lower your LDL cholesterol—through lifestyle changes alone, or through medication combined with lifestyle changes. Depending on your risk category, the use of these treatments will differ. Because of the recent studies that showed the benefit of more intensive cholesterol lowering, physicians have the option to start cholesterol medication—in addition to lifestyle therapy—at lower LDL levels than previously recommended for high-risk patients.

Lifestyle Changes. One important treatment approach is called the TLC Program. TLC stands for "Therapeutic Lifestyle Changes," a three-part treatment that uses diet, physical activity, and weight management. Every woman who needs to lower her LDL cholesterol should use the TLC Program.

Medication. If your LDL level stays too high even after making lifestyle changes, you may need to take medicine. If you need medication, be sure to use it along with the TLC approach. This will keep the dose of medicine as low as possible and lower your risk in other ways as well. You will also need to control all of your other heart disease risk factors, including high blood pressure, diabetes, and smoking.

As part of your cholesterol-lowering treatment plan, your doctor may recommend medication. The most commonly used medicines are listed below.

Statins. These are the most commonly prescribed drugs for people who need a cholesterol-lowering medicine. They lower LDL levels more than other types of drugs—about 20 to 55 percent. They also moderately lower triglycerides and raise HDL. Side effects are usually mild, although liver and muscle problems may occur rarely. If you experience muscle aches or weakness, you should contact your doctor promptly.

Ezetimibe. This is the first in a new class of cholesterol-lowering drugs that interferes with the absorption of cholesterol in the intestine. Ezetimbe lowers LDL by about 18 to 25 percent. It can be used alone or in combination with a statin to get more lowering of LDL. Side effects may include back and joint pain.

Bile acid resins. These medications lower LDL cholesterol by about 15 to 30 percent. Bile acid resins are often prescribed along with a statin to further decrease LDL cholesterol levels. Side effects may include constipation, bloating, nausea, and gas. However, long-term use of these medicines is considered safe.

Niacin. Niacin, or nicotinic acid, lowers total cholesterol, LDL cholesterol, and triglyceride levels, while also raising HDL cholesterol. It reduces LDL levels by about 5 to 15 percent, and up to 25 percent in some patients. Although niacin is available without a prescription, it is important to use it only under a doctor's care because of possibly serious side effects. In some people, it may worsen peptic ulcers or cause liver problems, gout, or high blood sugar.

Fibrates. These drugs can reduce triglyceride levels by 20 to 50 percent, while increasing HDL cholesterol by 10 to 15 percent. Fibrates are not very effective for lowering LDL cholesterol. The drugs can increase the chances of developing gallstones and heighten the effects of blood-thinning drugs.

Section 13.2

Preventing and Controlling High Blood Pressure

This section contains text excerpted from the following sources: Text in this section begins with excerpts from "High Blood Pressure (Hypertension)," U.S. Food and Drug Administration (FDA), September 28, 2015; Text under the heading "Preventing High Blood Pressure" is excerpted from "Preventing High Blood Pressure: Healthy Living Habits," Centers for Disease Control and Prevention (CDC), July 7, 2014; Text beginning with the heading "High Blood Pressure in the United States" is excerpted from "High Blood Pressure Facts," Centers for Disease Control and Prevention (CDC), November 30, 2016.

High blood pressure (also called hypertension) is a serious illness that affects nearly 65 million adults in the United States. High blood pressure is often called a "silent killer" because many people have it but don't know it. Over time, people who do not get treated for high blood pressure can get very sick or even die.

What Does High Blood Pressure Do to Your Body?

High blood pressure can cause life-threatening illnesses like kidney problems, stroke, heart failure, blindness, and heart attacks.

Who Is at Risk?

Anyone can have high blood pressure. Some people are more likely to have high blood pressure including:

- African Americans
- People over age 55
- People with a family history of high blood pressure

Your chances of having high blood pressure are higher if you:

- Are overweight

138

- Eat foods high in salt
- Do not get regular exercise
- Smoke
- Drink alcohol heavily

What Are the Signs of High Blood Pressure?

Many people with high blood pressure do not feel sick at first. The only way to know for sure is to get your blood pressure checked by a doctor or other health professional.

How Is High Blood Pressure Treated?

There are medicines people can take every day to control their high blood pressure. Only your doctor can tell if you need to take medicines.

Understanding Your Blood Pressure: What Do the Numbers Mean?

When you have your blood pressure taken at the doctor, you are told 2 numbers like 120/80. Both numbers are important.

The first number is your pressure when your heart beats (**systolic pressure**). The second number is your pressure when your heart relaxes (**diastolic pressure**).

Your blood pressure goes up and down during the day, depending on what you are doing. Brief rises in blood pressure are normal, but the higher your blood pressure stays, the more at risk you are.

If your blood pressure is often greater than **140/90,** you may need treatment.

If your blood pressure is greater than **120/80,** and you have other **risk factors, like diabetes,** you may need treatment.

How Does High Blood Pressure Affect Pregnant Women?

A few women will get high blood pressure when they are pregnant. When pregnant women get high blood pressure, it is called preeclampsia or toxemia.

How Do I Control My High Blood Pressure?

- Exercise often

- Eat foods low in salt

- Lose weight or keep weight at a healthy level

- Do not smoke

- Limit alcohol

- Talk to your doctor regularly about your pressure

Preventing High Blood Pressure

By living a healthy lifestyle, you can help keep your blood pressure in a healthy range and lower your risk for heart disease and stroke. A healthy lifestyle includes:

- Eating a healthy diet

- Maintaining a healthy weight

- Getting enough physical activity

- Not smoking

- Limiting alcohol use

Healthy Diet

Choosing healthful meal and snack options can help you avoid high blood pressure and its complications. Be sure to eat plenty of fresh fruits and vegetables.

Eating foods low in salt (sodium) and high in potassium can lower your blood pressure. The DASH (Dietary Approaches to Stop Hypertension) eating plan is one healthy diet that is proven to help people lower their blood pressure.

Healthy Weight

Being overweight or obese increases your risk for high blood pressure. To determine if your weight is in a healthy range, doctors often calculate your body mass index (BMI). Doctors sometimes also use waist and hip measurements to measure excess body fat.

Physical Activity

Physical activity can help you maintain a healthy weight and lower your blood pressure. For adults, the Surgeon General recommends 2 hours and 30 minutes of moderate-intensity exercise, like brisk walking or bicycling, every week. Children and adolescents should get 1 hour of physical activity every day.

No Smoking

Cigarette smoking raises your blood pressure and puts you at higher risk for heart attack and stroke. If you do not smoke, do not start. If you do smoke, quitting will lower your risk for heart disease. Your doctor can suggest ways to help you quit.

Limited Alcohol

Avoid drinking too much alcohol, which can raise your blood pressure. Men should have no more than 2 drinks per day, and women only 1.

High Blood Pressure in the United States

About 75 million American adults (29%) have high blood pressure—that's **1 of every 3 adults.**

Only about half (54%) of people with high blood pressure have their condition under control.

Nearly **1 of 3 American adults** has prehypertension—blood pressure numbers that are higher than normal, but not yet in the high blood pressure range.

High blood pressure costs the nation **$46 billion each year.** This total includes the cost of healthcare services, medications to treat high blood pressure, and missed days of work.

Blood Pressure Levels Vary by Age

Women are about as likely as men to develop high blood pressure during their lifetimes. However, for people younger than 45 years old, the condition affects more men than women. For people 65 years old or older, high blood pressure affects more women than men.

Table 13.4. Blood Pressure Levels Vary by Age

Age	Women (%)	Men (%)
20–34	6.8	11.1
35–44	19	25.1
45–54	35.2	37.1

Table 13.4. Continued

Age	Women (%)	Men (%)
55–64	53.3	54
65–74	69.3	64
75 and older	78.5	66.7
All	32.7	34.1

Blood Pressure Levels Vary by Race and Ethnicity

Blacks develop high blood pressure more often, and at an earlier age, than whites and Hispanics do. More black women than men have high blood pressure.

Table 13.5. Blood Pressure Levels Vary by Race and Ethnicity

Race of Ethnic Group	Women (%)	Men (%)
African Americans	45.7	43
Mexican Americans	28.9	27.8
Whites	31.3	33.9
All	32.7	34.1

Why Blood Pressure Matters

More than **360,000** American deaths in 2013 included high blood pressure as a primary or contributing cause. That is almost **1,000 deaths each day.**

High blood pressure increases your risk for dangerous health conditions:

- **First heart attack.** About 7 of every 10 people having their first heart attack have high blood pressure.

- **First stroke.** About 8 of every 10 people having their first stroke have high blood pressure.

- **Chronic (long lasting) heart failure.** About 7 of every 10 people with chronic heart failure have high blood pressure.

- **Kidney disease** is also a major risk factor for high blood pressure.

Although you cannot control all of your risk factors for high blood pressure, you can take steps to prevent or control high blood pressure and its complications.

Talk with Your Healthcare Team about Blood Pressure

Since 1999, more people with high blood pressure—especially those 60 years old or older—have become aware of their condition and gotten treatment. Unfortunately, about **1 of 5 U.S.** adults with high blood pressure still do not know that they have it.

About **7 in 10 U.S.** adults with high blood pressure use medications to treat the condition.

In 2009, Americans visited their healthcare providers more than **55 million times** to treat high blood pressure.

Using team-based care that includes the patient, primary care provider, and other healthcare providers is a recommended strategy to reduce and control blood pressure.

Reducing the average amount of salt or sodium that people eat from 3,400 milligrams (mg) to 2,300 mg per day—the level recommended in the Dietary Guidelines for Americans, may reduce cases of high blood pressure by **11 million** and save **18 billion healthcare dollars every year.**

Section 13.3

Health Risks of Smoking and How to Quit Smoking

This section contains text excerpted from the following sources: Text under the heading "Women's Health and Smoking" is excerpted from "Health Information—Women's Health and Smoking," U.S. Food and Drug Administration (FDA), April 19, 2017; Text under the heading "How to Quit Smoking" is excerpted from "How to Quit Smoking—Quit Tips," Centers for Disease Control and Prevention (CDC), September 15, 2016.

Women's Health and Smoking

Smoking continues to have a profound impact on the health and well-being of women and their families in the United States.

• About 14 percent of all women smoke cigarettes.

- Every day, nearly 1,400 girls under 18 years of age smoke their first cigarette.

- Nearly 8 percent of all high school aged girls smoke cigarettes.

Impacts of Smoking on Women and Their Families

There's abundant research about the many harms of smoking— whether it's the dangerous chemicals, the addictive properties, or the damage smoking causes to the body, these effects can have a profound impact on not only your own body, but also those around you. Here are some facts about smoking's effects on women, families, babies, and pregnant moms.

For Women

- Smoking causes coronary heart disease, cancer, and stroke—the first, second, and fourth leading causes of death for women in the United States.

- Smoking cigarettes causes chronic obstructive pulmonary disease (COPD). People with COPD have trouble breathing and slowly start to die from lack of air. Women who smoke cigarettes are up to 40 times more likely to develop COPD than female nonsmokers.

- Life expectancy for smokers—both male and female—is at least 10 years less than for nonsmokers.

For Families

- Secondhand smoke causes disease and premature death in nonsmoking adults and children.

- The U.S. Surgeon General estimates that living with a smoker increases a nonsmoker's chances of developing lung cancer by 20–30 percent.

- Exposure to secondhand smoke increases children's risk for ear infections, lower respiratory illnesses, more frequent and more severe asthma attacks, and slowed lung growth, and can cause coughing, wheezing, phlegm, and breathlessness.

- Teens are more likely to smoke if they have friends or family who smoke.

For Babies and Pregnant Moms

Smoking during pregnancy can affect the baby's health.

Infants born to mothers who smoked during pregnancy are at a higher risk of low birth weight, birth defects like cleft palate, lungs that don't develop in a normal way, and sudden infant death syndrome.

How to Quit Smoking

Are you one of the more than 70 percent of smokers who want to quit? Then try following this advice.

1. **Don't smoke any cigarettes.** Each cigarette you smoke damages your lungs, your blood vessels, and cells throughout your body. Even occasional smoking is harmful.

2. **Write down why you want to quit.** Do you want to—

   • Be around for your loved ones?

   • Have better health?

   • Set a good example for your children?

   • Protect your family from breathing other people's smoke?

   Really wanting to quit smoking is very important to how much success you will have in quitting.

3. **Know that it will take commitment and effort to quit smoking**. Nearly all smokers have some feelings of nicotine withdrawal when they try to quit. Nicotine is addictive. Knowing this will help you deal with withdrawal symptoms that can occur, such as bad moods and really wanting to smoke.

   There are many ways smokers quit, including using nicotine replacement products (gum and patches) or U.S. Food and Drug Administration (FDA) approved, nonnicotine cessation medications. Some people do not experience any withdrawal symptoms. For most people, symptoms only last a few days to a couple of weeks. Take quitting one day at a time, even one minute at a time—whatever you need to succeed.

4. **Get help if you want it.** Smokers can receive free resources and assistance to help them quit by calling the 800-QUIT-NOW quitline (800-784-8669). Your healthcare providers are also a good source for help and support.

Concerned about weight gain? It's a common concern, but not everyone gains weight when they stop smoking.

5. **Remember this good news!** More than half of all adult smokers have quit, and you can, too. Millions of people have learned to face life without a cigarette. Quitting smoking is the single most important step you can take to protect your health and the health of your family.

Section 13.4

Women's Alcohol Consumption and How It Affects Health

This section includes text excerpted from "Excessive Alcohol Use and Risks to Women's Health," Centers for Disease Control and Prevention (CDC), March 7, 2016.

Although men are more likely to drink alcohol and drink in larger amounts, gender differences in body structure and chemistry cause women to absorb more alcohol, and take longer to break it down and remove it from their bodies (i.e., to metabolize it). In other words, upon drinking equal amounts, women have higher alcohol levels in their blood than men, and the immediate effects of alcohol occur more quickly and last longer in women than men. These differences also make it more likely that drinking will cause long-term health problems in women than men.

Drinking Levels among Women

- Approximately 46 percent of adult women report drinking alcohol in the last 30 days.

- Approximately 12 percent of adult women report binge drinking 3 times a month, averaging 5 drinks per binge.

- Most (90%) people who binge drink are not alcoholics or alcohol dependent.

- About 2.5 percent of women and 4.5 percent of men met the diagnostic criteria for alcohol dependence in the past year.

Reproductive Health Outcomes

- National surveys show that about 1 in 2 women of child-bearing age (i.e., aged 18–44 years) drink alcohol, and 18 percent of women who drink alcohol in this age group binge drink.

- Excessive drinking may disrupt the menstrual cycle and increase the risk of infertility.

- Women who binge drink are more likely to have unprotected sex and multiple sex partners. These activities increase the risks of unintended pregnancy and sexually transmitted diseases.

Pregnancy Outcomes

- About 10 percent of pregnant women drink alcohol.

- Women who drink alcohol while pregnant increase their risk of having a baby with fetal alcohol spectrum disorders (FASD). The most severe form is fetal alcohol syndrome (FAS), which causes mental retardation and birth defects.

- FASD are completely preventable if a woman does not drink while pregnant or while she may become pregnant. It is not safe to drink at any time during pregnancy.

- Excessive drinking increases a woman's risk of miscarriage, stillbirth, and premature delivery.

- Women who drink alcohol while pregnant are also more likely to have a baby die from Sudden Infant Death Syndrome (SIDS). This risk substantially increases if a woman binge drinks during her first trimester of pregnancy.

Other Health Concerns

- **Liver Disease.** The risk of cirrhosis and other alcohol-related liver diseases is higher for women than for men.

- **Impact on the Brain.** Excessive drinking may result in memory loss and shrinkage of the brain. Research suggests that women are more vulnerable than men to the brain damaging effects of excessive alcohol use, and the damage tends to appear with shorter periods of excessive drinking for women than for men.

- **Impact on the Heart.** Studies have shown that women who drink excessively are at increased risk for damage to the heart muscle than men even for women drinking at lower levels.

- **Cancer.** Alcohol consumption increases the risk of cancer of the mouth, throat, esophagus, liver, colon, and breast among women. The risk of breast cancer increases as alcohol use increases.

- **Sexual Assault.** Binge drinking is a risk factor for sexual assault, especially among young women in college settings. Each year, about 1 in 20 college women are sexually assaulted. Research suggests that there is an increase in the risk of rape or sexual assault when both the attacker and victim have used alcohol prior to the attack.

Section 13.5

Sunscreen Use and Avoiding Tanning Decrease Skin Cancer Risk

This section contains text excerpted from the following sources: Text in this section begins with excerpts from "Tanning," girlshealth. gov, Office on Women's Health (OWH), April 15, 2014; Text under the heading "What Can I Do to Reduce My Risk of Skin Cancer?" is excerpted from "What Can I Do to Reduce My Risk of Skin Cancer?" Centers for Disease Control and Prevention (CDC), April 25, 2017.

Do you think tanning gives you a healthy glow? The truth is that a tan is a sign your skin has been hurt. The sun's ultraviolet (UV) rays damage your skin, cause wrinkles and spots, and play a big role in causing skin cancer. Recently, the deadliest kind of skin cancer has been rising in kids and teens.

Remember that people with darker skin definitely can still get sun damage and skin cancer.

Sun Safety Tips

- **Try to stay out of the sun when its rays are strongest.** The sun's rays are usually the most dangerous between 10 a.m. and 4 p.m. Keep in mind, though, that the sun can reach you even on cloudy days and in the shade.

- **Wear protective clothing**, such as a wide-brimmed hat, long-sleeved shirt, and long pants.

- **Wear a broad-spectrum sunscreen and lip screen with at least sun protection factor (SPF 15).** "Broad spectrum" means it protects against both ultraviolet A (UVA) and ultraviolet B (UVB) rays. This protection helps guard better against all kinds of skin concerns, from cancer to wrinkles. If you are worried about acne, use an oil-free sunscreen or one labeled for faces.

- **Follow the directions on your sunscreen**, and check the expiration date. Sunscreen without an expiration date will last no more than three years. Sunscreen will not last as long if it is stored in very hot or very cold temperatures.

- **You need 1 ounce of sunscreen**—about the size of a ping-pong ball—every time. Put it on 15 minutes before you go out. Rub sunscreen in well, and don't forget spots you might miss, like your ears, under bathing suit straps, and the back of your neck.

- **Reapply sunscreen after two hours and after swimming or sweating.** That means a tube of 3 to 5 ounces might be enough for you for just one day at the beach.

- **Don't think your skin worries end when the summer is over.** You still need protection every day. And be extra careful on snow days since the snow reflects sun back up onto our faces.

- **Look for a sunscreen that says it is water resistant for up to 40 or 80 minutes.** New labeling rules mean sunscreens can't say they are completely waterproof.

- **Wear sunglasses.** You want ones that provide 100 percent UVA and UVB protection. Wraparound sunglasses prevent rays from sneaking in on the side.

You may have heard that the sun helps people get vitamin D, and that many people may not get enough vitamin D. Ask your doctor how best to protect your skin and get enough of this important vitamin.

Find out if you need to get more vitamin D from your diet or in the form of a supplement.

What about Tanning Beds and Sunless Tanning?

Trying to get that tan is dangerous both outside and inside. Indoor tanning salons use light bulbs in the beds and booths that give off dangerous UV rays. People who use indoor tanning have an increased risk of skin cancer. The risk is even higher if you start before age 25. And some research shows that frequent tanning can even be addictive.

Have you heard that indoor tanning sometimes is good for you? That's just not true. In fact, anyone under 18 should not use tanning beds and booths at all, according to the government group in charge of the safety of these products.

Spray tans you can get at a salon and tanning lotions you can buy can be safe. Sunless tanning products have no known risk for skin cancer, but you do have to be careful. Spray tans, lotions, or gels use a color additive that makes your skin look tan called docosa-hexaenoic acid (DHA). DHA is considered safe for use on the outside of your body by the U.S. Food and Drug Administration (FDA). You need to make sure it doesn't get into your nose, eyes, or mouth, though.

Tanning pills are dangerous. Don't be tempted to take pills that say they can darken your skin. They come with some serious health risks.

What Can I Do to Reduce My Risk of Skin Cancer?

Protection from ultraviolet (UV) radiation is important all year round, not just during the summer or at the beach. UV rays from the sun can reach you on cloudy and hazy days, as well as bright and sunny days. UV rays also reflect off of surfaces like water, cement, sand, and snow. Indoor tanning (using a tanning bed, booth, or sunlamp to get tan) exposes users to UV radiation.

The hours between 10 a.m. and 4 p.m. Daylight Saving Time (9 a.m. to 3 p.m. standard time) are the most hazardous for UV exposure outdoors in the continental United States. UV rays from sunlight are the greatest during the late spring and early summer in North America.

The Centers for Disease Control and Prevention (CDC), recommends easy options for protection from UV radiation:

- Stay in the shade, especially during midday hours.

- Wear clothing that covers your arms and legs.

- Wear a hat with a wide brim to shade your face, head, ears, and neck.

- Wear sunglasses that wrap around and block both UVA and UVB rays.

- Use sunscreen with a sun protection factor (SPF) of 15 or higher, and both UVA and UVB (broad spectrum) protection.

- Avoid indoor tanning.

Section 13.6

Safe Use of Cosmetics

This section contains text excerpted from the following sources: Text in this section begins with excerpts from "Makeup," girlshealth.gov, Office on Women's Health (OWH), April 15, 2014; Text beginning with the heading "Eye Cosmetic Safety" is excerpted from "Eye Cosmetic Safety," U.S. Food and Drug Administration (FDA), January 11, 2016.

Some girls think wearing makeup is creative and cool. Others think it's just a big cover-up. You may be wondering whether makeup is right for you. If so, you can think about why you'd want to do it and what your makeup "look" might say about you. And don't forget to talk to your parents and check out your school's rules.

Whatever you decide about makeup, remember that real beauty comes from the true you inside!

If you do wear makeup, don't just think about how it looks. It's a good idea to think about what's in it and how to use it safely. Here are some makeup issues worth a closer look:

- **Avoid infections.** It's easy for germs to get into makeup. If germs cause an infection, you could lose your eyelashes or have other nasty problems.

- Make sure to wash your hands before putting on makeup.

- Don't share makeup, because you'll also be sharing germs.

- Remember that lots of people use the testers at department stores, so always use a new cotton swab or sponge.

- Don't put eyeliner on the inner side of your eyelashes, right next to your eye.

- **Be careful about mascara.** If your mascara wand is dry, make it disappear into the trash! Don't add spit or water, because they might add germs that can cause an infection. It's also a good idea to toss your mascara after two to four months. And take off mascara before you go to bed at night. Otherwise, flakes can fall into your eyes while you sleep and—you guessed it—cause an infection.

- **Don't apply makeup on the road**. It's easy for your hand to slip in a car or bus, for example. A wand or brush could scratch your eye or put germs into it. If you drive, never put makeup on while you are behind the wheel. It can be very dangerous and even illegal.

- **Make sure that your makeup does not have kohl in it.** Look at the list of contents to make sure the color ingredient kohl is not listed. Kohl isn't allowed in makeup in the United States because it can cause health problems. (It is okay, though, if the word "kohl" is in the name of a product or used to describe the color or shade.)

- **Remember that "hypoallergenic" makeup can still cause an allergic reaction.** "Hypoallergenic" only means that the maker says the product is less likely to cause an allergic reaction. It's also possible to have an allergic reaction to products that say "all natural," "organic," or "dermatologist tested."

  - To figure out if you may be allergic, rub a small amount of the makeup on the inside of your elbow or behind your ear. Wait two days. If you get a rash, don't use the product.

  - Sometimes, you can have an allergic reaction even if you've used a product before without any problems. If that happens, stop using makeup until you can get help from your doctor.

- **Don't dye your eyebrows or eyelashes.** If you want to jazz up your lashes and brows, use mascara or eyebrow pencils.

Using dyes on your lashes or brows can really hurt your eyes—and even cause blindness.

- **Permanent makeup isn't a great idea either.** These tattoos that look like makeup are made by injecting inks or dyes into the skin. There's always the risk of an infection or allergic reaction with a tattoo. Also, makeup styles change, so you may not want to be locked into a look you choose now.

- **If you're concerned about acne, try makeup labeled "oil-free" or "nonacneogenic."** These products are made without some items that can clog pores, which means they may be less likely to cause acne. You might also skip foundation and use oil-free concealer to cover blemishes.

- **If you are worried about animal safety, check out labels**. If a product says "cruelty-free," though, the company just may not be testing on animals now. It's possible that the ingredients may have been tested on animals in the past. You can always call the company to find out what their testing methods are.

- **Think about phthalates.** These are chemicals that are sometimes found in nail polish, hairspray, perfume, lotion, and other beauty products. Scientists are studying these chemicals, and research suggests that they may act like the hormones in your body and may be connected to health problems. You can try to avoid phthalates by looking for names like di-n-butyl phthalate (DBP), diethyl phthalate (DEP), and butylbenzyl phthalate (BBP) on labels.

Eye Cosmetic Safety

Most eye cosmetics are safe when used properly. However, it's important to be careful about the risk of infection, injury from the applicator, and use of unapproved color additives.

Keep It Clean!

Eye cosmetics are usually safe when you buy them, but misusing them can allow dangerous bacteria or fungi to grow in them. Then, when applied to the eye area, a cosmetic can cause an infection. In rare cases, women have been temporarily or permanently blinded by an infection from an eye cosmetic.

Don't Share! Don't Swap!

Don't share or swap eye cosmetics—not even with your best friend. Another person's germs may be hazardous to you. The risk of contamination may be even greater with "testers" at retail stores, where a number of people are using the same sample product. If you feel you must sample cosmetics at a store, make sure they are applied with single-use applicators, such as clean cotton swabs.

Hold Still!

It may seem like efficient use of your time to apply makeup in the car or on the bus, but resist that temptation, even if you're not in the driver's seat. If you hit a bump, come to a sudden stop, or are hit by another vehicle, you risk injuring your eye (scratching your cornea, for example) with a mascara wand or other applicator. Even a slight scratch can result in a serious infection.

What's in It?

As with any cosmetic product sold on a retail basis to consumers, eye cosmetics are required to have an ingredient declaration on the label, according to regulations implemented under the Fair Packaging and Labeling Act, or FPLA—an important consumer protection law. If you wish to avoid certain ingredients or compare the ingredients in different brands, you can check the ingredient declaration.

If a cosmetic sold on a retail basis to consumers does not have an ingredient declaration, it is considered misbranded and is illegal in interstate commerce. Very small packages in tightly compartmented display racks may have copies of the ingredient declaration available on tear-off sheets accompanying the display. If neither the package nor the display rack provides the ingredient declaration, you aren't getting the information you're entitled to. Don't hesitate to ask the store manager or the manufacturer why not.

What's That Shade You're Wearing?

In the United States, the use of color additives is strictly regulated. A number of color additives approved for cosmetic use in general are not approved for use in the area of the eye. An import alert for cosmetics containing illegal colors lists several eye cosmetics.

Keep Away from Kohl—and Keep Kohl Away from Kids!

One color additive of particular concern is kohl. Also known as al-kahl, kajal, or surma, kohl is used in some parts of the world to enhance the appearance of the eyes, but is unapproved for cosmetic use in the United States. Kohl consists of salts of heavy metals, such as antimony and lead. It may be tempting to think that because kohl has been used traditionally as an eye cosmetic in some parts of the world, it must be safe. However, there have been reports linking the use of kohl to lead poisoning in children.

An U.S. Food and Drug Administration (FDA) Import Alert cites three main reasons for detaining imports of kohl:

1. For containing an unsafe color additive, which makes the product adulterated.

2. For labeling that describes the product falsely as "FDA Approved."

3. For lack of an ingredient declaration.

Some eye cosmetics may be labeled with the word "kohl" only to indicate the shade, not because they contain true kohl. If the product is properly labeled, you can check to see whether the color additives declared on the label are in FDA's list of color additives approved for use in cosmetics, then make sure they are listed as approved for use in the area of the eye.

Dying to Dye Your Eyelashes?

Permanent eyelash and eyebrow tints and dyes have been known to cause serious eye injuries, including blindness. There are no color additives approved by FDA for permanent dyeing or tinting of eyelashes and eyebrows.

Thinking of False Eyelashes or Extensions?

FDA considers false eyelashes, eyelash extensions, and their adhesives to be cosmetic products, and as such they must adhere to the safety and labeling requirements for cosmetics. False eyelashes and eyelash extensions require adhesives to hold them in place. Remember that the eyelids are delicate, and an allergic reaction, irritation, or other injury in the eye area can be particularly troublesome. Check the ingredients before using these adhesives.

Safety Checklist

If you use eye cosmetics, FDA urges you to follow these safety tips:

- If any eye cosmetic causes irritation, stop using it immediately. If irritation persists, see a doctor.

- Avoid using eye cosmetics if you have an eye infection or the skin around the eye is inflamed. Wait until the area is healed. Discard any eye cosmetics you were using when you got the infection.

- Be aware that there are bacteria on your hands that, if placed in the eye, could cause infections. Wash your hands before applying eye cosmetics.

- Make sure that any instrument you place in the eye area is clean.

- Don't share your cosmetics. Another person's bacteria may be hazardous to you.

- Don't allow cosmetics to become covered with dust or contaminated with dirt or soil. Keep containers clean.

- Don't use old containers of eye cosmetics. Manufacturers usually recommend discarding mascara two to four months after purchase.

- Discard dried-up mascara. Don't add saliva or water to moisten it. The bacteria from your mouth may grow in the mascara and cause infection. Adding water may introduce bacteria and will dilute the preservative that is intended to protect against microbial growth.

- When applying or removing eye cosmetics, be careful not to scratch the eyeball or other sensitive area. Never apply or remove eye cosmetics in a moving vehicle.

- Don't use any cosmetics near your eyes unless they are intended specifically for that use. For instance, don't use a lip liner as an eyeliner. You may be exposing your eyes to contamination from your mouth, or to color additives that are not approved for use in the area of the eye.

- Avoid color additives that are not approved for use in the area of the eye, such as "permanent" eyelash tints and kohl. Be especially careful to keep kohl away from children, since reports have linked it to lead poisoning.

Chapter 14

Recommended Screenings for Women

Chapter Contents

Section 14.1

Preventive Healthcare Screenings for Women

This section includes text excerpted from "Women: Stay Healthy at Any Age," Agency for Healthcare Research and Quality (AHRQ), U.S. Department of Health and Human Services (HHS), May 2014.

Women: Stay Healthy at Any Age—Get the Screenings You Need

Screenings are tests that look for diseases before you have symptoms. Blood pressure checks and mammograms are examples of screenings. You can get some screenings, such as blood pressure readings, in your doctor's office. Others, such as mammograms, need special equipment, so you may need to go to a different office.

After a screening test, ask when you will see the results and who to talk to about them.

Breast Cancer. Talk with your healthcare team about whether you need a mammogram.

BRCA 1 **and** *2* **Genes.** If you have a family member with breast, ovarian, or peritoneal cancer, talk with your doctor or nurse about your family history. Women with a strong family history of certain cancers may benefit from genetic counseling and BRCA genetic testing.

Cervical Cancer. Starting at age 21, get a Pap smear every 3 years until you are 65 years old. Women 30 years of age or older can choose to switch to a combination Pap smear and human papillomavirus (HPV) test every 5 years until the age of 65. If you are older than 65 or have had a hysterectomy, talk with your doctor or nurse about whether you still need to be screened.

Colon Cancer. Between the ages of 50 and 75, get a screening test for colorectal cancer. Several tests—for example, a stool test or a colonoscopy—can detect this cancer. Your healthcare team can help you decide which is best for you. If you are between the ages of 76 and

85, talk with your doctor or nurse about whether you should continue to be screened.

Depression. Your emotional health is as important as your physical health. Talk to your healthcare team about being screened for depression, especially if during the last 2 weeks:

- You have felt down, sad, or hopeless.
- You have felt little interest or pleasure in doing things.

Diabetes. Get screened for diabetes (high blood sugar) if you have high blood pressure or if you take medication for high blood pressure. Diabetes can cause problems with your heart, brain, eyes, feet, kidneys, nerves, and other body parts.

Hepatitis C Virus (HCV). Get screened one time for HCV infection if:

- You were born between 1945 and 1965.
- You have ever injected drugs.
- You received a blood transfusion before 1992.

If you currently are an injection drug user, you should be screened regularly.

High Blood Cholesterol. Have your blood cholesterol checked regularly with a blood test if:

- You use tobacco.
- You are overweight or obese.
- You have a personal history of heart disease or blocked arteries.
- A male relative in your family had a heart attack before age 50 or a female relative, before age 60.

High Blood Pressure. Have your blood pressure checked at least every 2 years. High blood pressure can cause strokes, heart attacks, kidney and eye problems, and heart failure.

Human Immunodeficiency Virus (HIV). If you are 65 or younger, get screened for HIV. If you are older than 65, talk to your doctor or nurse about whether you should be screened.

Lung Cancer. Talk to your doctor or nurse about getting screened for lung cancer if you are between the ages of 55 and 80, have a 30 pack-year smoking history, and smoke now or have quit within the past 15 years. (Your pack-year history is the number of packs of cigarettes smoked per day times the number of years you have smoked.) Know that quitting smoking is the best thing you can do for your health.

Overweight and Obesity. The best way to learn if you are overweight or obese is to find your body mass index (BMI). You can find your BMI by entering your height and weight into a BMI calculator, such as the one available at: www.nhlbi.nih.gov/guidelines/obesity/BMI/bmicalc.htm.

A BMI between 18.5 and 25 indicates a normal weight. Persons with a BMI of 30 or higher may be obese. If you are obese, talk to your doctor or nurse about getting intensive counseling and help with changing your behaviors to lose weight. Overweight and obesity can lead to diabetes and cardiovascular disease.

Osteoporosis (Bone Thinning). Have a screening test at age 65 to make sure your bones are strong. The most common test is a Dual Energy X-ray Absorptiometry (DEXA) Scan—a low-dose X-ray of the spine and hip. If you are younger than 65 and at high risk for bone fractures, you should also be screened. Talk with your healthcare team about your risk for bone fractures.

Sexually Transmitted Infections. Sexually transmitted infections can make it hard to get pregnant, may affect your baby, and can cause other health problems.

- Get screened for chlamydia and gonorrhea infections if you are 24 years or younger and sexually active. If you are older than 24 years, talk to your doctor or nurse about whether you should be screened.

- Ask your doctor or nurse whether you should be screened for other sexually transmitted infection.

Get Preventive Medicines If You Need Them

Aspirin. If you are 55 or older, ask your healthcare team if you should take aspirin to prevent strokes. Your healthcare team can help you decide whether taking aspirin to prevent stroke is right for you.

Breast Cancer Drugs. Talk to your doctor about your risks for breast cancer and whether you should take medicines that may reduce those risks. Medications to reduce breast cancer have some potentially serious harms, so think through both the potential benefits and harms.

Folic Acid. If you of an age at which you can get pregnant, you should take a daily supplement containing 0.4 to 0.8 mg of folic acid.

Vitamin D to Avoid Falls. If you are 65 or older and have a history of falls, mobility problems, or other risks for falling, ask your doctor about taking a vitamin D supplement to help reduce your chances of falling. Exercise and physical therapy may also help.

Immunizations

- Get a flu shot every year.

- Get shots for tetanus, diphtheria, and whooping cough. Get tetanus booster if it has been more than 10 years since your last shot.

- If you are 60 or older, get a shot to prevent shingles.

- If you are 65 or older, get a pneumonia shot.

- Talk with your healthcare team about whether you need other vaccinations. You can also find which ones you need by going to: www.cdc.gov/vaccines.

Take Steps to Good Health

- **Be physically active and make healthy food choices.**

- **Get to a healthy weight and stay there.** Balance the calories you take in from food and drink with the calories you burn off by your activities.

- **Be tobacco free.** For tips on how to quit, go to www.smokefree. gov. To talk to someone about how to quit, call the National Quitline: 1-800-QUITNOW (1-800-784-8669).

- **If you drink alcohol, have no more than one drink per day.** A standard drink is one 12-ounce bottle of beer or wine cooler, one 5-ounce glass of wine, or 1.5 ounces of 80-proof distilled spirits.

Section 14.2

What Are Mammograms (Breast Cancer Screening)?

This section includes text excerpted from documents published by two public domain sources. Text under heading marked 1 is excerpted from "Mammograms," Office on Women's Health (OWH), U.S. Department of Health and Human Services (HHS), February 6, 2017; Text under headings marked 2 are excerpted from "Breast Cancer—Mammograms," National Cancer Institute (NCI), December 7, 2016.

What Is a Mammogram?[1]

A mammogram is a low-dose X-ray exam of the breasts to look for changes that are not normal. The results are recorded on X-ray film or directly into a computer for a doctor called a radiologist to examine.

A mammogram allows the doctor to have a closer look for changes in breast tissue that cannot be felt during a breast exam. It is used for women who have no breast complaints and for women who have breast symptoms, such as a change in the shape or size of a breast, a lump, nipple discharge, or pain. Breast changes occur in almost all women. In fact, most of these changes are not cancer and are called "benign," but only a doctor can know for sure. Breast changes can also happen monthly, due to your menstrual period.

What Is the Best Method of Detecting Breast Cancer as Early as Possible?[1]

A high-quality mammogram plus a clinical breast exam, an exam done by your doctor, is the most effective way to detect breast cancer early. Finding breast cancer early greatly improves a woman's chances for successful treatment.

Like any test, mammograms have both benefits and limitations. For example, some cancers can't be found by a mammogram, but they may be found in a clinical breast exam.

Checking your own breasts for lumps or other changes is called a breast self-exam (BSE). Studies so far have not shown that BSE alone helps reduce the number of deaths from breast cancer. BSE should not take the place of routine clinical breast exams and mammograms.

If you choose to do BSE, remember that breast changes can occur because of pregnancy, aging, menopause, menstrual cycles, or from taking birth control pills or other hormones. It is normal for breasts to feel a little lumpy and uneven. Also, it is common for breasts to be swollen and tender right before or during a menstrual period. If you notice any unusual changes in your breasts, contact your doctor.

How Is a Mammogram Done?[1]

You stand in front of a special X-ray machine. The person who takes the X-rays, called a radiologic technician, places your breasts, one at a time, between an X-ray plate and a plastic plate. These plates are attached to the X-ray machine and compress the breasts to flatten them. This spreads the breast tissue out to obtain a clearer picture. You will feel pressure on your breast for a few seconds. It may cause you some discomfort; you might feel squeezed or pinched. This feeling only lasts for a few seconds, and the flatter your breast, the better the picture. Most often, two pictures are taken of each breast—one from the side and one from above. A screening mammogram takes about 20 minutes from start to finish.

Are There Different Types of Mammograms?[1]

- **Screening mammograms** are done for women who have no symptoms of breast cancer. It usually involves two X-rays of each breast. Screening mammograms can detect lumps or tumors that cannot be felt. They can also find microcalcifications or tiny deposits of calcium in the breast, which sometimes mean that breast cancer is present.

- **Diagnostic mammograms** are used to check for breast cancer after a lump or other symptom or sign of breast cancer has been found. Signs of breast cancer may include pain, thickened skin on the breast, nipple discharge, or a change in breast size or shape. This type of mammogram also can be used to find out more about breast changes found on a screening mammogram, or to view breast tissue that is hard to see on a screening mammogram. A diagnostic mammogram takes longer than a screening mammogram because it involves more X-rays in order to obtain views of the breast from several angles. The technician can magnify a problem area to make a more detailed picture, which helps the doctor make a correct diagnosis.

163

A digital mammogram also uses X-rays to produce an image of the breast, but instead of storing the image directly on film, the image is stored directly on a computer. This allows the recorded image to be magnified for the doctor to take a closer look. Current research has not shown that digital images are better at showing cancer than X-ray film images in general. But, women with dense breasts who are pre- or perimenopausal, or who are younger than age 50, may benefit from having a digital rather than a film mammogram. Digital mammography may offer these benefits:

- Long-distance consultations with other doctors may be easier because the images can be shared by computer.

- Slight differences between normal and abnormal tissues may be more easily noted.

- The number of follow-up tests needed may be fewer.

- Fewer repeat images may be needed, reducing exposure to radiation.

How Are Screening and Diagnostic Mammograms Different?[2]

The same machines are used for both types of mammograms. However, diagnostic mammography takes longer to perform than screening mammography and the total dose of radiation is higher because more X-ray images are needed to obtain views of the breast from several angles. The technologist may magnify a suspicious area to produce a detailed picture that can help the doctor make an accurate diagnosis.

What Are the Benefits and Potential Harms of Screening Mammograms?[2]

Early detection of breast cancer with screening mammography means that treatment can be started earlier in the course of the disease, possibly before it has spread. Results from randomized clinical trials and other studies show that screening mammography can help reduce the number of deaths from breast cancer among women ages 40 to 74, especially for those over age 50. However, studies to date have not shown a benefit from regular screening mammography in women under age 40 or from baseline screening mammograms (mammograms used for comparison) taken before age 40.

What Is the Best Method of Screening for Breast Cancer?[2]

Regular high-quality screening mammograms and clinical breast exams are the most sensitive ways to screen for breast cancer.

Regular breast self-exam, or BSE—that is, checking one's own breasts for lumps or other unusual changes—is not specifically recommended for breast cancer screening. In clinical trials, BSE alone was not found to help reduce the number of deaths from breast cancer.

However, many women choose to examine their own breasts. Women who do so should remember that breast changes can occur because of pregnancy, aging, or menopause; during menstrual cycles; or when taking birth control pills or other hormones. It is normal for breasts to feel a little lumpy and uneven. Also, it is common for breasts to be swollen and tender right before or during a menstrual period. Whenever a woman notices any unusual changes in her breasts, she should contact her healthcare provider.

How Often Should I Get a Mammogram?[1]

The United States Preventive Services Task Force (USPSTF) recommends:

- Women ages 50 to 74 years should get a mammogram every 2 years.

- Women younger than age 50 should talk to a doctor about when to start and how often to have a mammogram.

What Can Mammograms Show?[1]

The radiologist will look at your X-rays for breast changes that do not look normal and for differences in each breast. He or she will compare your past mammograms with your most recent one to check for changes. The doctor will also look for lumps and calcifications.

- **Lump or mass.** The size, shape, and edges of a lump sometimes can give doctors information about whether or not it may be cancer. On a mammogram, a growth that is benign often looks smooth and round with a clear, defined edge. Breast cancer often has a jagged outline and an irregular shape.

- **Calcification.** A calcification is a deposit of the mineral calcium in the breast tissue. Calcifications appear as small white spots on a mammogram. There are two types:

165

- *Macrocalcifications* are large calcium deposits often caused by aging. These usually are not a sign of cancer.

- *Microcalcifications* are tiny specks of calcium that may be found in an area of rapidly dividing cells.

If calcifications are grouped together in a certain way, it may be a sign of cancer. Depending on how many calcium specks you have, how big they are, and what they look like, your doctor may suggest that you have other tests. Calcium in the diet does not create calcium deposits, or calcifications, in the breast.

What If My Screening Mammogram Shows a Problem?[1]

If you have a screening test result that suggests cancer, your doctor must find out whether it is due to cancer or to some other cause. Your doctor may ask about your personal and family medical history. You may have a physical exam. Your doctor also may order some of these tests:

- **Diagnostic mammogram,** to focus on a specific area of the breast

- **Ultrasound,** an imaging test that uses sound waves to create a picture of your breast. The pictures may show whether a lump is solid or filled with fluid. A cyst is a fluid-filled sac. Cysts are not cancer. But a solid mass may be cancer. After the test, your doctor can store the pictures on video or print them out. This exam may be used along with a mammogram.

- **Magnetic resonance imaging (MRI),** which uses a powerful magnet linked to a computer. MRI makes detailed pictures of breast tissue. Your doctor can view these pictures on a monitor or print them on film. MRI may be used along with a mammogram.

- **Biopsy,** a test in which fluid or tissue is removed from your breast to help find out if there is cancer. Your doctor may refer you to a surgeon or to a doctor who is an expert in breast disease for a biopsy.

How Do I Get Ready for My Mammogram?[1]

First, check with the place you are having the mammogram for any special instructions you may need to follow before you go. Here are some general guidelines to follow:

- If you are still having menstrual periods, try to avoid making your mammogram appointment during the week before your period. Your breasts will be less tender and swollen. The mammogram will hurt less and the picture will be better.

- If you have breast implants, be sure to tell your mammography facility that you have them when you make your appointment.

- Wear a shirt with shorts, pants, or a skirt. This way, you can undress from the waist up and leave your shorts, pants, or skirt on when you get your mammogram.

- Don't wear any deodorant, perfume, lotion, or powder under your arms or on your breasts on the day of your mammogram appointment. These things can make shadows show up on your mammogram.

- If you have had mammograms at another facility, have those X-ray films sent to the new facility so that they can be compared to the new films.

Section 14.3

Breast Self-Examination

"Breast Self-Exam," © 2018 Omnigraphics.
Reviewed August 2017.

Breast self-examination is a technique people can use to visually and manually check their own breast tissue for lumps or other changes. Many healthcare practitioners and cancer-prevention organizations recommend performing monthly breast self-examinations beginning at age 18 as a method of early detection for breast cancer. People who conduct regular self-exams become familiar with the normal appearance and feel of their breast tissue, which enables them to recognize changes and discover lumps that may require medical attention. Some of the changes that should be checked by a doctor include:

- new lumps or areas of thickness, which may or may not be painful

- discharge of fluid from the nipples

- dimpling, puckering, rashes, or other changes to the skin
- changes to the size or shape of the breast

Finding lumps or noticing changes should not be a cause for alarm, however. An estimated 80 percent of lumps found in self-examinations are not cancerous, and most breast problems are caused by something other than cancer. In fact, some experts do not recommend self-examinations by people over 40 with no increased risk of breast cancer. They argue that the potential benefits of early detection are outweighed by the risks of undergoing tests and treatments that are unnecessary. Instead, they recommend regular checkups at a doctor's office as well as annual mammograms.

Self-Examination Procedures

Ideally, breast self-examinations should be performed on a monthly basis. For women who are menstruating, the best time is usually toward the end of the monthly period, when the breasts are less likely to be tender. For those who no longer have periods, experts recommend choosing a certain day of the month. Performing self-examinations on a regular schedule makes it easier to compare the results and recognize changes in breast tissue.

The first part of the process involves a visual examination of the breasts. This examination should be conducted while standing in front of a mirror in three different positions: with your arms hanging naturally at your sides; with your arms raised above your head; and with your hands on your hips and your upper body leaning forward from the waist. Be sure to look from the right and left sides as well as from the front. Check carefully for any changes to the following:

- **Size and shape:** Make sure your breasts appear to be their usual size and shape, and that no sudden changes have occurred. Although one breast may normally be larger than the other, you should not see any visible swelling or bulging.

- **Skin and veins:** Check the skin on your breasts for anything that appears unusual, such as puckering, dimpling, or distortion. Also look for areas of redness, soreness, rashes, or texture changes. Make sure that the veins beneath the skin appear as they usually do. You should not see a noticeable increase in the size or number of veins in one breast as compared to the other breast.

- **Nipples:** Check for any physical changes to the appearance or position of the nipples, such as a sudden inversion. Also check the skin for redness, itching, scaliness, or swelling. Look for any fluid discharge, which may appear watery, milky, sticky, or bloody.

Manual Examination

The second part of the process involves a manual examination of each breast using the fingers of the opposite hand. It should cover the entire surface area of each breast, from the collarbone down to the abdomen, and from the armpit across to the cleavage. This examination should be conducted while lying down, and then again while standing up. The main steps are as follows:

1. Lie down on your back and place a pillow beneath your right shoulder.

2. Place your right arm on top of your head.

3. Use the pads of the three middle fingers on your left hand to examine your right breast.

4. Move your fingers in small circles, about the size of a quarter.

5. Vary the amount of pressure you apply in order to feel all levels of your breast tissue. Use light pressure to feel just beneath the skin, and firm pressure to feel the deep tissue against the ribcage.

6. Begin under the armpit and work from top to bottom along the outer part of your breast.

7. After completing one vertical strip, move over one finger width and begin a new strip, working from bottom to top. Do not lift the fingers between rows.

8. Check the entire breast area in an up-and-down pattern, as if mowing a lawn.

9. Repeat the process by using the left hand to examine the right breast.

10. Examine both breasts again while standing. Many women find it convenient to perform this part of the self-examination in the shower, while the skin is wet and soapy.

If you discover a lump in one breast, check to see if the same kind of lump exists in the other breast. If so, the lumps are probably normal. Many women have fibrocystic lumps that occur throughout both breasts, which may make self-examination difficult. By performing regular self-examinations, women can become familiar with the normal appearance of their breast tissue and consult with medical professionals if they notice any changes.

References

1. "Breast Self-Examination," Healthwise, February 20, 2015.

2. "The Five Steps of a Breast Self-Exam," Breastcancer.org, 2016.

3. "How to Do a Breast Self-Exam," Maurer Foundation, March 26, 2016.

Section 14.4

Pap Tests (Cervical Cancer Screening)

This section includes text excerpted from "Cervical Cancer—Pap and HPV Testing," National Cancer Institute (NCI), September 9, 2014.

What Causes Cervical Cancer?

Nearly all cases of cervical cancer are caused by infection with oncogenic, or high-risk, types of human papillomavirus, or HPV. There are about 12 high-risk HPV types. Infections with these sexually transmitted viruses also cause most anal cancers; many vaginal, vulvar, and penile cancers; and some oropharyngeal cancers.

Although HPV infection is very common, most infections will be suppressed by the immune system within 1 to 2 years without causing cancer. These transient infections may cause temporary changes in cervical cells. If a cervical infection with a high-risk HPV type persists, the cellular changes can eventually develop into more severe precancerous lesions. If precancerous lesions are not treated, they can progress to cancer. It can take 10 to 20 years or more for a persistent infection with a high-risk HPV type to develop into cancer.

What Is Cervical Cancer Screening?

Cervical cancer screening is an essential part of a woman's routine healthcare. It is a way to detect abnormal cervical cells, including precancerous cervical lesions, as well as early cervical cancers. Both precancerous lesions and early cervical cancers can be treated very successfully. Routine cervical screening has been shown to greatly reduce both the number of new cervical cancers diagnosed each year and deaths from the disease.

Cervical cancer screening includes two types of screening tests: cytology-based screening, known as the Pap test or Pap smear, and HPV testing. The main purpose of screening with the Pap test is to detect abnormal cells that may develop into cancer if left untreated. The Pap test can also find noncancerous conditions, such as infections and inflammation. It can also find cancer cells. In regularly screened populations, however, the Pap test identifies most abnormal cells before they become cancer.

HPV testing is used to look for the presence of high-risk HPV types in cervical cells. These tests can detect HPV infections that cause cell abnormalities, sometimes even before cell abnormalities are evident. Several different HPV tests have been approved for screening. Most tests detect the deoxyribonucleic acid (DNA) of high-risk HPV, although one test detects the ribonucleic acid (RNA) of high-risk HPV. Some tests detect any high-risk HPV and do not identify the specific type or types that are present. Other tests specifically detect infection with HPV types 16 and 18, the two types that cause most HPV-associated cancers.

How Is Cervical Cancer Screening Done?

Cervical cancer screening can be done in a medical office, a clinic, or a community health center. It is often done during a pelvic examination.

While a woman lies on an exam table, a healthcare professional inserts an instrument called a speculum into her vagina to widen it so that the upper portion of the vagina and the cervix can be seen. This procedure also allows the healthcare professional to take a sample of cervical cells. The cells are taken with a wooden or plastic scraper and/ or a cervical brush and are then prepared for Pap analysis in one of two ways. In a conventional Pap test, the specimen (or smear) is placed on a glass microscope slide and a fixative is added. In an automated liquid-based Pap cytology test, cervical cells collected with a brush or other instrument are placed in a vial of liquid preservative. The slide or vial is then sent to a laboratory for analysis.

In the United States, automated liquid-based Pap cytology testing has largely replaced conventional Pap tests. One advantage of liquid-based testing is that the same cell sample can also be tested for the presence of high-risk types of HPV, a process known as "Pap and HPV cotesting." In addition, liquid-based cytology appears to reduce the likelihood of an unsatisfactory specimen. However, conventional and liquid-based Pap tests appear to have a similar ability to detect cellular abnormalities.

When Should a Woman Begin Cervical Cancer Screening, and How Often Should She Be Screened?

Women should talk with their doctor about when to start screening and how often to be screened. The updated screening guidelines were released by the United States Preventive Services Task Force (USPSTF) and jointly by the American Cancer Society (ACS), the American Society for Colposcopy and Cervical Pathology (ASCCP), and the American Society for Clinical Pathology (ASCP). These guidelines recommend that women have their first Pap test at age 21. Although previous guidelines recommended that women have their first Pap test 3 years after they start having sexual intercourse, waiting until age 21 is now recommended because adolescents have a very low risk of cervical cancer and a high likelihood that cervical cell abnormalities will go away on their own.

According to the updated guidelines, women ages 21 through 29 should be screened with a Pap test every 3 years. Women ages 30 through 65 can then be screened every 5 years with Pap and HPV cotesting or every 3 years with a Pap test alone.

The guidelines also note that women with certain risk factors may need to have more frequent screening or to continue screening beyond age 65. These risk factors include being infected with the human immunodeficiency virus (HIV), being immunosuppressed, having been exposed to diethylstilbestrol before birth, and having been treated for a precancerous cervical lesion or cervical cancer.

Women who have had a hysterectomy (surgery to remove the uterus and cervix) do not need to have cervical screening, unless the hysterectomy was done to treat a precancerous cervical lesion or cervical cancer.

What Are the Benefits of Pap and HPV Cotesting?

For women age 30 and older, Pap and HPV cotesting is less likely to miss an abnormality (i.e., has a lower false negative rate) than Pap testing alone. Therefore, a woman with a negative HPV test and normal Pap test has very little risk of a serious abnormality developing over the next several years. In fact, researchers have found that, when Pap and HPV cotesting is used, lengthening the screening interval to 5 years still allows abnormalities to be detected in time to treat them while also reducing the detection of HPV infections that would have gone away on their own.

Adding HPV testing to Pap testing may also improve the detection of glandular cell abnormalities, including adenocarcinoma of the cervix (cancer of the glandular cells of the cervix). Glandular cells are mucus-producing cells found in the endocervical canal (the opening in the center of the cervix) or in the lining of the uterus. Glandular cell abnormalities and adenocarcinoma of the cervix are much less common than squamous cell abnormalities and squamous cell carcinoma. There is some HPV evidence that Pap testing is not as good at detecting adenocarcinoma and glandular cell abnormalities as it is at detecting squamous cell abnormalities and cancers.

Can HPV Testing Be Used Alone for Cervical Cancer Screening?

On April 24, 2014, the U.S. Food and Drug Administration (FDA) approved the use of one HPV deoxyribonucleic acid (DNA) test (cobas HPV test, Roche Molecular Systems, Inc.) as a first-line primary screening test for use alone for women age 25 and older. This test detects each of HPV types 16 and 18 and gives pooled results for 12 additional high-risk HPV types.

The new approval was based on long-term findings from the ATHENA trial, a clinical trial that included more than 47,000 women. The results showed that the HPV test used in the study performed better than the Pap test at identifying women at risk of developing severe cervical cell abnormalities.

The greater assurance against future cervical cancer risk with HPV testing has also been demonstrated by a cohort study of more than a million women, which found that, after 3 years, women who tested negative on the HPV test had an extremely low risk of developing cervical cancer—about half the already low risk of women who tested negative on the Pap test.

First-line HPV testing has not yet been incorporated into the current professional cervical cancer screening guidelines. Professional societies are developing interim guidance documents, and some medical practices might incorporate primary HPV screening.

Do Women Who Have Been Vaccinated against HPV Still Need to Be Screened for Cervical Cancer?

Yes. Because current HPV vaccines do not protect against all HPV types that cause cervical cancer, it is important for vaccinated women to continue to undergo routine cervical cancer screening.

What Are the Limitations of Cervical Cancer Screening?

Although cervical cancer screening tests are highly effective, they are not completely accurate. Sometimes a patient can be told that she has abnormal cells when the cells are actually normal (a false positive result), or she can be told that her cells are normal when in fact there is an abnormality that was not detected (a false negative result).

Cervical cancer screening has another limitation, caused by the nature of HPV infections. Because most HPV infections are transient and produce only temporary changes in cervical cells, overly frequent cervical screening could detect HPV infections or cervical cell changes that would never cause cancer. Treating abnormalities that would have gone away on their own can cause needless psychological stress. In addition, follow-up tests and treatments can be uncomfortable, and some treatments that remove cervical tissue, such as LEEP and conization, have the potential to weaken the cervix and may affect fertility or slightly increase the rate of premature delivery, depending on how much tissue is removed.

The screening intervals in the guidelines are intended to minimize the harms caused by treating abnormalities that would never progress to cancer while also limiting false negative results that would delay the diagnosis and treatment of a precancerous condition or cancer. With these intervals, if an HPV infection or abnormal cells are missed at one screen, chances are good that abnormal cells will be detected at the next screening exam, when they can still be treated successfully.

Section 14.5

Colorectal Cancer Screening

This section includes text excerpted from
"Colorectal Cancer Screening (PDQ®)–Patient Version,"
National Cancer Institute (NCI), February 3, 2017.

Some screening tests are used because they have been shown to be helpful both in finding colorectal cancers early and decreasing the chance of dying from these cancers. Other tests are used because they have been shown to find colorectal cancer in some people; however, it has not been proven in clinical trials that use of these tests will decrease the risk of dying from cancer.

Scientists study screening tests to find those with the fewest risks and most benefits. Colorectal cancer screening trials also are meant to show whether early detection (finding cancer before it causes symptoms) decreases a person's chance of dying from the disease. For some types of cancer, finding and treating the disease at an early stage may result in a better chance of recovery.

Studies show that some screening tests for colorectal cancer help find cancer at an early stage and may decrease the number of deaths from the disease.

Five Types of Tests Are Used to Screen for Colorectal Cancer

Fecal Occult Blood Test

A fecal occult blood test (FOBT) is a test to check stool (solid waste) for blood that can only be seen with a microscope. A small sample of stool is placed on a special card or in a special container and returned to the doctor or laboratory for testing. Blood in the stool may be a sign of polyps, cancer, or other conditions.

There are two types of FOBTs:

- **Guaiac FOBT.** The sample of stool on the special card is tested with a chemical. If there is blood in the stool, the special card changes color.

- **Immunochemical FOBT.** A liquid is added to the stool sample. This mixture is injected into a machine that contains antibodies that can detect blood in the stool. If there is blood in the stool, a line appears in a window in the machine. This test is also called fecal immunochemical test or FIT.

Sigmoidoscopy

Sigmoidoscopy is a procedure to look inside the rectum and sigmoid (lower) colon for polyps, abnormal areas, or cancer. A sigmoidoscope is inserted through the rectum into the sigmoid colon. A sigmoidoscope is a thin, tube-like instrument with a light and a lens for viewing. It may also have a tool to remove polyps or tissue samples, which are checked under a microscope for signs of cancer.

Colonoscopy

Colonoscopy is a procedure to look inside the rectum and colon for polyps, abnormal areas, or cancer. A colonoscope is inserted through the rectum into the colon. A colonoscope is a thin, tube-like instrument with a light and a lens for viewing. It may also have a tool to remove polyps or tissue samples, which are checked under a microscope for signs of cancer.

Virtual Colonoscopy

Virtual colonoscopy is a procedure that uses a series of X-rays called computed tomography to make a series of pictures of the colon. A computer puts the pictures together to create detailed images that may show polyps and anything else that seems unusual on the inside surface of the colon. This test is also called computed tomography colonography or CTC.

Clinical trials are comparing virtual colonoscopy with other colorectal cancer screening tests. Some clinical trials are testing whether drinking a contrast material that coats the stool, instead of using laxatives to empty the colon, shows polyps clearly.

Deoxyribonucleic Acid (DNA) Stool Test

This test checks DNA in stool cells for genetic changes that may be a sign of colorectal cancer.

Studies have shown that screening for colorectal cancer using digital rectal exam does not decrease the number of deaths from the disease.

A digital rectal exam (DRE) is an exam of the rectum that may be done as part of a routine physical exam. A doctor or nurse inserts a lubricated, gloved finger into the lower part of the rectum to feel for lumps or anything else that seems unusual. Study results have shown that DRE does not work as a screening method for colorectal cancer.

Section 14.6

Osteoporosis Screening (Bone Density Testing)

This section includes text excerpted from "Bone Mass Measurement: What the Numbers Mean," National Institute of Arthritis and Musculoskeletal and Skin Diseases (NIAMS), June 2015.

What Is a Bone Density Test?

A bone mineral density (BMD) test is can provide a snapshot of your bone health. The test can identify osteoporosis, determine your risk for fractures (broken bones), and measure your response to osteoporosis treatment. The most widely recognized BMD test is called a central dual-energy X-ray absorptiometry, or central DXA test. It is painless—a bit like having an X-ray. The test can measure bone density at your hip and spine.

Peripheral bone density tests measure bone density in the lower arm, wrist, finger, or heel. These tests are often used for screening purposes and can help identify people who might benefit from additional bone density testing.

What Does the Test Do?

A BMD test measures your bone mineral density and compares it to that of an established norm or standard to give you a score. Although no bone density test is 100-percent accurate, the BMD test is an important predictor of whether a person will have a fracture in the future.

The T-Score

Most commonly, your BMD test results are compared to the ideal or peak bone mineral density of a healthy 30-year-old adult, and you are given a T-score. A score of 0 means your BMD is equal to the norm for a healthy young adult. Differences between your BMD and that of the healthy young adult norm are measured in units called standard deviations (SDs). The more standard deviations below 0, indicated as negative numbers, the lower your BMD and the higher your risk of fracture.

As shown in the table below, a T-score between +1 and −1 is considered normal or healthy. A T-score between −1 and −2.5 indicates that you have low bone mass, although not low enough to be diagnosed with osteoporosis. A T-score of −2.5 or lower indicates that you have osteoporosis. The greater the negative number, the more severe the osteoporosis.

Table 14.1. World Health Organization Definitions Based on Bone Density Levels

Level	Definition
Normal	Bone density is within 1 SD (+1 or −1) of the young adult mean.
Low bone mass	Bone density is between 1 and 2.5 SD below the young adult mean (−1 to −2.5 SD).
Osteoporosis	Bone density is 2.5 SD or more below the young adult mean (−2.5 SD or lower).
Severe (established) osteoporosis	Bone density is more than 2.5 SD below the young adult mean, and there have been one or more osteoporotic fractures.

Low Bone Mass versus Osteoporosis

The information provided by a BMD test can help your doctor decide which prevention or treatment options are right for you.

If you have low bone mass that is not low enough to be diagnosed as osteoporosis, this is sometimes referred to as osteopenia. Low bone mass can be caused by many factors such as:

- heredity

- the development of less-than-optimal peak bone mass in your youth

- a medical condition or medication to treat such a condition that negatively affects bone

- abnormally accelerated bone loss

Although not everyone who has low bone mass will develop osteoporosis, everyone with low bone mass is at higher risk for the disease and the resulting fractures.

As a person with low bone mass, you can take steps to help slow down your bone loss and prevent osteoporosis in your future. Your doctor will want you to develop—or keep—healthy habits such as eating foods rich in calcium and vitamin D and doing weight-bearing exercise such as walking, jogging, or dancing. In some cases, your doctor may recommend medication to prevent osteoporosis.

If you are diagnosed with osteoporosis, these healthy habits will help, but your doctor will probably also recommend that you take medication. Several effective medications are available to slow—or even reverse—bone loss. If you do take medication to treat osteoporosis, your doctor can advise you concerning the need for future BMD tests to check your progress.

Who Should Get a Bone Density Test?

The U.S. Preventive Services Task Force (USPSTF) recommends that all women over age 65 should have a bone density test. Women who are younger than age 65 and at high risk for fractures should also have a bone density test.

Due to a lack of available evidence, the Task Force did not make recommendations regarding osteoporosis screening in men.

Various professional medical societies have established guidelines concerning when a person should get a BMD test. Many of these guidelines can be found by conducting a search in an online database established by the National Guideline Clearinghouse at www.guideline.gov.

Section 14.7

How to Spot Skin Cancer

This section includes text excerpted from "Skin Cancer Screening (PDQ®)–Patient Version," National Cancer Institute (NCI), June 21, 2017.

Skin cancer is a disease in which malignant (cancer) cells form in the tissues of the skin. Skin cancer begins in the epidermis, which is made up of three kinds of cells:

- Squamous cells: Thin, flat cells that form the top layer of the epidermis. Cancer that forms in squamous cells is called squamous cell carcinoma.

- Basal cells: Round cells under the squamous cells. Cancer that forms in basal cells is called basal cell carcinoma.

- Melanocytes: Found in the lower part of the epidermis, these cells make melanin, the pigment that gives skin its natural color. When skin is exposed to the sun, melanocytes make more pigment and cause the skin to tan, or darken. Cancer that forms in melanocytes is called melanoma.

Nonmelanoma skin cancer is the most common cancer in the United States. Basal cell carcinoma and squamous cell carcinoma are also called nonmelanoma skin cancer and are the most common forms of skin cancer. Most basal cell and squamous cell skin cancers can be cured.

Melanoma is more likely to spread to nearby tissues and other parts of the body and can be harder to cure. Melanoma is easier to cure if the tumor is found before it spreads to the dermis (inner layer of skin). Melanoma is less likely to cause death when it is found and treated early.

Skin Cancer Screening

Tests are used to screen for different types of cancer. Some screening tests are used because they have been shown to be helpful both in finding cancers early and in decreasing the chance of dying from these cancers. Other tests are used because they have been shown to find cancer in some people; however, it has not been proven in clinical trials that use of these tests will decrease the risk of dying from cancer.

Scientists study screening tests to find those with the fewest risks and most benefits. Cancer screening trials also are meant to show whether early detection (finding cancer before it causes symptoms) decreases a person's chance of dying from the disease. For some types of cancer, finding and treating the disease at an early stage may result in a better chance of recovery.

Clinical trials that study cancer screening methods are taking place in many parts of the country. Information about ongoing clinical trials is available from the NCI website.

Having a skin exam to screen for skin cancer has not been shown to decrease your chance of dying from skin cancer.

During a skin exam a doctor or nurse checks the skin for moles, birthmarks, or other pigmented areas that look abnormal in color, size, shape, or texture. Skin exams to screen for skin cancer have not been shown to decrease the number of deaths from the disease.

Regular skin checks by a doctor are important for people who have already had skin cancer. If you are checking your skin and find a worrisome change, you should report it to your doctor.

If an area on the skin looks abnormal, a biopsy is usually done. The doctor will remove as much of the suspicious tissue as possible with a local excision. A pathologist then looks at the tissue under a microscope to check for cancer cells. Because it is sometimes difficult to tell if a skin growth is benign (not cancer) or malignant (cancer), you may want to have the biopsy sample checked by a second pathologist.

Most melanomas in the skin can be seen by the naked eye. Usually, melanoma grows for a long time under the top layer of skin (the epidermis) but does not grow into the deeper layer of skin (the dermis). This allows time for skin cancer to be found early. Melanoma is easier to cure if it is found before it spreads.

Risks of Skin Cancer Screening Tests

Screening may not improve your health or help you live longer if you have advanced skin cancer. Some cancers never cause symptoms or become life-threatening, but if found by a screening test, the cancer may be treated. Treatments for cancer may have serious side effects.

False negative test results can occur.

Screening test results may appear to be normal even though cancer is present. A person who receives a false negative test result (one that shows there is no cancer when there really is) may delay getting medical care even if there are symptoms.

False positive test results can occur.

Screening test results may appear to be abnormal even though no cancer is present. A false positive test result (one that shows there is cancer when there really isn't) can cause anxiety and is usually followed by more tests (such as a biopsy), which also have risks.

A biopsy may cause scarring.

When a skin biopsy is done, the doctor will try to leave the smallest scar possible, but there is a risk of scarring and infection. Talk to your doctor about your risk for skin cancer and your need for screening tests.

Chapter 15

Immunizations for Women

Chapter Contents

Section 15.1

Recommended Immunizations for Women of Reproductive Age

This section includes text excerpted from "Immunization," Centers for Disease Control and Prevention (CDC), September 2, 2014.

All women of reproductive age should have their immunization status for tetanus-diphtheria toxoid/diphtheria-tetanus-pertussis; measles, mumps, and rubella; and varicella reviewed annually and updated as indicated. All women should be assessed annually for health, lifestyle, and occupational risks for other infections and be offered indicated immunizations.

Hepatitis B

The hepatitis B vaccine prevents transmission of infection to infants and eliminates the risks to the woman of hepatic failure, liver carcinoma, cirrhosis, and death due to HBV infection.

All women who are at high risk and who have not been vaccinated previously should receive the hepatitis B vaccine before pregnancy; women who are chronic carriers should be instructed on ways to prevent transmission to close contacts and how to prevent vertical transmission to their babies.

Human Papillomavirus (HPV)

Women should be screened routinely for human papillomavirus (HPV)-associated abnormalities of the cervix with cytologic (Papanicolaou) screening. Recommended subgroups should receive the HPV vaccine for the purpose of decreasing the incidence of cervical abnormalities and cancer. By avoiding procedures of the cervix because of abnormalities caused by HPV, the vaccine could help maintain cervical competency during pregnancy.

Influenza

Influenza vaccination is recommended for everyone 6 months of age and older. It is especially important for women who will be pregnant during influenza season and for any woman with an increased risk for influenza-related complications, such as cardiopulmonary disease or metabolic disorders, before influenza season begins. To prevent influenza, encourage your pregnant patients to get the trivalent inactivated seasonal influenza vaccine during any trimester.

Measles, Mumps, and Rubella

The rubella vaccine provides protection against congenital rubella syndrome.

All women of reproductive age should be screened for rubella immunity. Immunization should be offered to women who have not been vaccinated or who are not immune and who are not pregnant. Women should be counseled not to become pregnant for 3 months after receiving the vaccination. This vaccination will provide protection against measles, mumps, and rubella.

Tetanus, Diphtheria, and Pertussis

Women of reproductive age should be up to date for tetanus toxoid because passive immunity probably is protective against neonatal tetanus. If a tetanus and diphtheria booster vaccination is indicated during pregnancy for a woman who has previously not received Tdap (i.e., more than 10 years since previous Td), then healthcare providers should administer Tdap during pregnancy, preferably during the third or late second trimester (after 20 weeks' gestation)

Varicella

Because the varicella vaccine is contraindicated during pregnancy, screening for varicella immunity (by either a history of previous vaccination, previous varicella infection verified by a healthcare provider, or laboratory evidence of immunity) should be done as part of a pre-conception visit. All non-pregnant women of childbearing age who do not have evidence of varicella immunity should be vaccinated against varicella.

Section 15.2

Vaccinations for Women with Chronic Conditions

This section includes text excerpted from "Adults with Chronic Conditions: Get Vaccinated," Centers for Disease Control and Prevention (CDC), August 1, 2016.

Vaccines are recommended for all women to help prevent getting and spreading diseases. Vaccines are especially important for those with chronic conditions, who are more likely to develop complications from certain vaccine-preventable diseases. Find out which vaccines are recommended for you.

Vaccines are an important step in protecting women against serious, sometimes deadly, diseases. Even if you were vaccinated at a younger age, the protection from some vaccines can wear off or the viruses or bacteria that the vaccines protect against change so your resistance is not as strong. As you get older, you may also be at risk for vaccine-preventable diseases due to your age, job, hobbies, travel, or health conditions.

CDC recommends that all women get the following vaccines:

- Influenza vaccine every year to protect against seasonal flu

- Td vaccine every 10 years to protect against tetanus

- Tdap vaccine once instead of Td vaccine to protect against tetanus and diphtheria plus pertussis (whooping cough) and during each pregnancy for women

- Other vaccines you need as an adult are determined by factors such as age, lifestyle, job, health condition and vaccines you have had in the past. Vaccines you need may include those that protect against: shingles, human papillomavirus (which can cause certain cancers), pneumococcal disease, meningococcal disease, hepatitis A and B, chickenpox (varicella), measles, mumps, and rubella

Women with chronic conditions are more likely to develop complications, including long-term illness, hospitalization, and even death, from certain vaccine-preventable diseases. Talk to your doctor to make sure you are up to date on the vaccines that are recommended for you.

Heart Disease

Women with heart disease, or those who have had a stroke, have a higher risk of serious medical complications from the flu, including worsening of their heart disease. Women with heart disease are at almost three times higher risk of being hospitalized with flu than those without heart disease.

Centers for Disease Control and Prevention (CDC) recommends women with heart disease get a yearly influenza (flu) vaccine. They should also get pneumococcal vaccines, once as an adult before 65 years of age and then two more doses at 65 years or older.

Lung Disease

Women with asthma, chronic obstructive pulmonary disease (COPD), or other conditions that affect the lungs have a higher risk of complication from influenza (the flu) even if the condition is mild and symptoms are controlled. Since women with asthma and COPD have sensitive airways, inflammation from the flu can cause asthma attacks or make asthma and COPD symptoms worse. Those with asthma, COPD, or other conditions that affect the lungs are more likely to develop pneumonia and other respiratory diseases after getting sick with the flu than those without these conditions.

CDC recommends women with asthma, COPD, or other conditions that affect the lungs get a yearly flu vaccine. If you have a lung condition, you should also get pneumococcal vaccines—once as an adult before 65 years of age, and then two more doses at 65 years or older. Your doctor may recommend additional vaccines based on your lifestyle, travel habits, and other factors.

Diabetes

Women with type 1 or type 2 diabetes have a higher risk of hepatitis B virus infection. Hepatitis B can be spread through sharing of blood glucose meters, fingerstick devices, or other diabetes care equipment such as insulin pens. Diabetes, either type 1 or type 2, can also weaken the immune system's ability to fight the flu. Women with diabetes, even if well managed, are more likely than those without diabetes to have complications from the flu such as pneumonia, which can lead to hospitalization.

CDC recommends women with diabetes get pneumococcal vaccines, once as an adult before 65 years of age and then two more doses at 65 years or older, a yearly influenza (flu) vaccine, and a hepatitis B vaccine series if they're between the ages of 19 and 59. If you are 60 years or older, talk to your doctor to see if you should get hepatitis B vaccine.

Section 15.3

Human Papillomavirus (HPV) Vaccine

This section includes text excerpted from "Human Papillomavirus," Office on Women's Health (OWH), U.S. Department of Health and Human Services (HHS), April 28, 2017.

Human papillomavirus, or HPV, is the most common sexually transmitted infection (STI) in the United States. About 80% of women will get at least one type of HPV at some point in their lifetime. It is usually spread through vaginal, oral, or anal sex. Many women do not know they have HPV, because it usually has no symptoms and usually goes away on its own. Some types of HPV can cause illnesses such as genital warts or cervical cancer. There is a vaccine to help you prevent HPV.

What Is Human Papillomavirus (HPV)?

HPV is the name for a group of viruses that includes more than 100 types. More than 40 types of HPV can be passed through sexual contact. The types that infect the genital area are called genital HPV.

Who Gets HPV?

Genital HPV is the most common STI in the United States for both women and men. About 79 million Americans have HPV. It is so common that 80% of women will get at least one type of HPV at some point in their lifetime.

How Do You Get HPV?

HPV is spread through:

- Vaginal, oral, or anal sex. HPV can be spread even if there are no symptoms. This means you can get HPV from someone who has no signs or symptoms.

- Genital touching. A man does not need to ejaculate (come) for HPV to spread. HPV can also be passed between women who have sex with women.

- Childbirth from a woman to her baby.

What Are the Symptoms of HPV?

Most women with HPV do not have any symptoms. This is one reason why women need regular Pap tests. Experts recommend that you get your first Pap test at age 21. The Pap test can find changes on the cervix caused by HPV. If you are a woman between ages 30 and 65, your doctor might also do an HPV test with your Pap test every five years. This is a DNA test that detects most types of HPV.

Another way to tell if you have an HPV infection is if you have genital warts. Genital warts usually appear as a small bump or group of bumps in the genital area. They can be small or large, raised or flat, or shaped like a cauliflower. Doctors can usually diagnose warts by looking at the genital area.

What Health Problems Can HPV Cause?

HPV usually goes away on its own and does not cause any health problems. But when HPV does not go away, it can cause health problems including:

- Cervical cancer

- Other genital cancers (such as cancers of the vulva, vagina, penis, or anus)

- Oropharyngeal cancer (cancer of the back of the throat, including the base of the tongue and tonsils)

- Genital warts

- Recurrent respiratory papillomatosis (a rare condition that causes warts to grow in the respiratory tract)

189

Do I Need to Get Tested for HPV?

- If you are 21 to 29 years old, your doctor might suggest the HPV test if you have had an unusual or unclear Pap test result. The test will help determine if HPV caused the abnormal cells on your cervix. Most women younger than 30 do not need the HPV test, because the immune system fights off HPV within two years in 90% of cases in that age group.

- If you are 30 years or older, you may choose to have the HPV test along with the Pap test to screen for cervical cancer.

- If results of both tests are normal, your chance of getting cervical cancer in the next few years is very low. Your doctor might then say that you can wait up to five years for your next HPV screening.

How Does HPV Affect Pregnancy?

HPV does not affect your chances of getting pregnant, but it may cause problems during pregnancy.

Some possible problems during pregnancy include:

- **Cervical cell changes.** Continue to get regular cervical cancer screening during and after pregnancy to help your doctor find any changes.

- **Genital warts that bleed and grow.** Hormonal changes during pregnancy can cause any genital warts that you had before getting pregnant or that you get during pregnancy to bleed and grow (in size and number).

- **Cesarean section.** If genital warts block the birth canal, you may need to have a cesarean section.

- **Health problems in the baby.** A woman with genital HPV can—very rarely—pass it on to her baby. Babies and children may develop growths in their airways from HPV. This rare but potentially serious condition is called recurrent respiratory papillomatosis.

How Can I Prevent HPV?

There are two ways to prevent HPV. One way is get an HPV vaccine. The other way to prevent HPV or any STI is to not have sexual contact with another person.

If you do have sex, lower your risk of getting an STI with the following steps:

Use condoms. Condoms are the best way to prevent STIs when you have sex. Although HPV can also happen in female and male genital areas that are not protected by condoms, research shows that condom use is linked to lower cervical cancer rates. The HPV vaccine does not replace or decrease the need to wear condoms. Make sure to put the condom on before the penis touches the vagina, mouth, or anus. Also, other methods of birth control, like birth control pills, shots, implants, or diaphragms, will not protect you from STIs.

Get tested. Be sure you and your partner are tested for STIs. Talk to each other about the test results before you have sex.

Be monogamous. Having sex with just one partner can lower your risk for STIs. After being tested for STIs, be faithful to each other. That means that you have sex only with each other and no one else.

Limit your number of sex partners. Your risk of getting STIs goes up with the number of partners you have.

Do not douche. Douching removes some of the normal bacteria in the vagina that protects you from infection. This may increase your risk of getting STIs.

Do not abuse alcohol or drugs. Drinking too much alcohol or using drugs increases risky behavior and may put you at risk of sexual assault and possible exposure to STIs.

The steps work best when used together. No single step can protect you from every single type of STI.

What Is the HPV Vaccine?

The HPV vaccine prevents cervical cancer in women. The U.S. Food and Drug Administration (FDA) approved the HPV vaccine to prevent HPV and related diseases, including cervical cancer.

When Can I Get the HPV Vaccine?

Experts recommend the HPV vaccine for 11 or 12 year olds. The HPV vaccine works best when you get it before you have any type of sexual contact with anyone else. The FDA approved the HPV vaccine for girls and women from 9 through 26.

If you are 26 or younger and never had the HPV vaccine, or did not get all of the HPV shots, ask your doctor or nurse about getting vaccinated.

The HPV vaccine is given in two or three doses, over a 6 to 12-month period. Spacing out the HPV shots helps your immune system develop the antibodies against HPV. The schedule for HPV vaccine shots depend on the age and health history of the person getting it.

Talk to your doctor to find out if getting vaccinated is recommended for you based on your age and health history.

Do I Need the HPV Vaccine If I Have Already Had Sexual Contact?

Yes. You can still benefit from the HPV vaccine if you have already had sexual contact. The vaccine can protect you from HPV types you haven't gotten yet. However, the vaccine is recommended for most women only if you are 26 years old or younger.

If I Get the HPV Vaccine, Do I Still Need to Use a Condom?

Yes. The vaccine does not replace or decrease the need to wear condoms. Using condoms lowers your risk of getting other types of HPV and other STIs.

Do I Still Need a Pap Test If I got the HPV Vaccine?

Yes. There are three reasons why:

- Although the HPV vaccine protects against many of the HPV types that cause cervical cancer, it does not prevent all HPV types that cause cervical cancer.

- You might not be fully protected if you did not get all the vaccine doses (or at the recommended ages).

- You might not fully benefit from the vaccine if you were vaccinated after getting one or more types of HPV before vaccination.

Can HPV Be Cured?

No, HPV has no cure. Most often, HPV goes away on its own. If HPV does not go away on its own, there are treatments for the genital warts and cervical cell changes caused by HPV.

Part Three

Breast and Gynecological Concerns

Chapter 16

Nonmalignant Breast Conditions

Chapter Contents

Section 16.1

Breast Changes

This section includes text excerpted from "Understanding Breast Changes," National Cancer Institute (NCI), February 2014.

What Are Breast Changes?

Many breast changes are changes in how your breast or **nipple** looks or feels. You may notice a lump or firmness in your breast or under your arm. Or perhaps the size or shape of your breast has changed. Your nipple may be pointing or facing inward (inverted) or feeling tender. The skin on your breast, **areola**, or nipple may be scaly, red, or swollen. You may have **nipple discharge**, which is an **abnormal** fluid coming from the nipple.

If you have these or other breast changes, talk with your healthcare provider to get these changes checked as soon as possible.

Breast and Lymphatic System Basics

To better understand breast changes, it helps to know what the breasts and lymphatic system are made of.

What Are Breasts Made of?

Breasts are made of **connective tissue, glandular tissue, and fatty tissue**. Connective tissue and glandular tissue look dense, or white on a mammogram. Fatty tissue is non-dense, or black on a mammogram. **Dense breasts** can make mammograms harder to interpret.

Breasts have **lobes, lobules, ducts,** an areola, and a nipple.

- Lobes are sections of the glandular tissue. Lobes have smaller sections called lobules that end in tiny bulbs that can make milk.

- Ducts are thin tubes that connect the lobes and lobules. Milk flows from the lobules through the ducts to the nipple.

- The nipple is the small raised area at the tip of the breast. Milk flows through the nipple. The areola is the area of darker-colored skin around the nipple. Each breast also has **lymph vessels**.

What Is the Lymphatic System Made of?

The lymphatic system, which is a part of your body's defense system, contains lymph vessels and lymph nodes.

- Lymph vessels are thin tubes that carry a fluid called lymph and white blood cells.

- Lymph vessels lead to small, bean-shaped organs called lymph nodes. Lymph nodes are found near your breast, under your arm, above your collarbone, in your chest, and in other parts of your body.

- Lymph nodes filter substances in lymph to help fight infection and disease. They also store disease-fighting white blood cells called lymphocytes.

Check with Your Healthcare Provider about Breast Changes

Check with your healthcare provider if you notice that your breast looks or feels different. No change is too small to ask about. In fact, the best time to call is when you first notice a breast change.

Breast changes to see your healthcare provider about:

A Lump (Mass) or a Firm Feeling

- A lump in or near your breast or under your arm

- Thick or firm tissue in or near your breast or under your arm

- A change in the size or shape of your breast

Lumps come in different shapes and sizes. Most lumps are not cancer.

If you notice a lump in one breast, check your other breast. If both breasts feel the same, it may be normal. Normal breast tissue can sometimes feel lumpy.

Some women do regular **breast self-exams.** Doing breast self-exams can help you learn how your breasts normally feel and make it easier to notice and find any changes. Breast self-exams are not a substitute for mammograms.

Always get a lump checked. Don't wait until your next mammogram. You may need to have tests to be sure that the lump is not cancer.

Nipple Discharge or Changes

- Nipple discharge (fluid that is not breast milk)

- Nipple changes, such as a nipple that points or faces inward (inverted) into the breast

Nipple discharge may be different colors or textures. Nipple discharge is not usually a sign of cancer. It can be caused by birth control pills, some medicines, and infections.

Get nipple discharge checked, especially fluid that comes out by itself or fluid that is bloody.

Skin Changes

- Itching, redness, scaling, dimples, or puckers on your breast.

If the skin on your breast changes, get it checked as soon as possible.

Breast Changes during Your Lifetime That Are Not Cancer

Most women have changes in their breasts during their lifetime. Many of these changes are caused by hormones. For example, your breasts may feel more lumpy or tender at different times in your menstrual cycle.

Other breast changes can be caused by the normal aging process. As you near menopause, your breasts may lose tissue and fat. They may become smaller and feel lumpy. Most of these changes are not cancer; they are called benign changes. However, if you notice a breast change, don't wait until your next mammogram. Make an appointment to get it checked.

Young women who have not gone through menopause often have more dense tissue in their breasts. Dense tissue has more glandular and connective tissue and less fat tissue. This kind of tissue makes mammograms harder to interpret—because both dense tissue and tumors show up as solid white areas on X-ray images. Breast tissue gets less dense as women get older.

Before or during your menstrual periods, your breasts may feel swollen, tender, or painful. You may also feel one or more lumps during this time because of extra fluid in your breasts. These changes usually go away by the end of your menstrual cycle. Because some lumps are caused by normal hormone changes, your healthcare provider may have you come back for a return visit, at a different time in your menstrual cycle.

During pregnancy, your breasts may feel lumpy. This is usually because the glands that produce milk are increasing in number and getting larger.

While breastfeeding, you may get a condition called mastitis. This happens when a milk duct becomes blocked. Mastitis causes the breast to look red and feel lumpy, warm, and tender. It may be caused by an infection and it is often treated with antibiotics. Sometimes the duct

may need to be drained. If the redness or mastitis does not go away with treatment, call your healthcare provider.

As you approach menopause, your menstrual periods may come less often. Your hormone levels also change. This can make your breasts feel tender, even when you are not having your menstrual period. Your breasts may also feel more lumpy than they did before.

If you are taking hormones (such as menopausal hormone therapy, birth control pills, or injections) your breasts may become more dense. This can make a mammogram harder to interpret. Be sure to let your healthcare provider know if you are taking hormones.

When you stop having menstrual periods (menopause), your hormone levels drop, and your breast tissue becomes less dense and more fatty. You may stop having any lumps, pain, or nipple discharge that you used to have. And because your breast tissue is less dense, mammograms may be easier to interpret.

Finding Breast Changes

Here are some ways your healthcare provider can find breast changes:

- Clinical Breast Exam
- Magnetic resonance imaging (MRI)
- Mammogram

Follow-Up Tests to Diagnose Breast Changes

An ultrasound exam, an MRI, a biopsy, or other follow-up tests may be needed to learn more about a breast change.

Getting the Support You Need

It can be upsetting to notice a breast change, to get an abnormal test result, or to learn about a new condition or disease.

Many women choose to get extra help and support for themselves. It may help to think about people who have been there for you during challenging times in the past.

- Ask friends or loved ones for support. Take someone with you while you are learning about your testing and treatment choices.

- Ask your healthcare provider to:

  - Explain medical terms that are new or confusing.

  - Share with you how other people have handled the types of feelings that you are having.

  - Tell you about specialists that you can talk with to learn more.

Section 16.2

Common Breast Infections Due to Breastfeeding

This section contains text excerpted from the following sources:
Text beginning with the heading "Mastitis" is excerpted from
"Common Breastfeeding Challenges," Office on Women's
Health (OWH), U.S. Department of Health and Human
Services (HHS), February 1, 2017; Text under the heading
"Breast Injury and Infection Due to Breast Pumps" is excerpted
from "Injury and Infection," U.S. Food and Drug
Administration (FDA), October 7, 2014.

Mastitis

Mastitis is soreness or a lump in the breast. It can cause symptoms such as:

- Fever and/or flu-like symptoms, such as feeling run down or very achy

- Nausea

- Vomiting

- Yellowish discharge from the nipple that looks like colostrum

- Breasts that feel warm or hot to the touch and appear pink or red

A breast infection can happen when other family members have a cold or the flu. It usually happens in only one breast. It is not always easy to tell the difference between a breast infection and a plugged duct, because both have similar symptoms and can get better within 24 to 48 hours. Some breast infections that do not get better on their own need to be treated with prescription medicine from a doctor.

What You Can Do

- Breastfeed on the infected side every two hours or more often. This will keep the milk moving freely and your breast from becoming too full.

- Massage the area, starting behind the sore spot. Move your fingers in a circular motion and massage toward the nipple.

- Apply heat to the sore area with a warm, wet cloth.

- Rely on others to help you get extra sleep, or relax with your feet up to help speed healing. Often a breast infection is a sign that you are doing too much and becoming overly tired.

- Wear a well-fitting, supportive bra that is not too tight, since a tight bra can constrict milk ducts.

Ask your doctor for help if you do not feel better within 24 hours of trying these tips, if you have a fever, or if your symptoms get worse. You might need medicine. See your doctor right away if:

- You have a breast infection in which both breasts look affected

- There is pus or blood in your breastmilk

- You have red streaks near the affected area of the breast

- Your symptoms came on severely and suddenly

Fungal Infections

A fungal infection, also called a yeast infection or thrush, can form on your nipples or in your breast. This type of infection thrives on milk and is an overgrowth of the Candida organism. Candida lives in our bodies and is kept healthy and at the correct levels by the natural bacteria in our bodies. When the natural balance of bacteria is upset, Candida can overgrow, causing an infection.

A key sign of a fungal infection is sore nipples that last more than a few days, even after your baby has a good latch. Or you may suddenly get sore nipples after several weeks of pain-free breastfeeding. Other signs are pink, flaky, shiny, itchy, or cracked nipples or deep pink and blistered nipples. You could also have achy breasts or shooting pains deep in the breast during or after feedings.

Causes of fungal infection include:

- Thrush in your baby's mouth, which can pass to you

- Nipples that are sore or cracked

- Receiving or taking antibiotics or steroids (often given to mothers during labor)

- A chronic illness like HIV, diabetes, or anemia

What You Can Do

Fungal infections are treated with a medicine you rub on your breasts several times a day for about a week. It may take several weeks to clear up, so it is important to follow these tips to avoid spreading the infection:

- Change disposable nursing pads often.

- Wash any towels or clothing that comes in contact with the yeast in very hot water (above 122°F).

- Wear a clean bra every day.

- Wash your hands often.

Breast Injury and Infection due to Breast Pumps

The first few times you pump may feel uncomfortable but pumping should not be painful, result in sore nipples, or cause bleeding. Pain, sore nipples, and nipple irritation or bleeding may be signs of an injury.

Signs of infection can include soreness, yellowish discharge, a fever, and/or flu-like symptoms, such as feeling run down or very achy. Check with your healthcare provider if your symptoms do not improve within 24 to 48 hours.

If you are injured or experience persistent pain or bleeding when using your breast pump, contact your doctor, lactation consultant or other healthcare professional for advice.

If you are having trouble using your pump, a qualified healthcare professional may be able to help you.

If your pump is not working, contact the manufacturer. Check the box your breast pump came in or call directory assistance for the manufacturer's contact information.

Reporting an Injury or Infection from a Breast Pump to the FDA

Reporting of injuries and other adverse events can help the U.S. Food and Drug Administration (FDA) identify and better understand potential risks associated with medical devices, like breast pumps. If you suspect a problem with a breast pump, FDA encourages you to file a voluntary report with the FDA through MedWatch (www.fda.gov/Safety/MedWatch/HowToReport/ucm2007306.htm), the FDA Safety Information and Adverse Event Reporting program.

Things you might not think to report, that should be reported:

- Pump problems (breaking, not working right)

- Infections that might be related to the pump

- Presence of mold or mold-like substances in a pump

Section 16.3

Fibrocystic Breast Disease

"Fibrocystic Breast Disease," © 2018 Omnigraphics.
Reviewed August 2017.

What Is Fibrocystic Breast Disease?

A common condition, fibrocystic breast disease is a term that refers to the presence of painful, thickened areas in one or both breasts, which may feel lumpy or rope-like. The term fibrocystic breast disease is used less frequently now than other terms to describe the condition, primarily "fibrocystic breasts" or "fibrocystic breast changes," since such changes in breasts are now considered normal and not caused by a disease. The condition is not harmful or dangerous but can cause discomfort. Only physicians can identify if changes in the breast are fibrocystic in nature or whether they are related to some other specific problem, such as breast cancer. Fibrocystic lumps themselves, however, are not cancerous.

What Causes Fibrocystic Breast Disease?

The exact cause of fibrocystic breast disease is unknown. However, hormonal changes, such as those associated with the menstrual cycle, are considered a possible contributor. Fibrocystic breast changes commonly are seen in women anywhere in age from their 20s to their 50s. Such changes are rare in postmenopausal women unless they are undergoing hormone therapy.

What Are the Signs and Symptoms of Fibrocystic Breast Disease?

Symptoms of fibrocystic breast disease include:

• Lumps in the breast that move freely from the surrounding tissue

• Pain or tenderness in the breasts

• Change in the size of lumps along with the menstrual cycle

The symptoms generally are worse before the start of your monthly periods, but become better once it starts. The symptoms tend to be worse for women with heavy and irregular periods. If you are using birth control pills, your symptoms may be better.

You may have a lump in your breast that becomes bigger before your periods and shrink afterwards. The lump also moves when pushed with your finger. These kinds of lumps are common in fibrocystic breast changes.

When Should You Consult a Doctor?

Since the appearance of lumps in the breast can signal a more serious condition than fibrocystic breast changes, such as breast cancer, you should consult a doctor when:

• you find any lump in the breast with thickened surrounding tissue

• you have areas in the breast with continuous or worsening pain

- pain in the breast continues after periods
- discharge from the nipples that are dark brown or green in color. The discharge happens without squeezing or application of pressure.
- lump in the breast is increasing in size

What Are the Tests and Exams Used for Diagnosis?

Inform your healthcare provider of any changes you've noticed in your breast. The healthcare provider will try to determine if the lumps are cancerous or benign, initially conducting an ultrasound or mammogram. Ultrasound works best for young women since breast tissue in young women is dense. If the imaging test indicated that the lump may be cancerous, the doctor will order a biopsy to collect tissue samples for analysis. The results of the biopsy will show if the growth is cancerous or benign.

What Is the Treatment for Fibrocystic Breast Disease?

No treatment is required for fibrocystic breasts that have little or no pain. Lumps that are large or very painful could be cysts that can be treated with fine-needle aspiration or surgical excision.

The pain experienced by women with fibrocystic breast disease can be managed:

- With pain medications such as acetaminophen, nonsteroidal anti-inflammatory drugs (NSAIDs), such as ibuprofen and other prescription medications
- With oral contraceptives that regulate the hormone levels associated with the menstrual cycle
- By applying heat or cold compressions on the breast
- By wearing a well-fitting and supportive bra all the time when symptoms are worse
- By avoiding coffee, tea, soda, and chocolate, which have been associated with the occurrence of increased fibrocystic breast changes

Complementary and Alternative Medicine

Some food supplements (like evening primrose oil) and vitamins (like vitamin E) are associated with alleviating pain in women. Talk to your healthcare provider about which ones you should consume along with dosage recommendations and possible side effects.

What Are the Risk Factors?

Alcohol consumption in women between the ages of 18 and 22 is linked to increased risk of fibrocystic breast changes. It is thought that caffeine contributes to severity of pain in fibrocystic breast disease, though this is being debated in the medical community.

What Is the Relationship between Fibrocystic Breast Disease and Cancer?

Women with fibrocystic breast disease are not at risk for breast cancer but healthcare providers have a difficult time identifying lumps that are cancerous during breast exams and diagnostic imaging tests.

The U.S. Preventive Services Task Force (USPSTF) recommends that women between the ages of 50 and 75 should have a mammogram every two years. Regular breast self-examination is also recommended. Women should be familiar with how their breast looks and feels so that they can identify changes immediately upon self-examination.

What Is the Outlook for Women with Fibrocystic Breast Changes?

Fibrocystic breast changes are not harmful to women in general. But it is essential that changes in the breast are screened by a medical practitioner to rule out cancer.

References

1. "Fibrocystic Breasts," Mayo Foundation for Medical Education and Research (MFMER), March 12, 2016.

2. Mancini, Mary C., MD, PhD. "Fibrocystic Breast Disease," A.D.A.M., Inc., November 11, 2016.

3. "Fibrocystic Breast Disease," The Cleveland Clinic Foundation, 2017.

4. Cafasso, Jacquelyn. "Fibrocystic Breast Disease," July 19, 2016.

Chapter 17

Premenstrual Syndrome and Premenstrual Dysphoric Disorder

What Is Premenstrual Syndrome (PMS)?

Premenstrual syndrome (PMS) is a group of symptoms linked to the menstrual cycle. PMS symptoms occur 1 to 2 weeks before your period (menstruation or monthly bleeding) starts. The symptoms usually go away after you start bleeding. PMS can affect menstruating women of any age and the effect is different for each woman. For some people, PMS is just a monthly bother. For others, it may be so severe that it makes it hard to even get through the day. PMS goes away when your monthly periods stop, such as when you get pregnant or go through menopause.

This chapter contains text excerpted from the following sources: Text beginning with the heading "What Is Premenstrual Syndrome (PMS)?" is excerpted from "Premenstrual Syndrome," Office on Women's Health (OWH), U.S. Department of Health and Human Services (HHS), December 23, 2014; Text under the heading "Sensitive Gene Complex Linked to Premenstrual Mood Disorder" is excerpted from "Sex Hormone–Sensitive Gene Complex Linked to Premenstrual Mood Disorder," National Institute of Mental Health (NIMH), January 3, 2017.

What Causes PMS?

The causes of PMS are not clear, but several factors may be involved. Changes in hormones during the menstrual cycle seem to be an important cause. These changing hormone levels may affect some women more than others. Chemical changes in the brain may also be involved. Stress and emotional problems, such as depression, do not seem to cause PMS, but they may make it worse. Some other possible causes include:

- Low levels of vitamins and minerals

- Eating a lot of salty foods, which may cause you to retain (keep) fluid

- Drinking alcohol and caffeine, which may alter your mood and energy level

What Are the Symptoms of PMS?

PMS often includes both physical and emotional symptoms, such as:

- Acne
- Swollen or tender breasts
- Feeling tired
- Trouble sleeping
- Upset stomach, bloating, constipation, or diarrhea
- Headache or backache
- Appetite changes or food cravings
- Joint or muscle pain
- Trouble with concentration or memory
- Tension, irritability, mood swings, or crying spells
- Anxiety or depression

Symptoms vary from woman to woman.

How Do I Know If I Have PMS?

Your doctor may diagnose PMS based on which symptoms you have, when they occur, and how much they affect your life. If you think you have PMS, keep track of which symptoms you have and how severe they are for a few months. Record your symptoms each day on a calendar or PMS symptom tracker. Take this form with you when you see your doctor about your PMS.

Your doctor will also want to make sure you don't have one of the following conditions that shares symptoms with PMS:

- Depression

- Anxiety

- Menopause

- Chronic fatigue syndrome (CFS)

- Irritable bowel syndrome (IBS)

- Problems with the endocrine system, which makes hormones

How Common Is PMS?

There's a wide range of estimates of how many women suffer from PMS. The American College of Obstetricians and Gynecologists (ACOG) estimates that at least 85 percent of menstruating women have at least 1 PMS symptom as part of their monthly cycle. Most of these women have fairly mild symptoms that don't need treatment. Others (about 3 to 8 percent) have a more severe form of PMS, called premenstrual dysphoric disorder (PMDD).

PMS occurs more often in women who:

- Are between their late 20s and early 40s

- Have at least 1 child

- Have a family history of depression

- Have a past medical history of either postpartum depression or a mood disorder

What Is the Treatment for PMS?

Many things have been tried to ease the symptoms of PMS. No treatment works for every woman. You may need to try different ones to see what works for you. Some treatment options include:

- Lifestyle changes

- Medications

- Alternative therapies

Lifestyle Changes

If your PMS isn't so bad that you need to see a doctor, some lifestyle changes may help you feel better. Below are some steps you can take that may help ease your symptoms.

- Exercise regularly. Each week, you should get:
  - Two hours and 30 minutes of moderate-intensity physical activity;
  - One hour and 15 minutes of vigorous-intensity aerobic physical activity; or
  - A combination of moderate and vigorous-intensity activity; and
  - Muscle-strengthening activities on 2 or more days.
- Eat healthy foods, such as fruits, vegetables, and whole grains.
- Avoid salt, sugary foods, caffeine, and alcohol, especially when you're having PMS symptoms.
- Get enough sleep. Try to get about 8 hours of sleep each night.
- Find healthy ways to cope with stress. Talk to your friends, exercise, or write in a journal.
- Some women also find yoga, massage, or relaxation therapy helpful.
- Don't smoke.

Medications

Over-the-counter pain relievers may help ease physical symptoms, such as cramps, headaches, backaches, and breast tenderness. These include:

- Ibuprofen (for instance, Advil, Motrin, Midol Cramp)
- Ketoprofen (for instance, Orudis KT)
- Naproxen (for instance, Aleve)
- Aspirin

In more severe cases of PMS, prescription medicines may be used to ease symptoms. One approach has been to use drugs that stop ovulation, such as birth control pills. Women on the pill report fewer PMS symptoms, such as cramps and headaches, as well as lighter periods.

Researchers continue to search for new ways to treat PMS. Talk to your doctor about whether taking part in a clinical trial might be right for you.

Alternative Therapies

Certain vitamins and minerals have been found to help relieve some PMS symptoms. These include:

- Folic acid (400 micrograms)
- Calcium with vitamin D (see Table 17.1 below for amounts)
- Magnesium (400 milligrams)
- Vitamin B-6 (50 to 100 mg)
- Vitamin E (400 international units)

Table 17.1. Amounts of Calcium You Need Each Day

Ages	Milligrams Per Day
9–18	1300
19–50	1000
51 and older	1200

Pregnant or nursing women need the same amount of calcium as other women of the same age.

Some women find their PMS symptoms relieved by taking supplements such as:

- Black cohosh
- Chasteberry
- Evening primrose oil

Talk with your doctor before taking any of these products. Many have not been proven to work and they may interact with other medicines you are taking.

What Is Premenstrual Dysphoric Disorder (PMDD)?

A brain chemical called serotonin may play a role in premenstrual dysphoric disorder (PMDD), a severe form of PMS. The main symptoms, which can be disabling, include:

- Feelings of sadness or despair, or even thoughts of suicide

- Feelings of tension or anxiety

- Panic attacks

- Mood swings or frequent crying

- Lasting irritability or anger that affects other people

- Lack of interest in daily activities and relationships

- Trouble thinking or focusing

- Tiredness or low energy

- Food cravings or binge eating

- Trouble sleeping

- Feeling out of control

- Physical symptoms, such as bloating, breast tenderness, headaches, and joint or muscle pain

You must have 5 or more of these symptoms to be diagnosed with PMDD. Symptoms occur during the week before your period and go away after bleeding starts.

Making some lifestyle changes may help ease PMDD symptoms.

Antidepressants called selective serotonin reuptake inhibitors (SSRIs) have also been shown to help some women with PMDD. These drugs change serotonin levels in the brain. The U.S. Food and Drug Administration (FDA) has approved 3 SSRIs for the treatment of PMDD:

- Sertraline (Zoloft)

- Fluoxetine (Sarafem)

- Paroxetine HCl (Paxil CR)

Yaz (drospirenone and ethinyl estradiol) is the only birth control pill approved by the FDA to treat PMDD. Individual counseling, group counseling, and stress management may also help relieve symptoms.

Sensitive Gene Complex Linked to Premenstrual Mood Disorder

National Institutes of Health (NIH) researchers have discovered molecular mechanisms that may underlie a woman's susceptibility to disabling irritability, sadness, and anxiety in the days leading up to her menstrual period. Such premenstrual dysphoric disorder (PMDD) affects 2 to 5 percent of women of reproductive age, whereas less severe premenstrual syndrome (PMS) is much more common.

"We found dysregulated expression in a suspect gene complex which adds to evidence that PMDD is a disorder of cellular response to estrogen and progesterone," explained Peter Schmidt, M.D. of the NIH's National Institute of Mental Health, Behavioral Endocrinology Branch. "Learning more about the role of this gene complex holds hope for improved treatment of such prevalent reproductive endocrine-related mood disorders."

"This is a big moment for women's health, because it establishes that women with PMDD have an intrinsic difference in their molecular apparatus for response to sex hormones—not just emotional behaviors they should be able to voluntarily control," said David Goldman, M.D., of the NIH's National Institute on Alcohol Abuse and Alcoholism (NIAAA).

By the late 1990s, the NIMH team had demonstrated that women who regularly experience mood disorder symptoms just prior to their periods were abnormally sensitive to normal changes in sex hormones—even though their hormone levels were normal. But the cause remained a mystery.

In women with PMDD, experimentally turning off estrogen and progesterone eliminated PMDD symptoms, while experimentally adding back the hormones triggered the re-emergence of symptoms. This confirmed that they had a biologically-based behavioral sensitivity to the hormones that might be reflected in molecular differences detectable in their cells.

Following up on clues—including the fact that PMS is 56 percent heritable—the NIH researchers studied the genetic control of gene expression in cultured white blood cell lines from women with PMDD and controls. These cells express many of the same genes expressed in brain cells—potentially providing a window into genetically-influenced differences in molecular responses to sex hormones.

An analysis of all gene transcription in the cultured cell lines turned up a large gene complex in which gene expression differed conspicuously in cells from patients compared to controls. Notably, this ESC/E(Z) (Extra Sex Combs/Enhancer of Zeste) gene complex regulates epigenetic mechanisms that govern the transcription of genes into proteins in response to the environment—including sex hormones and stressors.

More than half of the ESC/E(Z) genes were over-expressed in PMDD patients' cells, compared to cells from controls. But paradoxically, protein expression of four key genes was decreased in cells from women with PMDD. In addition, progesterone boosted expression of several of these genes in controls, while estrogen decreased expression in cell lines derived from PMDD patients. This suggested dysregulated cellular response to the hormones in PMDD.

"For the first time, we now have cellular evidence of abnormal signaling in cells derived from women with PMDD, and a plausible biological cause for their abnormal behavioral sensitivity to estrogen and progesterone," explained Schmidt.

Using cutting edge "disease in a dish" technologies, the researchers are now following up the leads discovered in blood cell lines in neurons induced from stem cells derived from the blood of PMDD patients—in hopes of gaining a more direct window into the ESC/E(Z) complex's role in the brain.

Chapter 18

Menstrual Irregularities

Chapter Contents

Section 18.1

Abnormal Uterine Bleeding (AUB)

"Abnormal Uterine Bleeding (AUB),"
© 2018 Omnigraphics. Reviewed August 2017.

What Is Abnormal Uterine Bleeding (AUB)?

Abnormal uterine bleeding (AUB) is irregular bleeding from the uterus that is heavier, lighter, or longer than normal. Sometimes bleeding can be frequent, random, or absent. Bleeding during pregnancy is a different complication and should be brought to the attention of a medical practitioner immediately.

What Causes AUB?

AUB signals that the normal changes in hormonal levels associated with ovulation have been disrupted or altered. Ovulation, the physiological process by which the ovaries release an egg, is regulated by the hormones estrogen and progesterone. Changes in the levels of these hormones can cause abnormal uterine bleeding. Anovulation, a condition in which the ovaries fail to release an egg, is a common cause for change in hormone levels. Sometimes hormonal changes can be triggered by compulsive exercise, excessive weight gain or loss, unhealthy eating patterns, or stress. Abnormal uterine bleeding could also be a result of thyroid disease, polycystic ovarian syndrome (PCOS), uterine fibroids and polyps, or cancer in the female reproductive organs. Use of birth control methods such as birth control pills and intrauterine devices (IUD) could be a cause. Diseases such as von Willebrand disease could lead to severe cases of abnormal uterine bleeding.

What Are the Symptoms of AUB?

Abnormal uterine bleeding is characterized by:

- Bleeding or spotting between periods
- Bleeding or spotting after sex

- Heavy bleeding during periods

- Menstrual cycles that are more than 38 days or lesser than 24 days

- Irregular periods with the length of the menstrual cycle varying by more than 7 to 9 days

- Absence of periods for more than 3 months

- Bleeding after menopause

Use the 1-10-20 rule of thumb to alert yourself to abnormal uterine bleeding.

- Requiring more than 1 sanitary pad or tampon per hour.

- Your periods last for more than 10 days.

- There are less than 20 days in between periods.

If you note any of the above signs and symptoms, contact your healthcare provider.

How Is AUB Diagnosed?

A medical practitioner will rule out the existence of other diseases such as von Willebrand disease before diagnosing abnormal uterine bleeding. Vaginal bleeding because of pregnancy and miscarriage will also be ruled out. The doctor will seek information about periods and bleeding such as the last time a period occurred.

Questions pertaining to recent changes in weight and sexual activity help the doctor rule out conditions such as polycystic ovarian syndrome, sexually transmitted diseases (STDs), or an ectopic pregnancy, all of which could cause the bleeding.

A pelvic examination and a series of tests such as urine and blood tests as well as an ultrasound may also be ordered.

How Is AUB Treated?

Treatment is largely meant to restore the normal cycle of menstruation. The effectiveness of treatment varies depending on the patient and her medical history. The following treatment methods may be used:

- Prescribing progestin hormone pills or birth control pills with progestin and estrogen

- Implanting an IUD (intrauterine device) that releases progestin
- If caused by fibroid tumors, prescribing of gonadotropin-releasing hormone (GnRH) agonists to stop the menstrual cycle and reduce the size of fibroids
- Surgery to remove polyps or fibroids
- Tranexamic acid to control excessive bleeding

Doctors may also prescribe the following:

- NSAIDs (nonsteroidal anti-inflammatory drugs) such as ibuprofen to relieve menstrual cramps
- Antibiotics to control infection
- Special medications to control blood clots in case a bleeding disorder exists
- Iron pills if the patient is anemic

If symptoms do not improve after initial treatment procedures, other steps may be taken, including:

- Surgical removal of the endometrial lining
- Removal of the uterus (hysterectomy)

What Are the Possible Complications of AUB?

The following complications are seen in women with abnormal uterine bleeding.

- Anemia
- Infertility
- Increased risk of endometrial cancer

What Is the Outlook for Treatment of AUB?

Symptoms are usually relieved with hormone therapy. Treatment may be unnecessary if the underlying cause is not serious and you do not become anemic in spite of blood loss.

References

1. "Abnormal Uterine Bleeding—Topic Overview," WebMD, LLC, n.d.

2. John D. Jacobson, MD. "Abnormal Uterine Bleeding," A.D.A.M. Inc., December 8, 2016.

3. "Abnormal Uterine Bleeding (AUB)," The Nemours Foundation, August 2016.

4. "Abnormal Uterine Bleeding," The American College of Obstetricians and Gynecologists, March 2017.

Section 18.2

Amenorrhea (Absent Menstrual Periods)

This section includes text excerpted from "Amenorrhea," *Eunice Kennedy Shriver* National Institute of Child Health and Human Development (NICHD), June 5, 2017.

What Is Amenorrhea?

Amenorrhea is the absence of a menstrual period. Amenorrhea is sometimes categorized as:

- **Primary amenorrhea**. This describes a young woman who has not had a period by age 16.

- **Secondary amenorrhea**. This occurs when a woman who once had regular periods experiences an absence of more than three cycles. Causes of secondary amenorrhea include pregnancy.

Having regular periods is an important sign of overall health. Missing a period, when not caused by pregnancy, breastfeeding, or menopause, is generally a sign of another health problem. If you miss your period, talk to your healthcare provider about possible causes, including pregnancy.

What Are the Symptoms of Amenorrhea?

Missing a period is the main sign of amenorrhea.

Depending on the cause, a woman might have other signs or symptoms as well, such as:

- Excess facial hair
- Hair loss
- Headache
- Lack of breast development
- Milky discharge from the breasts
- Vision changes

Who Is at Risk of Amenorrhea?

According to the American Society for Reproductive Medicine (ASRM), amenorrhea that is not caused by pregnancy, breastfeeding, or menopause occurs in 3 percent to 4 percent of women during their lifetime. Secondary amenorrhea is more common than primary amenorrhea.

The risk factors for amenorrhea include:

- Excessive exercise

- Obesity

- Eating disorders, such as anorexia nervosa

- A family history of amenorrhea or early menopause

- Genetics, such as having a change to the *FMR1* gene, which also causes Fragile X syndrome

What Causes Amenorrhea?

Amenorrhea is often a sign of another health problem rather than a disease itself, and it can happen for many reasons. It can occur as a natural part of life, such as during pregnancy or breastfeeding. It can also be a sign of a health problem, such as polycystic ovary syndrome (PCOS). Because amenorrhea is associated with health conditions that are also linked to infertility, understanding amenorrhea is an important part of *Eunice Kennedy Shriver* National Institute of Child Health and Human Development's (NICHD) research on infertility and fertility.

Common characteristics of women with hypothalamic amenorrhea include:

- Low body weight

- Low percentage of body fat

- Very low intake of calories or fat

- Emotional stress

- Strenuous exercise that burns more calories than are taken in through food

- Deficiency of leptin, a protein hormone that regulates appetite and metabolism

- Some medical conditions or illnesses

- **Gynecological conditions,** specifically those that lead to or result from hormone imbalances, may also have secondary amenorrhea as a main symptom.

  - Polycystic ovary syndrome (PCOS). PCOS occurs when a woman's body produces more androgens (a type of hormone) than normal. High levels of androgens can cause fluid-filled sacs or cysts to grow in the ovaries, interfering with the release of eggs (ovulation). Most women with PCOS either have amenorrhea or experience irregular periods, called oligomenorrhea.

  - Fragile X-associated primary ovarian insufficiency (FXPOI). The term FXPOI describes a condition in which a woman's ovaries stop functioning before normal menopause, sometimes around age 40. FXPOI results from certain changes to a gene on the X chromosome. As many as 10 percent of women who seek treatment for amenorrhea have FXPOI.

- **Thyroid problems.** The thyroid is a small butterfly-shaped gland at the base of the neck, just below the Adam's apple. The thyroid produces hormones that control metabolism and play a role in puberty and menstruation. A thyroid gland that is overactive (called hyperthyroidism) or underactive (hypothyroidism) can cause menstrual irregularities, including amenorrhea.

- **Pituitary tumors.** The pituitary gland in the brain regulates the production of hormones that affect many body functions, including metabolism and the reproductive cycle. Tumors on the

pituitary gland are usually noncancerous (benign) but can interfere with the body's hormonal regulation of menstruation.

How Is Amenorrhea Diagnosed?

A healthcare provider will usually ask a series of questions to begin
diagnosing amenorrhea, including:

- How old were you when you started your period?

- What are your menstrual cycles like? (What is the typical length
  of your cycle? How heavy or light are your periods?)

- Are you sexually active?

- Could you be pregnant?

- Have you gained or lost weight recently?

- How often and how much do you exercise?

Primary Amenorrhea

If you are older than 16 and have never had a period, your healthcare provider will do a thorough medical history and physical exam,
including a pelvic exam, to see if you are experiencing other signs
of puberty. Depending on the findings and on your answers to the
questions above, other tests may be ordered to determine the cause
of your amenorrhea.

Secondary Amenorrhea

If you are sexually active, your healthcare provider will likely order
a pregnancy test. He or she will also perform a complete physical exam,
including a pelvic exam.

You should contact your healthcare provider as soon as possible
after you miss a period.

Other Tests You May Need

- **Thyroid function test.** This test measures the amount of thy-
  roid-stimulating hormone (TSH) in your blood, which can help
  determine if your thyroid is working properly. A thyroid gland
  that is overactive (hyperthyroidism) or underactive (hypothyroidism) can cause menstrual irregularities, including amenorrhea.

- **Ovary function test.** This test measures the amount of follicle-stimulating hormone (FSH) or luteinizing hormone (LH)—hormones made by the pituitary gland—in your blood to determine if your ovaries are working properly. Your healthcare provider may also evaluate the level of anti-Mullerian hormone (AMH), which is produced by the ovarian follicles. Higher levels of AMH may be associated with polycystic ovary syndrome (PCOS). Low or undetectable amounts of AMH may be associated with menopause or primary ovarian insufficiency.

- **Androgen test.** Androgens are sometimes called "male hormones" because men need higher levels of these hormones than women do for overall health. However, both women and men need androgens to stay healthy. Your healthcare provider may want to check the level of androgens in your blood.

- High levels of androgens may indicate a woman has PCOS.

- **Hormone challenge test.** With this test, you will take a hormonal medication for seven to 10 days in an effort to trigger a menstrual cycle. Results from the test can tell your healthcare provider whether your periods have stopped because of a lack of estrogen.

- **Screening for a premutation of the *FMR1* gene.** Changes in this gene can cause the ovaries to stop functioning properly, leading to amenorrhea.

- **Chromosome evaluation.** This test, also known as a karyotype, involves counting and evaluating the chromosomes from cells in the body to identify any missing, extra, or rearranged cells. Results from this evaluation can help determine the cause of the chromosomal abnormality causing primary or secondary amenorrhea.

- **Ultrasound.** This painless test uses sound waves to produce images of internal organs. This test can help determine if your reproductive organs are all present and shaped normally.

- **Computed tomography (CT).** CT scans combine many X-ray images taken from different directions to create cross-sectional views of internal structures. A CT scan can indicate whether your uterus, ovaries, and kidneys look normal.

- **Magnetic resonance imaging (MRI).** MRI uses radio waves with a strong magnetic field to produce detailed images of soft tissues within the body. Your healthcare provider may order an MRI to check for a pituitary tumor or to examine your reproductive organs.

- **Hysteroscopy.** In this procedure a thin, lighted camera is passed through your vagina and cervix to allow your healthcare provider to look at the inside of your uterus.

Your healthcare provider might use several of these tests to attempt to diagnose the cause of amenorrhea. In some cases, no specific cause for the amenorrhea can be found. This situation is called idiopathic amenorrhea.

What Are the Treatments for Amenorrhea?

The treatment for amenorrhea depends on the underlying cause, as well as the health status and goals of the individual.

If primary or secondary amenorrhea is caused by lifestyle factors, your healthcare provider may suggest changes in the areas below:

- **Weight.** Being overweight or severely underweight can affect your menstrual cycle. Attaining and maintaining a healthy weight often helps balance hormone levels and restore your menstrual cycle.

- **Stress.** Assess the areas of stress in your life and reduce the things that are causing stress. If you can't decrease stress on your own, ask for help from family, friends, your healthcare provider, or a professional listener such as a counselor.

- **Level of physical activity.** You may need to change or adjust your physical activity level to help restart your menstrual cycle. Talk to your healthcare provider and your coach or trainer about how to train in a way that maintains your health and menstrual cycles.

Be aware of changes in your menstrual cycle and check with your healthcare provider if you have concerns. Keep a record of when your periods occur. Note the date your period starts, how long it lasts, and any problems you experience. The first day of bleeding is considered the first day of your menstrual cycle.

For **primary amenorrhea**, depending on your age and the results of the ovary function test, healthcare providers may recommend watchful waiting. If an ovary function test shows low follicle-stimulating hormone (FSH) or luteinizing hormone (LH) levels, menstruation may just be delayed. In females with a family history of delayed menstruation, this kind of delay is common.

Primary amenorrhea caused by chromosomal or genetic problems may require surgery. Women with a genetic condition called 46, XY gonadal dysgenesis have one X and one Y chromosome, but their ovaries do not develop normally. This condition increases the risk for cancer developing in the ovaries. The gonads (ovaries) are often removed through laparoscopic surgery to prevent or reduce the risk of cancer.

Treatment for **secondary amenorrhea**, depending on the cause, may include medical or surgical treatments or a combination of the two.

Medical Treatments for Secondary Amenorrhea

Common medical treatments for secondary amenorrhea include:

- **Birth control pills or other types of hormonal medication.** Certain oral contraceptives may help restart the menstrual cycle.

- **Medications to help relieve the symptoms of PCOS.** Clomiphene citrate (CC) therapy is often prescribed to help trigger ovulation.

- **Estrogen replacement therapy (ERT).** ERT may help balance hormonal levels and restart the menstrual cycle in women with primary ovarian insufficiency (POI) or Fragile X-associated primary ovarian insufficiency (FXPOI). Women with FXPOI often experience symptoms of menopause, such as hot flashes and night sweats. ERT replaces the estrogen a woman's body should be making naturally for a normal menstrual cycle. In addition, ERT may help women with FXPOI lower their risk for the bone disease osteoporosis. ERT can increase the risk for uterine cancer, so your healthcare provider may also prescribe progestin or progesterone to reduce this risk.

In general, medications are safe, but they can have side effects, some of which may be serious. You should discuss side effects and risks with your healthcare provider before deciding on any specific medical treatment.

Surgical Treatments for Secondary Amenorrhea

Surgical treatment for amenorrhea is not common, but may be recommended in certain conditions.

These include:

- **Uterine scarring.** This scarring sometimes occurs after removal of uterine fibroids, a cesarean section, or a dilation and curettage (D&C), a procedure in which tissue is removed from the uterus to diagnose or treat heavy bleeding or to clear the uterine lining after a miscarriage. Removal of the scar tissue during a procedure called a hysteroscopic resection can help restore the menstrual cycle.

- **Pituitary tumor**. Medications may be recommended to shrink the tumor. If this does not work, surgery may be necessary to remove the tumor. Pituitary tumors are not cancerous, but they can cause problems as they grow. Pituitary tumors can put pressure on surrounding blood vessels and nerves such as the optic nerve and may result in loss of vision.

Most of the time, pituitary tumors are removed through the nose and sinuses. Radiation therapy may be used to shrink the tumor, either in combination with surgery or, for those who cannot have surgery, by itself.

Section 18.3

Dysmenorrhea (Painful Menstrual Periods)

This section includes text excerpted from "Period Pain," National Institutes of Health (NIH), November 15, 2016.

What Are Painful Periods?

Menstruation, or period, is normal vaginal bleeding that happens as part of a woman's monthly cycle. Many women have painful periods, also called dysmenorrhea. The pain is most often menstrual cramps, which are a throbbing, cramping pain in your lower abdomen. You may also have other symptoms, such as lower back pain, nausea, diarrhea, and headaches. Period pain is not the same as premenstrual syndrome (PMS). PMS causes many different symptoms, including weight gain, bloating, irritability, and fatigue. PMS often starts one to two weeks before your period starts.

What Causes Painful Periods?

There are two types of dysmenorrhea: primary and secondary. Each type has different causes.

- **Primary dysmenorrhea** is the most common kind of period pain. It is period pain that is not caused by another condition. The cause is usually having too many prostaglandins, which are chemicals that your uterus makes. These chemicals make the muscles of your uterus tighten and relax, and this causes the cramps.

The pain can start a day or two before your period. It normally lasts for a few days, though in some women it can last longer.

You usually first start having period pain when you are younger, just after you begin getting periods. Often, as you get older, you have less pain. The pain may also get better after you have given birth.

- **Secondary dysmenorrhea** often starts later in life. It is caused by conditions that affect your uterus or other reproductive organs, such as endometriosis and uterine fibroids. This kind of pain often gets worse over time. It may begin before your period starts, and continue after your period ends.

What Can I Do about Period Pain?

To help ease your period pain, you can try:

- Using a heating pad or hot water bottle on your lower abdomen

- Getting some exercise

- Taking a hot bath

- Doing relaxation techniques, including yoga and meditation

You might also try taking over-the-counter pain relievers such as nonsteroidal anti-inflammatory drugs (NSAIDs). NSAIDs include ibuprofen and naproxen. Besides relieving pain, NSAIDs reduce the amount of prostaglandins that your uterus makes, and lessen their effects. This helps to lessen the cramps. You can take NSAIDs when you first have symptoms, or when your period starts. You can keep taking them for a few days. You should not take NSAIDs if you have ulcers or other stomach problems, bleeding problems, or liver disease. You should also not take them if you are allergic to aspirin. Always check with your healthcare provider if you are not sure whether or not you should take NSAIDs.

It may also help to get enough rest and avoid using alcohol and tobacco.

When Should I Get Medical Help for My Period Pain?

For many women, some pain during your period is normal. However, you should contact your healthcare provider if:

- NSAIDs and self-care measures don't help, and the pain interferes with your life

- Your cramps suddenly get worse

- You are over 25 and you get severe cramps for the first time

- You have a fever with your period pain

- You have the pain even when you are not getting your period

How Is the Cause of Severe Period Pain Diagnosed?

To diagnose severe period pain, your healthcare provider will ask you about your medical history and do a pelvic exam. You may also have an ultrasound or other imaging test. If your healthcare provider thinks you have secondary dysmenorrhea, you might have laparoscopy. It is a surgery that that lets your healthcare provider look inside your body.

What Are Treatments for Severe Period Pain?

If your period pain is primary dysmenorrhea and you need medical treatment, your healthcare provider might suggest using hormonal birth control, such as the pill, patch, ring, or intrauterine device (IUD). Another treatment option might be prescription pain relievers.

If you have secondary dysmenorrhea, your treatment depends upon the condition that is causing the problem. In some cases, you may need surgery.

Section 18.4

Menorrhagia (Heavy Menstrual Bleeding)

This section includes text excerpted from "Heavy Menstrual Bleeding," Centers for Disease Control and Prevention (CDC), November 28, 2016.

Menorrhagia is menstrual bleeding that lasts more than 7 days. It can also be bleeding that is very heavy. How do you know if you have heavy bleeding? If you need to change your tampon or pad after less than 2 hours or you pass clots the size of a quarter or larger, that is heavy bleeding. If you have this type of bleeding, you should see a doctor.

Untreated heavy or prolonged bleeding can stop you from living your life to the fullest. It also can cause *anemia*. Anemia is a common blood problem that can leave you feeling tired or weak. If you have a bleeding problem, it could lead to other health problems. Sometimes treatments, such as dilation and curettage (D&C) or a hysterectomy, might be done when these procedures could have been avoided.

Who Is Affected

Heavy bleeding (menorrhagia) is one of the most common problems women report to their doctors. It affects more than 10 million American women each year. This means that about one out of every five women has it.

Causes

Possible causes fall into the following three areas:

1. Uterine-related problems

    *   Growths or tumors of the uterus that are not cancer; these can be called uterine fibroids or polyps.

    *   Cancer of the uterus or cervix.

    *   Certain types of birth control—for example, an intrauterine device (IUD).

229

- Problems related to pregnancy, such as a miscarriage or ectopic pregnancy, can cause abnormal bleeding. A miscarriage is when an unborn baby (also called a fetus) dies in the uterus. An ectopic pregnancy is when a baby starts to grow outside the womb (uterus), which is not safe.

2. Hormone-related problems

3. Other illnesses or disorders:

- Bleeding-related disorders, such as von Willebrand disease (VWD) or platelet function disorder.

- Nonbleeding-related disorders such as liver, kidney, or thyroid disease; pelvic inflammatory disease; and cancer.

In addition, certain drugs, such as aspirin, can cause increased bleeding. Doctors have not been able to find the cause in half of all women who have this problem. If you have bleeding such as this, and your gynecologist has not found any problems during your routine visit, you should be tested for a bleeding disorder.

Signs

You might have menorrhagia if you:

- Have a menstrual flow that soaks through one or more pads or tampons every hour for several hours in a row.
- Need to double up on pads to control your menstrual flow.
- Need to change pads or tampons during the night.
- Have menstrual periods lasting more than 7 days.
- Have a menstrual flow with blood clots the size of a quarter or larger.
- Have a heavy menstrual flow that keeps you from doing the things you would do normally.
- Have constant pain in the lower part of the stomach during your periods.
- Are tired, lack energy, or are short of breath.

Diagnosis

Finding out if a woman has heavy menstrual bleeding often is not easy because each person might think of "heavy bleeding" in a different way. Usually, menstrual bleeding lasts about 4 to 5 days and the amount of blood lost is small (2 to 3 tablespoons). However, women who have menorrhagia usually bleed for more than 7 days and lose twice as much blood. If you have bleeding that lasts longer than 7 days per period, or is so heavy that you have to change your pad or tampon nearly every hour, you need to talk with your doctor.

To find out if you have menorrhagia, your doctor will ask you about your medical history and menstrual cycles.

He or she may ask you questions like the following:

- How old were you when you got your first period?

- How long is your menstrual cycle?

- How many days does your period usually last?

- How many days do you consider your period to be heavy?

- How do your periods affect your quality of life?

Your doctor may also ask if any of your family members have had heavy menstrual bleeding. He or she may also have you complete this questionnaire to help determine if you need to be tested for a possible bleeding disorder.

You might want to track your periods by writing down the dates of your periods and how heavy you think your flow is (maybe by counting how many pads or tampons you use). Do this before you visit the doctor so that you can give the doctor as much information as possible. Your doctor also will do a pelvic exam and might tell you about other tests that can be done to help find out if you have menorrhagia.

Tests

Your doctor might tell you that one or more of the following tests will help find out if you have a bleeding problem:

- **Blood test.** In this test, your blood will be taken using a needle. It will then be looked at to check for anemia, problems with the thyroid, or problems with the way the blood clots.

- **Pap test.** For this test, cells from your cervix are removed and then looked at to find out if you have an infection, inflammation, or changes in your cells that might be cancer or might cause cancer.

- **Endometrial biopsy.** Tissue samples are taken from the inside lining of your uterus or "endometrium" to find out if you have cancer or other abnormal cells. You might feel as if you were having a bad menstrual cramp while this test is being done. But, it does not take long, and the pain usually goes away when the test ends.

- **Ultrasound.** This is a painless test using sound waves and a computer to show what your blood vessels, tissues, and organs look like. Your doctor then can see how they are working and check your blood flow.

Using the results of these first tests, the doctor might recommend more tests, including,

- **Sonohysterogram.** This ultrasound scan is done after fluid is injected through a tube into the uterus by way of your vagina and cervix. This lets your doctor look for problems in the lining of your uterus. Mild to moderate cramping or pressure can be felt during this procedure.

- **Hysteroscopy.** This is a procedure to look at the inside of the uterus using a tiny tool to see if you have fibroids, polyps, or other problems that might be causing bleeding. You might be given drugs to put you to sleep (this is known as "general anesthesia) or drugs simply to numb the area being looked at (this is called "local anesthesia").

- **Dilation and Curettage (D&C).** This is a procedure (or test) that can be used to find and treat the cause of bleeding. During a D&C, the inside lining of your uterus is scraped and looked at to see what might be causing the bleeding. A D&C is a simple procedure. Most often it is done in an operating room, but you will not have to stay in the hospital afterwards. You might be given drugs to make you sleep during the procedure, or you might be given something that will numb only the area to be worked on.

Treatment

The type of treatment you get will depend on the cause of your bleeding and how serious it is. Your doctor also will look at things such as your age, general health, and medical history; how well you respond to certain medicines, procedures, or therapies; and your wants and needs. For example, some women do not want to have a period, some want to know when they can usually expect to have their period, and some want just to reduce the amount of bleeding. Some women want to make sure they can still have children in the future. Others want to lessen the pain more than they want to reduce the amount of bleeding. Some treatments are ongoing and others are done one time. You should discuss all of your options with your doctor to decide which is best for you. Following is a list of the more common treatments.

Drug Therapy

- **Iron supplements.** To get more iron into your blood to help it carry oxygen if you show signs of anemia.

- **Ibuprofen (Advil).** To help reduce pain, menstrual cramps, and the amount of bleeding. In some women, nonsteroidal anti-inflammatory drugs (NSAIDs) can increase the risk of bleeding.

- **Birth control pills.** To help make periods more regular and reduce the amount of bleeding.

- **Intrauterine contraception (IUC).** To help make periods more regular and reduce the amount of bleeding through drug-releasing devices placed into the uterus.

- **Hormone therapy (drugs that contain estrogen and/or progesterone).** To reduce the amount of bleeding.

- **Desmopressin Nasal Spray (Stimate®).** To stop bleeding in people who have certain bleeding disorders, such as von Willebrand disease and mild hemophilia, by releasing a clotting protein or "factor," stored in the lining of the blood vessels that helps the blood to clot and temporarily increasing the level of these proteins in the blood.

- **Antifibrinolytic medicines (tranexamic acid, aminocaproic acid).** To reduce the amount of bleeding by stopping a clot from breaking down once it has formed.

Surgical Treatment

- **Dilation and Curettage (D&C).** A procedure in which the top layer of the uterus lining is removed to reduce menstrual bleeding. This procedure might need to be repeated over time.

- **Operative hysteroscopy.** A surgical procedure, using a special tool to view the inside of the uterus, that can be used to help remove polyps and fibroids, correct abnormalities of the uterus, and remove the lining of the uterus to manage heavy menstrual flow.

- **Endometrial ablation or resection.** Two types of surgical procedures using different techniques in which all or part of the lining of the uterus is removed to control menstrual bleeding. While some patients will stop having menstrual periods altogether, others may continue to have periods but the menstrual flow will be lighter than before. Although the procedures do not remove the uterus, they will prevent women from having children in the future.

- **Hysterectomy.** A major operation requiring hospitalization that involves surgically removing the entire uterus. After having this procedure, a woman can no longer become pregnant and will stop having her period.

Menorrhagia is common among women. But, many women do not know that they can get help for it. Others do not get help because they are too embarrassed to talk with a doctor about their problem. Talking openly with your doctor is very important in making sure you are diagnosed properly and get the right treatment.

Chapter 19

Menopausal Concerns

Chapter Contents

Section 19.1

Premature Menopause
(Premature Ovarian Failure)

This section includes text excerpted from "Primary Ovarian
Insufficiency (POI): Condition Information," *Eunice Kennedy Shriver*
National Institute of Child Health and Human Development
(NICHD), December 4, 2012. Reviewed August 2017.

What Is Primary Ovarian Insufficiency (POI)?

Healthcare providers use the term primary ovarian insufficiency
(POI) when a woman's ovaries stop working normally before she is 40
years of age.

Many women naturally experience reduced fertility when they are
around 40 years old. This age may mark the start of irregular menstrual periods that signal the onset of menopause. For women with
POI, irregular periods and reduced fertility occur before the age of 40,
sometimes as early as the teenage years.

In the past, POI used to be called "premature menopause" or "premature ovarian failure," but those terms do not accurately describe
what happens in a woman with POI. A woman who has gone through
menopause will never have another normal period and cannot get
pregnant. A woman with POI may still have periods, even though they
might not come regularly, and she may still get pregnant.

What Are the Symptoms of POI?

The first sign of POI is usually menstrual irregularities or missed
periods, which is sometimes called amenorrhea.

In addition, some women with POI have symptoms similar to those
experienced by women who are going through natural menopause,
including:

- Hot flashes
- Night sweats
- Irritability

- Poor concentration

- Decreased sex drive

- Pain during sex

- Vaginal dryness

For many women with POI, trouble getting pregnant or infertility is the first symptom they experience and is what leads them to visit their healthcare provider. This is sometimes called "occult" (hidden) or early POI.

How Many People Are Affected by or at Risk for POI?

Estimates suggest that about 1 percent of women and teenage girls in the United States have POI. Researchers estimate that, categorized by age, POI affects:

- 1 in 10,000 women by age 20

- 1 in 1,000 women by age 30

- 1 in 250 women by age 35

- 1 in 100 women by age 40

Several factors can affect a woman's risk for POI:

- **Family history.** Women who have a mother or sister with POI are more likely to have the disorder. About 10 percent to 20 percent of women with POI have a family history of the condition.

- **Genes.** Some changes to genes and genetic conditions put women at higher risk for POI. Research suggests that these disorders and conditions cause as much as 28 percent of POI cases. For example:

  - Women who carry a variation of the gene for Fragile X syndrome are at higher risk for Fragile X-Associated POI (FXPOI). Fragile X syndrome is the most common inherited form of intellectual and developmental disability, but women with FXPOI do not have Fragile X syndrome itself. Instead, they have a change or mutation in the same gene that causes Fragile X syndrome, and this change is linked to FXPOI.

  - Most women who have Turner syndrome develop POI. Turner syndrome is a condition in which a girl or woman

237

is partially or completely missing an X chromosome. Most women are XX, meaning they have two X chromosomes. Women with Turner syndrome are X0, meaning one of the X chromosomes is missing.

- **Other factors.** Autoimmune diseases, viral infections, chemotherapy, and other treatments also may put a woman at higher risk of POI.

What Causes POI?

In about 90 percent of cases, the exact cause of POI is a mystery.

Research shows that POI is related to problems with the follicles—the small sacs in the ovaries in which eggs grow and mature.

Follicles start out as microscopic seeds called primordial follicles. These seeds are not yet follicles, but they can grow into them. Normally, a woman is born with approximately 2 million primordial follicles, typically enough to last until she goes through natural menopause, usually around age 50.

For a woman with POI, there are problems with the follicles:

- **Follicle depletion.** A woman with follicle depletion runs out of working follicles earlier than normal or expected. In the case of POI, the woman runs out of working follicles before natural menopause occurs around age 50. Presently there is no safe way for scientists today to make primordial follicles.

- **Follicle dysfunction.** A woman with follicle dysfunction has follicles remaining in her ovaries, but the follicles are not working properly. Scientists do not have a safe and effective way to make follicles start working normally again.

Although the exact cause is unknown in a majority of cases, some causes of follicle depletion and dysfunction have been identified:

- **Genetic and chromosomal disorders.** Disorders such as Fragile X syndrome and Turner syndrome can cause follicle depletion.

- **Low number of follicles.** Some women are born with fewer primordial follicles, so they have a smaller pool of follicles to use throughout their lives. Even though only one mature follicle releases an egg each month, less mature follicles usually develop along with that mature follicle and egg. Scientists don't understand exactly why this happens, but these "supporting" follicles seem to help the mature follicle function normally. If these extra follicles are missing, the main follicle will not mature and release an egg properly.

- **Autoimmune diseases.** Typically, the body's immune cells protect the body from invading bacteria and viruses. However, in autoimmune diseases, immune cells turn on healthy tissue. In the case of POI, the immune system may damage developing follicles in the ovaries. It could also damage the glands that make the hormones needed for the ovaries and follicles to work properly. Recent studies suggest that about 20 percent of women with POI have an autoimmune disease.

- Thyroiditis is the autoimmune disorder most commonly associated with POI. It is an inflammation of the thyroid gland, which makes hormones that control metabolism, or the pace of body processes.

- Addison disease is also associated with POI. Addison disease affects the adrenal glands, which produce hormones that help the body respond to physical stress, such as illness and injury; the hormones also affect ovary function. About 3 percent of women with POI have Addison disease.

- **Chemotherapy or radiation therapy.** These strong treatments for cancer may damage the genetic material in cells, including follicle cells.

- **Metabolic disorders.** These disorders affect the body's ability to create, store, and use the energy it needs. For example, galactosemia affects how your body processes galactose, a type of sugar. More than 80 percent of women and girls with galactosemia also have POI.

- **Toxins.** Cigarette smoke, chemicals, and pesticides can speed up follicle depletion. In addition, viruses have been shown to affect follicle function.

How Do Healthcare Providers Diagnose POI?

The key signs of POI are:

- Missed or irregular periods for 4 months, typically after having had regular periods for a while

- High levels of follicle-stimulating hormone (FSH)

- Low levels of estrogen

If a woman is younger than age 40 and begins having irregular periods or stops having periods for 4 months or longer, her healthcare provider may take these steps to diagnose the problem:

- **Do a pregnancy test.** This test will rule out an unexpected pregnancy as the reason for missed periods.

- **Do a physical exam.** During the physical exam, the healthcare provider looks for signs of other disorders. In some cases, the presence of these other disorders will rule out POI. Or, if the other disorders are associated with POI, such as Addison disease, a healthcare provider will know that POI may be present.

- **Collect blood.** The healthcare provider will collect your blood and send it to a lab, where a technician will run several tests, including:

  - **Follicle-Stimulating Hormone (FSH) test.** FSH signals the ovaries to make estrogen, sometimes called the "female hormone" because women need high levels of it for fertility and overall health. If the ovaries are not working properly, as is the case in POI, the level of FSH in the blood increases. The healthcare provider may do two FSH tests, at least a month apart. If the FSH level in both tests is as high as it is in women who have gone through menopause, then POI is likely.

  - **Luteinizing hormone (LH) test.** LH signals a mature follicle to release an egg. Women with POI have high LH levels, more evidence that the follicles are not functioning normally.

  - **Estrogen test.** In women with POI, estrogen levels are usually low, because the ovaries are not functioning properly in their role as estrogen producers.

  - **Karyotype test.** This test looks at all 46 of your chromosomes to check for abnormalities. The karyotype test could reveal genetic changes in the structure of chromosomes that might be associated with POI and other health problems.

- **Do a pelvic ultrasound.** In this test, the healthcare provider uses a sound wave (sonogram) machine to create and view pictures of the inside of a woman's pelvic area. A sonogram can show whether or not the ovaries are enlarged or have multiple follicles.

The healthcare provider will also ask questions about a woman's medical history. He or she may ask about:

- A blood relative with POI or its symptoms

- A blood relative with Fragile X syndrome or an unidentified intellectual or developmental disability

- Ovarian surgery

- Radiation or chemotherapy treatment

- Pelvic inflammatory disease or other sexually transmitted infections

- An endocrine disorder, such as diabetes

If they do not do tests to rule out POI, some healthcare providers might assume missed periods are related to stress. However, this approach is problematic because it will lead to a delay in diagnosis; further evaluation is needed.

Are There Disorders or Conditions Associated with POI?

Because POI results in lower levels of certain hormones, women with POI are at greater risk for a number of health conditions, including:

- **Osteoporosis.** The hormone estrogen helps keep bones strong. Without enough estrogen, women with POI often develop osteoporosis. Osteoporosis is a bone disease that causes weak, brittle bones that are more likely to break and fracture.

- **Low thyroid function.** This problem also is called hypothyroidism. The thyroid is a gland that makes hormones that control your body's metabolism and energy level. Low levels of the hormones made by the thyroid can affect your metabolism and can cause very low energy and mental sluggishness. Cold feet and constipation are also features of low thyroid function. Researchers estimate that between 14 percent and 27 percent of women with POI also have low thyroid function.

- **Anxiety and depression.** Hormonal changes caused by POI can contribute to anxiety or lead to depression. Women diagnosed with POI can be shy, anxious in social settings, and may have low self-esteem more often than women without POI. It is possible that depression may contribute to POI.

241

- **Cardiovascular (heart) disease.** Lower levels of estrogen, as seen in POI, can affect the muscles lining the arteries and can increase the buildup of cholesterol in the arteries. Both factors increase the risk of atherosclerosis—or hardening of the arteries—which can slow or block the flow of blood to the heart. Women with POI have higher rates of illness and death from heart disease than do women without POI.

- **Dry eye syndrome and ocular (eye) surface disease.** Some women with POI have one of these conditions, which cause discomfort and may lead to blurred vision. If not treated, these conditions can cause permanent eye damage.

Addison disease is also associated with POI. Addison disease is a life-threatening condition that affects the adrenal glands, which produce hormones that help the body respond to physical stress, such as illness and injury. These hormones also affect ovary function. About 3 percent of women with POI have Addison disease.

What Are the Treatments for POI?

Currently, there is no proven treatment to restore normal function to a woman's ovaries. But there are treatments for some of the symptoms of POI, as well as treatments and behaviors to reduce health risks and conditions associated with POI.

It is also important to note that between 5 percent and 10 percent of women with POI get pregnant without medical intervention after they are diagnosed with POI. Some research suggests that these women go into what is known as "spontaneous remission" of POI, meaning that the ovaries begin to function normally on their own. When the ovaries are working properly, fertility is restored and the women can get pregnant.

- Hormone replacement therapy (HRT)

- Calcium and vitamin D supplements

- Regular physical activity and healthy body weight

- Treatments for associated conditions

- Emotional support

Section 19.2

Treating the Symptoms of Menopause

This section includes text excerpted from "Menopause Symptom Relief and Treatments," Office on Women's Health (OWH), U.S. Department of Health and Human Services (HHS), September 22, 2010. Reviewed August 2017.

Menopause Treatment Options

Most women do not need treatment of menopausal symptoms. Some women find that their symptoms go away by themselves, and some women just don't find the symptoms very uncomfortable. But if you are bothered by symptoms, there are many ways to deal with them, including medications and lifestyle changes.

You may find it hard to decide about treatment options like menopausal hormone therapy because of the possible side effects. Talk to your doctor about the possible risks and benefits so you can choose what's best for you. No one treatment is right for all women.

When you talk about treatment options with your doctor, discuss issues like:

- Your symptoms and how much they bother you

- Your personal risks based on your age, your overall health, and your risk for diseases such as heart disease or cancer

- Whether you have used a treatment like menopausal hormone therapy (MHT) before

- Whether you have already gone through menopause and, if so, how long ago

Dealing with Specific Menopause Symptoms

Below are some symptoms that women may have around the time of menopause and tips for dealing with them.

Hot Flashes

- Try to notice what triggers your hot flashes and avoid those things. Possible triggers to consider include spicy foods, alcohol, caffeine, stress, or being in a hot place.

- Dress in layers and remove some when you feel a flash starting.

- Use a fan in your home or workplace.

- If you still have menstrual periods, ask your doctor if you might take low-dose oral contraceptives (birth control pills). These may help symptoms and prevent pregnancy.

- Menopausal hormone therapy (MHT) is the most effective treatment for hot flashes and night sweats. Ask your doctor if the benefits of MHT outweigh the risks for you.

- If MHT is not an option for you, ask your doctor about prescription medicines that are usually used for other conditions. These include antidepressants, epilepsy medicine, and blood pressure medicine.

- Try taking slow, deep breaths when a flash starts.

- If you're overweight, losing weight might help with hot flashes, according to one recent study.

Vaginal Dryness

- A water-based, over-the-counter vaginal lubricant like K-Y Jelly or Astroglide can help make sex more comfortable.

- An over-the-counter vaginal moisturizer like Replens can help keep needed moisture in your vagina if used every few days and can make sex more comfortable.

Problems Sleeping

- One of the best ways to get a good night's sleep is to be physically active. You might want to avoid exercise close to bedtime, though, since it might make you more awake.

- Avoid large meals, smoking, and working right before bedtime. Avoid caffeine after noon, and avoid alcohol close to bedtime.

- Try drinking something warm before bedtime, such as caffeine-free tea or warm milk.

- Keep your bedroom dark, quiet, and cool. Use your bedroom only for sleep and sex.

- Avoid napping during the day, and try to go to bed and get up at the same times every day.

- If you wake during the night and can't get back to sleep, get up and do something relaxing until you're sleepy.

- Talk to your doctor about your sleep problems.

- If hot flashes are the cause of sleep problems, treating the hot flashes will usually improve sleep.

Mood Swings

- Getting enough sleep and staying physically active will help you feel your best.

- Avoid taking on too many duties. Look for positive ways to ease your stress.

- Talk to your doctor. He or she can look for signs of depression, which is a serious illness that needs treatment. You also could consider seeing a therapist to talk about your problems.

- Try a support group for women who are going through the same things as you.

- If you are using MHT for hot flashes or another menopause symptom, your mood swings may get better too.

Memory Problems

- Some women complain of memory problems or trouble focusing in midlife. But studies suggest that natural menopause has little effect on these functions. Women should not use MHT to protect against memory loss or brain diseases, including dementia and Alzheimer disease.

- Getting enough sleep and keeping physically active might help improve symptoms. Mental exercises may help too, so ask your doctor about them.

- If forgetfulness or other mental problems are affecting your daily life, see your doctor.

245

Medications and Menopause

A number of medications can help with symptoms during the years around menopause.

- **Low-dose oral contraceptives (birth control pills)** are an option if you are in perimenopause (the years leading up to your final period). Low-dose contraceptives may stop or reduce hot flashes, vaginal dryness, and moodiness. They can also help with very heavy, frequent, or unpredictable periods. Your doctor may advise you not to take the pill, though, if you smoke or have a history of blood clots or certain types of cancer.

- **Prescription medications that are usually used for other conditions** may help with hot flashes and moodiness. These include medications for epilepsy, depression, and high blood pressure.

- **Menopausal hormone therapy (MHT)** can be very good at helping with moderate to severe symptoms of menopause. It has certain possible risks, though. Learn more about MHT and whether it may be right for you.

- **Over-the-counter medicines (OTC)** can treat vaginal discomfort. A water-based vaginal lubricant like K-Y Jelly can help make sex more comfortable. A vaginal moisturizer like Replens can provide lubrication and help keep needed moisture in vaginal tissues.

- **Prescription medicines for vaginal discomfort** may be an option if OTC treatments don't work. These include estrogen creams, tablets, or rings that you put in your vagina. If you have severe vaginal dryness, the most effective treatment may be an MHT pill or patch.

Section 19.3

Menopause and Sexuality

This section includes text excerpted from "Menopause and Sexuality,"
Office on Women's Health (OWH), U.S. Department of Health and
Human Services (HHS), September 22, 2010. Reviewed August 2017.

Sexual Issues and Menopause

In the years around menopause, you may experience changes in
your sexual life. Some women say they enjoy sex more after they don't
have to worry about getting pregnant. Other women find that they
think about sex less often or don't enjoy it as much.

Changes in sexuality at this time of life have several possible
causes, including:

- Decreased hormones can make vaginal tissues drier and thinner, which can make sex uncomfortable.

- Decreased hormones may reduce sex drive.

- Night sweats can disturb a woman's sleep and make her too tired for sex.

- Emotional changes can make a woman feel too stressed for sex.

Keep in mind that being less interested in sex as you get older is not
a medical condition that needs treatment. But if you are upset about
sexual changes, you can get help. Don't be shy about talking with your
doctor or nurse. They certainly have talked with many women about
these issues before.

Lifestyle Changes

Some simple steps may help with sexual issues you face at this
time:

- **Get treated for any medical problems.** Your overall health can affect your sexual health. For example, you need healthy arteries to supply blood to your vagina.

- **Try to exercise.** Physical activity can increase your energy, lift your mood, and improve your body image—all of which can help with sexual interest.

- **Don't smoke.** Cigarette smoking can reduce both the blood flow to the vagina and the effects of estrogen, which are important to sexual health.

- **Avoid drugs and alcohol.** They can slow down how your body responds.

- **Try to have sex more often.** Sex can increase blood flow to your vagina and help keep tissues healthy.

- **Allow time to become aroused during sex.** Moisture from being aroused protects tissues. Also, avoid sex if you have any vaginal irritation.

- **Practice pelvic floor exercises.** These can increase blood flow to the vagina and strengthen the muscles involved in orgasm.

- **Avoid products that irritate your vagina.** Bubble bath and strong soaps might cause irritation. Don't douche. If you're experiencing vaginal dryness, allergy and cold medicines may add to the problem.

Treatment Options

Discuss your symptoms and personal health issues with your doctor to decide whether one or more treatment options are right for you.
If vaginal dryness is an issue:

- Using an over-the-counter, water-based vaginal lubricant like K-Y Jelly or Astroglide when you have sex can lessen discomfort.

- An over-the-counter vaginal moisturizer like Replens can help put moisture back in vaginal tissues. You may need to use it every few days.

- Prescription medicines that are put into a woman's vagina may increase moisture and sensation. These include estrogen creams, tablets, or rings. If you have severe vaginal dryness, the most effective treatment may be menopausal hormone therapy.

If sexual interest is an issue:

- Treating vaginal dryness may help. Talking with your partner or making lifestyle changes also may help.

- You may wonder about Viagra. This medication has helped men with erection problems, but it has not proven effective in increasing women's sexual interest.

- Some women try products like pills or creams that contain the male hormone testosterone or similar products. The U.S. Food and Drug Administration (FDA) has not approved these products for treating reduced female sex drive because there is not enough research proving them safe and effective.

- The FDA has approved menopausal hormone therapy (MHT) for symptoms like hot flashes, but research has not proven that MHT increases sex drive.

Talking with Your Partner

Talking with your partner about your sexual changes can be very helpful. Some possible topics to discuss include:

- What feels good and what doesn't

- Times that you may feel more relaxed

- Which positions are more comfortable

- Whether you need more time to get aroused than you used to

- Concerns you have about the way your appearance may be changing

- Ways to enjoy physical connection other than intercourse, like massage

Talking with your partner can strengthen your sexual relationship and your overall connection. If you need help, consider meeting with a therapist or sex counselor for individual or couples therapy.

Section 19.4

Menopausal Hormone Therapy

This section includes text excerpted from "Menopausal Hormone
Therapy," Office on Women's Health (OWH), U.S.
Department of Health and Human Services (HHS),
September 22, 2010. Reviewed August 2017.

Some women can use menopausal hormone therapy (MHT) to help
control the symptoms of menopause. MHT, which used to be called
hormone replacement therapy (HRT), involves taking the hormones
estrogen and progesterone. (Women who don't have a uterus anymore
take just estrogen.)

MHT can be very good at helping with moderate to severe symptoms
of the menopausal transition and preventing bone loss. But MHT also
has some risks, especially if used for a long time.

MHT can help with menopause by:

- Reducing hot flashes, night sweats, and related problems such
  as poor sleep and irritability

- Treating vaginal symptoms, such as dryness and discomfort, and
  related effects, such as pain during sex

- Slowing bone loss

- Possibly easing mood swings and mild depressive symptoms
  (MHT is not an antidepressant medication—talk to your doctor
  if you are having signs of depression.)

For some women, MHT may increase their chances of:

- Blood clots
- Heart attack
- Stroke
- Breast cancer
- Gall bladder disease

Research into the risks and benefits of MHT continues. For example, a study suggests that the low-dose patch form of MHT may not
have the possible risk of stroke that other forms can have. Talk with

your doctor about the positives and negatives of MHT based on your medical history and age. Keep in mind, too, that you may have symptoms when you stop MHT.

Keep in mind when considering MHT that:

- Once a woman reaches menopause, MHT is recommended only as a short-term treatment.
- Doctors very rarely recommend MHT to prevent certain chronic diseases like osteoporosis.
- Women who have gone through menopause should not take MHT to prevent heart disease.
- MHT should not be used to prevent memory loss, dementia, or Alzheimer disease.

You should not use menopausal hormone therapy (MHT) if you:

- May be pregnant
- Have problems with vaginal bleeding
- Have had certain kinds of cancers (such as breast and uterine cancer)
- Have had a stroke or heart attack
- Have had blood clots
- Have liver disease
- Have heart disease

If you choose MHT, experts recommend that you:

- Use it at the lowest dose that helps
- Use it for the shortest time needed

MHT can cause side effects. Call your doctor if you develop any of these problems:

- Vaginal bleeding
- Bloating
- Breast tenderness or swelling
- Headaches
- Mood changes
- Nausea

Chapter 20

Ovarian Pain and Disorders of the Ovaries

Chapter Contents

Section 20.1

Ovarian Cysts

This section includes text excerpted from "Ovarian Cysts," Office on Women's Health (OWH), U.S. Department of Health and Human Services (HHS), August 18, 2014.

Ovarian cysts are fluid-filled sacs in the ovary. They are common and usually form during ovulation. Ovulation happens when the ovary releases an egg each month. Many women with ovarian cysts don't have symptoms. The cysts are usually harmless.

What Are Ovarian Cysts?

A cyst is a fluid-filled sac. It can form in many places in the body. Ovarian cysts form in or on the ovaries.

What Are the Different Types of Ovarian Cysts?

The most common types of ovarian cysts (called functional cysts) form during the menstrual cycle. They are usually benign (not cancerous).

The two most common types of cysts are:

- **Follicle cysts.** In a normal menstrual cycle, an ovary releases an egg each month. The egg grows inside a tiny sac called a follicle. When the egg matures, the follicle breaks open to release the egg. Follicle cysts form when the follicle doesn't break open to release the egg. This causes the follicle to continue growing into a cyst. Follicle cysts often have no symptoms and go away in one to three months.

- **Corpus luteum cysts.** Once the follicle breaks open and releases the egg, the empty follicle sac shrinks into a mass of cells called corpus luteum. Corpus luteum makes hormones to prepare for the next egg for the next menstrual cycle. Corpus luteum cysts form if the sac doesn't shrink. Instead, the sac reseals itself after the egg is released, and then fluid builds up inside. Most corpus luteum cysts go away after a few weeks. But, they can grow to almost four inches wide. They also may bleed or twist the ovary and cause pain. Some medicines used to cause ovulation can raise the risk of getting these cysts.

Other types of benign ovarian cysts are less common:

- **Endometriomas** are caused by endometriosis. Endometriosis happens when the lining of the uterus (womb) grows outside of the uterus.

- **Dermoids** come from cells present from birth and do not usually cause symptoms.

- **Cystadenomas** are filled with watery fluid and can sometimes grow large.

In some women, the ovaries make many small cysts. This is called polycystic ovary syndrome (PCOS). PCOS can cause problems with the ovaries and with getting pregnant.

Malignant (cancerous) cysts are rare. They are more common in older women. Cancerous cysts are ovarian cancer. For this reason, ovarian cysts should be checked by your doctor. Most ovarian cysts are not cancerous.

Who Gets Ovarian Cysts?

Ovarian cysts are common in women with regular periods. In fact, most women make at least one follicle or corpus luteum cyst every month. You may not be aware that you have a cyst unless there is a problem that causes the cyst to grow or if multiple cysts form. About 8 percent of premenopausal women develop large cysts that need treatment.

Ovarian cysts are less common after menopause. Postmenopausal women with ovarian cysts are at higher risk for ovarian cancer.

At any age, see your doctor if you think you have a cyst. See your doctor also if you have symptoms such as bloating, needing to urinate more often, pelvic pressure or pain, or abnormal (unusual) vaginal bleeding. These can be signs of a cyst or other serious problem.

What Causes Ovarian Cysts?

The most common causes of ovarian cysts include:

- **Hormonal problems.** Functional cysts usually go away on their own without treatment. They may be caused by hormonal problems or by drugs used to help you ovulate.

- **Endometriosis.** Women with endometriosis can develop a type of ovarian cyst called an endometrioma. The endometriosis tissue may attach to the ovary and form a growth. These cysts can be painful during sex and during your period.

- **Pregnancy.** An ovarian cyst normally develops in early pregnancy to help support the pregnancy until the placenta forms. Sometimes, the cyst stays on the ovary until later in the pregnancy and may need to be removed.

- **Severe pelvic infections.** Infections can spread to the ovaries and fallopian tubes and cause cysts to form.

What Are the Symptoms of Ovarian Cysts?

Most ovarian cysts are small and don't cause symptoms.

If a cyst does cause symptoms, you may have pressure, bloating, swelling, or pain in the lower abdomen on the side of the cyst. This pain may be sharp or dull and may come and go.

If a cyst ruptures, it can cause sudden, severe pain.

If a cyst causes twisting of an ovary, you may have pain along with nausea and vomiting.

Less common symptoms include:

- Pelvic pain
- Dull ache in the lower back and thighs
- Problems emptying the bladder or bowel completely
- Pain during sex
- Unexplained weight gain
- Pain during your period
- Unusual (not normal) vaginal bleeding
- Breast tenderness
- Needing to urinate more often

How Are Ovarian Cysts Found?

If you have symptoms of ovarian cysts, talk to your doctor. Your doctor may do a pelvic exam to feel for swelling of a cyst on your ovary.

If a cyst is found, your doctor will either watch and wait or order tests to help plan treatment. Tests include:

- **Ultrasound.** This test uses sound waves to create images of the body. With ultrasound, your doctor can see the cysts:
  - Shape
  - Size
  - Location
  - Mass (whether it is fluid-filled, solid, or mixed)
- **Pregnancy test** to rule out pregnancy
- **Hormone level tests** to see if there are hormone-related problems
- **Blood test.** If you are past menopause, your doctor may give you a test to measure the amount of cancer-antigen 125 (CA-125) in your blood. The amount of CA-125 is higher with ovarian cancer. In premenopausal women, many other illnesses or diseases besides cancer can cause higher levels of CA-125.

Are Ovarian Cysts Ever an Emergency?

Yes, sometimes. If your doctor told you that you have an ovarian cyst and you have any of the following symptoms, get medical help right away:

- Pain with fever and vomiting
- Sudden, severe abdominal pain
- Faintness, dizziness, or weakness
- Rapid breathing

These symptoms could mean that your cyst has broken open, or ruptured. Sometimes, large, ruptured cysts can cause heavy bleeding.

Will My Ovarian Cyst Require Surgery?

Maybe. The National Institutes of Health (NIH) estimates that 5 percent to 10 percent of women have surgery to remove an ovarian cyst. Only 13 percent to 21 percent of these cysts are cancerous.

Your cyst may require surgery if you are past menopause or if your cyst:

- Does not go away after several menstrual cycles

- Gets larger

- Looks unusual on the ultrasound

- Causes pain

If your cyst does not require surgery, your doctor may:

- Talk to you about pain medicine. Your doctor may recommend over-the-counter medicine or prescribe stronger medicine for pain relief.

- Prescribe hormonal birth control if you have cysts often. Hormonal birth control, such as the pill, vaginal ring, shot, or patch, help prevent ovulation. This may lower your chances of getting more cysts.

What Types of Surgeries Remove Ovarian Cysts?

If your cyst requires surgery, your doctor will either remove just the cyst or the entire ovary.

Surgery can be done in two different ways:

- **Laparoscopy.** With this surgery, the doctor makes a very small cut above or below your belly button to look inside your pelvic area and remove the cyst. This is often recommended for smaller cysts that look benign (not cancerous) on the ultrasound.

- **Laparotomy.** Your doctor may choose this method if the cyst is large and may be cancerous. This surgery uses a larger cut in the abdomen to remove the cyst. The cyst is then tested for cancer. If it is likely to be cancerous, it is best to see a gynecologic oncologist, who may need to remove the ovary and other tissues, like the uterus.

Can Ovarian Cysts Lead to Cancer?

Yes, some ovarian cysts can become cancerous. But most ovarian cysts are not cancerous.

The risk for ovarian cancer increases as you get older. Women who are past menopause with ovarian cysts have a higher risk for ovarian cancer. Talk to your doctor about your risk for ovarian cancer.

Screening for ovarian cancer is not recommended for most women. This is because testing can lead to "false positives." A false positive is a test result that says a woman has ovarian cancer when she does not.

Can Ovarian Cysts Make It Harder to Get Pregnant?

Typically, no. Most ovarian cysts do not affect your chances of getting pregnant. Sometimes, though, the illness causing the cyst can make it harder to get pregnant. Two conditions that cause ovarian cysts and affect fertility are:

- **Endometriosis,** which happens when the lining of the uterus (womb) grows outside of the uterus. Cysts caused by endometriosis are called endometriomas.

- **Polycystic ovary syndrome (PCOS),** one of the leading causes of infertility (problems getting pregnant). Women with PCOS often have many small cysts on their ovaries.

How Do Ovarian Cysts Affect Pregnancy?

Ovarian cysts are common during pregnancy. Typically, these cysts are benign (not cancerous) and harmless. Ovarian cysts that continue to grow during pregnancy can rupture or twist or cause problems during childbirth. Your doctor will monitor any ovarian cyst found during pregnancy.

Can I Prevent Ovarian Cysts?

No, you cannot prevent functional ovarian cysts if you are ovulating. If you get ovarian cysts often, your doctor may prescribe hormonal birth control to stop you from ovulating. This will help lower your risk of getting new cysts.

Section 20.2

Polycystic Ovary Syndrome (PCOS)

This section includes text excerpted from "Polycystic Ovary Syndrome," Office on Women's Health (OWH), U.S. Department of Health and Human Services (HHS), January 5, 2016.

Polycystic ovary syndrome (PCOS) is a health problem that affects one in 10 women of childbearing age. Women with PCOS have a hormonal imbalance and metabolism problems that may affect their overall health and appearance. PCOS is also a common and treatable cause of infertility.

What Is Polycystic Ovary Syndrome (PCOS)?

Polycystic ovary syndrome (PCOS), also known as polycystic ovarian syndrome, is a common health problem caused by an imbalance of reproductive hormones. The hormonal imbalance creates problems in the ovaries. The ovaries make the egg that is released each month as part of a healthy menstrual cycle. With PCOS, the egg may not develop as it should or it may not be released during ovulation as it should be.

PCOS can cause missed or irregular menstrual periods. Irregular periods can lead to:

- Infertility (inability to get pregnant). In fact, PCOS is one of the most common causes of female infertility.

- Development of cysts (small fluid-filled sacs) in the ovaries.

Who Gets PCOS?

Between 5 percent and 10 percent of women of childbearing age (between 15 and 44) have PCOS. Most often, women find out they have PCOS in their 20s and 30s, when they have problems getting pregnant and see their doctor. But PCOS can happen at any age after puberty.

Women of all races and ethnicities are at risk for PCOS, but your risk for PCOS may be higher if you are obese or if you have a mother, sister, or aunt with PCOS.

What Are the Symptoms of PCOS?

Some of the symptoms of PCOS include:

- **Irregular menstrual cycle.** Women with PCOS may miss periods or have fewer periods (fewer than eight in a year). Or, their periods may come every 21 days or more often. Some women with PCOS stop having menstrual periods.

- **Too much hair** on the face, chin, or parts of the body where men usually have hair. This is called "hirsutism." Hirsutism affects up to 70 percent of women with PCOS.

- **Acne on the face**, chest, and upper back.

- **Thinning hair** or hair loss on the scalp; male-pattern baldness.

- **Weight gain** or difficulty losing weight.

- **Darkening of skin**, particularly along neck creases, in the groin, and underneath breasts.

- **Skin tags**, which are small excess flaps of skin in the armpits or neck area.

What Causes PCOS?

The exact cause of PCOS is not known. Most experts think that several factors, including genetics, play a role:

- **High levels of androgens.** Androgens are sometimes called "male hormones," although all women make small amounts of androgens. Androgens control the development of male traits, such as male-pattern baldness. Women with PCOS have more androgens than estrogens. Estrogens are also called "female hormones." Higher than normal androgen levels in women can prevent the ovaries from releasing an egg (ovulation) during each menstrual cycle, and can cause extra hair growth and acne, two signs of PCOS.

- **High levels of insulin.** Insulin is a hormone that controls how the food you eat is changed into energy. Insulin resistance is when the body's cells do not respond normally to insulin. As a result, your insulin blood levels become higher than normal. Many women with PCOS have insulin resistance, especially those who are overweight or obese, have unhealthy eating habits, do not get enough physical activity, and have a family history of diabetes (usually type 2 diabetes). Over time, insulin resistance can lead to type 2 diabetes.

How Is PCOS Diagnosed?

There is no single test to diagnose PCOS. To help diagnose PCOS and rule out other causes of your symptoms, your doctor may talk to you about your medical history and do a physical exam and different tests:

- **Physical exam.** Your doctor will measure your blood pressure, body mass index (BMI), and waist size. He or she will also look at your skin for extra hair on your face, chest or back, acne, or skin discoloration. Your doctor may look for any hair loss or signs of other health conditions (such as an enlarged thyroid gland).

- **Pelvic exam.** Your doctor may do a pelvic exam for signs of extra male hormones (for example, an enlarged clitoris) and check to see if your ovaries are enlarged or swollen.

- **Pelvic ultrasound (sonogram).** This test uses sound waves to examine your ovaries for cysts and check the endometrium (lining of the uterus or womb).

- **Blood tests.** Blood tests check your androgen hormone levels, sometimes called "male hormones." Your doctor will also check for other hormones related to other common health problems that can be mistaken for PCOS, such as thyroid disease. Your doctor may also test your cholesterol levels and test you for diabetes.

Once other conditions are ruled out, you may be diagnosed with PCOS if you have at least two of the following symptoms:

- Irregular periods, including periods that come too often, not often enough, or not at all
- Signs that you have high levels of androgens:
  - Extra hair growth on your face, chin, and body (hirsutism)
  - Acne
  - Thinning of scalp hair
- Higher than normal blood levels of androgens
- Multiple cysts on one or both ovaries

How Is PCOS Treated?

There is no cure for PCOS, but you can manage the symptoms of PCOS. You and your doctor will work on a treatment plan based on your symptoms, your plans for children, and your risk for long-term health problems such as diabetes and heart disease. Many women will need a combination of treatments, including:

- Steps you can take at home to help relieve your symptoms

- Medicines

Can I Still Get Pregnant If I Have PCOS?

Yes. Having PCOS does not mean you can't get pregnant. PCOS is one of the most common, but treatable, causes of infertility in women. In women with PCOS, the hormonal imbalance interferes with the growth and release of eggs from the ovaries (ovulation). If you don't ovulate, you can't get pregnant.

Your doctor can talk with you about ways to help you ovulate and to raise your chance of getting pregnant.

What Are My Treatment Options for PCOS If I Want to Get Pregnant?

You have several options to help your chances of getting pregnant if you have PCOS:

- **Losing weight.** If you are overweight or obese, losing weight through healthy eating, including eating the right amount of calories for you, and regular physical activity can help make your menstrual cycle more regular and improve your fertility.

- **Medicine.** After ruling out other causes of infertility in you and your partner, your doctor might prescribe medicine to help you ovulate, such as clomiphene (Clomid).

- **In vitro fertilization (IVF).** IVF may be an option if medicine does not work. In IVF, your egg is fertilized with your partner's sperm in a laboratory and then placed in your uterus to implant and develop. Compared to medicine alone, IVF has higher pregnancy rates and better control over your risk for twins and triplets (by allowing your doctor to transfer a single fertilized egg into your uterus).

- **Surgery.** Surgery is also an option, usually only if the other options do not work. The outer shell (called the cortex) of ovaries is thickened in women with PCOS and thought to play a role in preventing spontaneous ovulation. Ovarian drilling is a surgery in which the doctor makes a few holes in the surface of your ovary using lasers or a fine needle heated with electricity. Surgery usually restores ovulation, but only for six to eight months.

How Does PCOS Affect Pregnancy?

PCOS can cause problems during pregnancy for you and for your baby. Women with PCOS have higher rates of:

- Miscarriage
- Gestational diabetes
- Preeclampsia
- Cesarean section (C-section)

Your baby also has a higher risk of being heavy (macrosomia) and of spending more time in a neonatal intensive care unit (NICU).

How Can I Prevent Problems from PCOS during Pregnancy?

You can lower your risk of problems during pregnancy by:

- Reaching a healthy weight before you get pregnant.
- Reaching healthy blood sugar levels before you get pregnant. You can do this through a combination of healthy eating habits, regular physical activity, weight loss, and medicines such as metformin.
- Taking folic acid. Talk to your doctor about how much folic acid you need.

Chapter 21

Endometriosis

Endometriosis happens when the lining of the uterus (womb) grows outside of the uterus. It may affect more than 11 percent of American women between 15 and 44. It is especially common among women in their 30s and 40s and may make it harder to get pregnant. Several different treatment options can help manage the symptoms and improve your chances of getting pregnant.

What Is Endometriosis?

Endometriosis, sometimes called "endo," is a common health problem in women. It gets its name from the word endometrium, the tissue that normally lines the uterus or womb. Endometriosis happens when this tissue grows outside of your uterus and on other areas in your body where it doesn't belong.

Most often, endometriosis is found on the:

- Ovaries
- Fallopian tubes
- Tissues that hold the uterus in place
- Outer surface of the uterus

This chapter includes text excerpted from "Endometriosis," Office on Women's Health (OWH), U.S. Department of Health and Human Services (HHS), August 18, 2014.

Other sites for growths can include the vagina, cervix, vulva, bowel, bladder, or rectum. Rarely, endometriosis appears in other parts of the body, such as the lungs, brain, and skin.

What Are the Symptoms of Endometriosis?

Symptoms of endometriosis can include:

- **Pain.** This is the most common symptom. Women with endometriosis may have many different kinds of pain. These include:
  - Very painful menstrual cramps. The pain may get worse over time.
  - Chronic (long-term) pain in the lower back and pelvis
  - Pain during or after sex. This is usually described as a "deep" pain and is different from pain felt at the entrance to the vagina when penetration begins.
  - Intestinal pain
  - Painful bowel movements or pain when urinating during menstrual periods. In rare cases, you may also find blood in your stool or urine.
- **Bleeding or spotting between menstrual periods.** This can be caused by something other than endometriosis. If it happens often, you should see your doctor.
- **Infertility,** or not being able to get pregnant.
- **Stomach (digestive) problems.** These include diarrhea, constipation, bloating, or nausea, especially during menstrual periods.

How Common Is Endometriosis?

Endometriosis is a common health problem for women. Researchers think that at least 11 percent of women, or more than 6 ½ million women in the United States, have endometriosis.

Who Gets Endometriosis?

Endometriosis can happen in any girl or woman who has menstrual periods, but it is more common in women in their 30s and 40s.

You might be more likely to get endometriosis if you have:

- Never had children
- Menstrual periods that last more than seven days
- Short menstrual cycles (27 days or fewer)
- A family member (mother, aunt, sister) with endometriosis
- A health problem that blocks the normal flow of menstrual blood from your body during your period

What Causes Endometriosis?

No one knows for sure what causes this disease. Researchers are studying possible causes:

- **Problems with menstrual period flow.** Retrograde menstrual flow is the most likely cause of endometriosis. Some of the tissue shed during the period flows through the fallopian tube into other areas of the body, such as the pelvis.
- **Genetic factors.** Because endometriosis runs in families, it may be inherited in the genes.
- **Immune system problems.** A faulty immune system may fail to find and destroy endometrial tissue growing outside of the uterus. Immune system disorders and certain cancers are more common in women with endometriosis.
- **Hormones.** The hormone estrogen appears to promote endometriosis. Research is looking at whether endometriosis is a problem with the body's hormone system.
- **Surgery.** During a surgery to the abdominal area, such as a cesarean (C-section) or hysterectomy, endometrial tissue could be picked up and moved by mistake. For instance, endometrial tissue has been found in abdominal scars.

How Can I Prevent Endometriosis?

You can't prevent endometriosis. But you can reduce your chances of developing it by lowering the levels of the hormone estrogen in your body. Estrogen helps to thicken the lining of your uterus during your menstrual cycle.

To keep lower estrogen levels in your body, you can:

- **Talk to your doctor about hormonal birth control methods**, such as pills, patches or rings with lower doses of estrogen.

- **Exercise regularly** (more than 4 hours a week). This will also help you **keep a low percentage of body fat**. Regular exercise and a lower amount of body fat help decrease the amount of estrogen circulating through the body.

- **Avoid large amounts of alcohol.** Alcohol raises estrogen levels. No more than one drink per day is recommended for women who choose to drink alcohol.

- **Avoid large amount of drinks with caffeine.** Studies show that drinking more than one caffeinated drink a day, especially sodas and green tea, can raise estrogen levels.

How Is Endometriosis Diagnosed?

If you have symptoms of endometriosis, talk with your doctor. The doctor will talk to you about your symptoms and do or prescribe one or more of the following to find out if you have endometriosis:

- **Pelvic exam.** During a pelvic exam, your doctor will feel for large cysts or scars behind your uterus. Smaller areas of endometriosis are harder to feel.

- **Imaging test.** Your doctor may do an **ultrasound** to check for ovarian cysts from endometriosis. The doctor or technician may insert a wand-shaped scanner into your vagina or move a scanner across your abdomen. Both kinds of ultrasound tests use sound waves to make pictures of your reproductive organs. **Magnetic resonance imaging (MRI)** is another common imaging test that can make a picture of the inside of your body.

- **Medicine.** If your doctor does not find signs of an ovarian cyst during an ultrasound, he or she may prescribe medicine:

  - **Hormonal birth control** can help lessen pelvic pain during your period.

  - **Gonadotropin-releasing hormone (GnRH)** agonists block the menstrual cycle and lower the amount of estrogen your body makes. GnRH agonists also may help pelvic pain.

- If your pain gets better with hormonal medicine, you probably have endometriosis. But, these medicines work only as long as you take them. Once you stop taking them, your pain may come back.

- **Laparoscopy.** Laparoscopy is a type of surgery that doctors can use to look inside your pelvic area to see endometriosis tissue.

Surgery is the only way to be sure you have endometriosis. Sometimes doctors can diagnose endometriosis just by seeing the growths. Other times, they need to take a small sample of tissue and study it under a microscope to confirm this.

How Is Endometriosis Treated?

There is no cure for endometriosis, but treatments are available for the symptoms and problems it causes. Talk to your doctor about your treatment options.

Medicine

If you are not trying to get pregnant, hormonal birth control is generally the first step in treatment. This may include:

- Extended-cycle (you have only a few periods a year) or continuous cycle (you have no periods) birth control. These types of hormonal birth control are available in the pill or the shot and help stop bleeding and reduce or eliminate pain.

- Intrauterine device (IUD) to help reduce pain and bleeding. The hormonal IUD protects against pregnancy for up to 7 years. But the hormonal IUD may not help your pain and bleeding due to endometriosis for that long.

Hormonal treatment works only as long as it is taken and is best for women who do not have severe pain or symptoms.

If you are trying to get pregnant, your doctor may prescribe a gonadotropin-releasing hormone (GnRH) agonist. This medicine stops the body from making the hormones responsible for ovulation, the menstrual cycle, and the growth of endometriosis. This treatment causes a temporary menopause, but it also helps control the growth of endometriosis. Once you stop taking the medicine, your menstrual cycle returns, but you may have a better chance of getting pregnant.

Surgery

Surgery is usually chosen for severe symptoms, when hormones are not providing relief or if you are having fertility problems. During the operation, the surgeon can locate any areas of endometriosis and may remove the endometriosis patches. After surgery, hormone treatment is often restarted unless you are trying to get pregnant.

Other treatments you can try, alone or with any of the treatments listed above, include:

- **Pain medicine.** For mild symptoms, your doctor may suggest taking over-the-counter medicines for pain. These include ibuprofen (Advil and Motrin) or naproxen (Aleve).

- **Complementary and alternative medicine (CAM) therapies.** Some women report relief from pain with therapies such as acupuncture, chiropractic care, herbs like cinnamon twig or licorice root, or supplements, such as thiamine (vitamin B1), magnesium, or omega-3 fatty acids.

Can I Get Pregnant If I Have Endometriosis?

Yes. Many women with endometriosis get pregnant. But, you may find it harder to get pregnant. Endometriosis affects about one-half (50%) of women with infertility.

No one knows exactly how endometriosis might cause infertility. Some possible reasons include:

- Patches of endometriosis block off or change the shape of the pelvis and reproductive organs. This can make it harder for the sperm to find the egg.

- The immune system, which normally helps defend the body against disease, attacks the embryo.

- The endometrium (the layer of the uterine lining where implantation happens) does not develop as it should.

If you have endometriosis and are having trouble getting pregnant, talk to your doctor. He or she can recommend treatments, such as surgery to remove the endometrial growths.

Chapter 22

Uterine Fibroids

What Are Fibroids?

Fibroids are muscular tumors that grow in the wall of the uterus (womb). Another medical term for fibroids is leiomyoma or just "myoma." Fibroids are almost always benign (not cancerous). Fibroids can grow as a single tumor, or there can be many of them in the uterus. They can be as small as an apple seed or as big as a grapefruit. In unusual cases they can become very large.

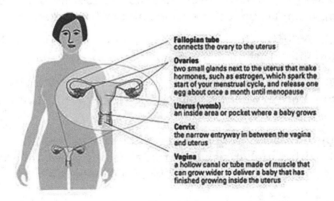

Figure 22.1. *The Female Reproductive System*

This chapter includes text excerpted from "Uterine Fibroids," Office on Women's Health (OWH), U.S. Department of Health and Human Services (HHS), January 15, 2015.

Not all women with fibroids have symptoms. Women who do have symptoms often find fibroids hard to live with. Some have pain and heavy menstrual bleeding. Treatment for uterine fibroids depends on your symptoms.

Why Should Women Know about Fibroids?

About 20 percent to 80 percent of women develop fibroids by the time they reach age 50. Fibroids are most common in women in their 40s and early 50s. Not all women with fibroids have symptoms. Women who do have symptoms often find fibroids hard to live with. Some have pain and heavy menstrual bleeding. Fibroids also can put pressure on the bladder, causing frequent urination, or the rectum, causing rectal pressure. Should the fibroids get very large, they can cause the abdomen (stomach area) to enlarge, making a woman look pregnant.

Who Gets Fibroids?

There are factors that can increase a woman's risk of developing fibroids.

- **Age.** Fibroids become more common as women age, especially during the 30s and 40s through menopause. After menopause, fibroids usually shrink.

- **Family history.** Having a family member with fibroids increases your risk. If a woman's mother had fibroids, her risk of having them is about three times higher than average.

- **Ethnic origin.** African-American women are more likely to develop fibroids than white women.

- **Obesity.** Women who are overweight are at higher risk for fibroids. For very heavy women, the risk is two to three times greater than average.

- **Eating habits.** Eating a lot of red meat (e.g., beef) and ham is linked with a higher risk of fibroids. Eating plenty of green vegetables seems to protect women from developing fibroids.

Where Can Fibroids Grow?

Most fibroids grow in the wall of the uterus. Doctors put them into three groups based on where they grow:

- **Submucosal** fibroids grow into the uterine cavity.

- **Intramural** fibroids grow within the wall of the uterus.

- **Subserosal** fibroids grow on the outside of the uterus.

Some fibroids grow on stalks that grow out from the surface of the uterus or into the cavity of the uterus. They might look like mushrooms. These are called **pedunculated** fibroids.

What Are Symptoms of Fibroids?

Most fibroids do not cause any symptoms, but some women with fibroids can have:

- Heavy bleeding (which can be heavy enough to cause anemia) or painful periods

- Feeling of fullness in the pelvic area (lower stomach area)

- Enlargement of the lower abdomen

- Frequent urination

- Pain during sex

- Lower back pain

- Complications during pregnancy and labor, including a six-time greater risk of cesarean section

- Reproductive problems, such as infertility, which is very rare

What Causes Fibroids?

No one knows for sure what causes fibroids. Researchers think that more than one factor could play a role. These factors could be:

- Hormonal (affected by estrogen and progesterone levels)

- Genetic (runs in families)

Because no one knows for sure what causes fibroids, we also don't know what causes them to grow or shrink. We do know that they are under hormonal control—both estrogen and progesterone. They grow rapidly during pregnancy, when hormone levels are high. They shrink when antihormone medication is used. They also stop growing or shrink once a woman reaches menopause.

Can Fibroids Turn Into Cancer?

Fibroids are almost always benign (not cancerous). Rarely (less than one in 1,000) a cancerous fibroid will occur. This is called leiomyosarcoma. Doctors think that these cancers do not arise from an already-existing fibroid. Having fibroids does not increase the risk of developing a cancerous fibroid. Having fibroids also does not increase a woman's chances of getting other forms of cancer in the uterus.

What If I Become Pregnant and Have Fibroids?

Women who have fibroids are more likely to have problems during pregnancy and delivery. This doesn't mean there will be problems. Most women with fibroids have normal pregnancies. The most common problems seen in women with fibroids are:

- **Cesarean section.** The risk of needing a c-section is six times greater for women with fibroids.

- **Baby is breech.** The baby is not positioned well for vaginal delivery.

- **Labor fails to progress.**

- **Placental abruption.** The placenta breaks away from the wall of the uterus before delivery. When this happens, the fetus does not get enough oxygen.

- **Preterm delivery.**

Talk to your obstetrician if you have fibroids and become pregnant. All obstetricians have experience dealing with fibroids and pregnancy. Most women who have fibroids and become pregnant do not need to see an OB who deals with high-risk pregnancies.

How Do I Know for Sure That I Have Fibroids?

Your doctor may find that you have fibroids when you see her or him for a regular pelvic exam to check your uterus, ovaries, and vagina. The doctor can feel the fibroid with her or his fingers during an ordinary pelvic exam, as a (usually painless) lump or mass on the uterus. Often, a doctor will describe how small or how large the fibroids are by comparing their size to the size your uterus would be if you were pregnant. For example, you may be told that your fibroids have made your uterus the size it would be if you were 16 weeks pregnant. Or the fibroid might be compared to fruits, nuts, or a ball, such as a grape or an orange, an acorn or a walnut, or a golf ball or a volleyball.

Your doctor can do imaging tests to confirm that you have fibroids. These are tests that create a "picture" of the inside of your body without surgery. These tests might include:

- **Ultrasound.** Uses sound waves to produce the picture. The ultrasound probe can be placed on the abdomen or it can be placed inside the vagina to make the picture.

- **Magnetic resonance imaging (MRI).** Uses magnets and radio waves to produce the picture

- **X-rays.** Uses a form of radiation to see into the body and produce the picture

- **Cat scan (CT).** Takes many X-ray pictures of the body from different angles for a more complete image

- **Hysterosalpingogram (HSG) or sonohysterogram.** An HSG involves injecting X-ray dye into the uterus and taking X-ray pictures. A sonohysterogram involves injecting water into the uterus and making ultrasound pictures.

You might also need surgery to know for sure if you have fibroids. There are two types of surgery to do this:

- **Laparoscopy.** The doctor inserts a long, thin scope into a tiny incision made in or near the navel. The scope has a bright light and a camera. This allows the doctor to view the uterus and other organs on a monitor during the procedure. Pictures also can be made.

- **Hysteroscopy.** The doctor passes a long, thin scope with a light through the vagina and cervix into the uterus. No incision is needed. The doctor can look inside the uterus for fibroids and other problems, such as polyps. A camera also can be used with the scope.

What Questions Should I Ask My Doctor If I Have Fibroids?

- How many fibroids do I have?

- What size is my fibroid(s)?

- Where is my fibroid(s) located (outer surface, inner surface, or in the wall of the uterus)?

- Can I expect the fibroid(s) to grow larger?

- How rapidly have they grown (if they were known about already)?

- How will I know if the fibroid(s) is growing larger?

- What problems can the fibroid(s) cause?

- What tests or imaging studies are best for keeping track of the growth of my fibroids?

- What are my treatment options if my fibroid(s) becomes a problem?

- What are your views on treating fibroids with a hysterectomy versus other types of treatments?

- A second opinion is always a good idea if your doctor has not answered your questions completely or does not seem to be meeting your needs.

How Are Fibroids Treated?

Most women with fibroids do not have any symptoms. For women who do have symptoms, there are treatments that can help. Talk with your doctor about the best way to treat your fibroids. She or he will consider many things before helping you choose a treatment. Some of these things include:

- Whether or not you are having symptoms from the fibroids

- If you might want to become pregnant in the future

- The size of the fibroids

- The location of the fibroids

- Your age and how close to menopause you might be

- If you have fibroids but do not have any symptoms, you may not need treatment. Your doctor will check during your regular exams to see if they have grown.

Chapter 23

Disorders of the Cervix

Chapter Contents

Section 23.1

Cervical Dysplasia

This section contains text excerpted from the following sources: Text in this section begins with excerpts from "Cervical Cancer Prevention (PDQ®)–Patient Version," National Cancer Institute (NCI), June 22, 2017; Text beginning with the heading "Grading of Cervical Dysplasia" is excerpted from "Understanding Cervical Changes," National Cancer Institute (NCI), May 2017; Text under the heading "How Can I Prevent Cervical Cancer?" is excerpted from "Cervical Cancer," Centers for Disease Control and Prevention (CDC), December 2016.

Cervical cancer usually develops slowly over time. Before cancer appears in the cervix, the cells of the cervix go through a series of changes in which cells that are not normal begin to appear in the cervical tissue. When cells change from being normal cells to abnormal cells, it is called dysplasia. The abnormal cervical cells may go away without treatment, stay the same, or turn into cancer cells over many years.

Grading of Cervical Dysplasia

AGC (Atypical Glandular Cells)

AGC means that some glandular cells were found that do not look normal. More testing is usually recommended.

LSIL (Low-Grade Squamous Intraepithelial Lesions)

LSIL is sometimes called mild dysplasia. It may also be called CIN 1. LSIL means that there are low-grade changes. LSIL changes are usually caused by HPV infection. Although the changes may go away on their own, further testing is usually done to find out whether there are more severe changes that need to be treated.

ASC-H (Atypical Squamous Cells, Cannot Exclude HSIL)

ASC-H means that some abnormal squamous cells were found that may be a high-grade squamous intraepithelial lesion (HSIL), although it's not certain. More testing is recommended.

HSIL (High-Grade Squamous Intraepithelial Lesions)

HSIL is sometimes called moderate or severe dysplasia. It may also be called CIN 2, CIN 2/3, or CIN 3. HSIL means that there are more serious changes than LSIL, in cervical cells. These changes are caused by HPV and may turn into cervical cancer if not treated.

AIS (Adenocarcinoma In Situ)

AIS means that an advanced lesion (area of abnormal growth) was found in the glandular tissue of the cervix. AIS lesions may become cancer (cervical adenocarcinoma) if not treated.

Follow-Up Testing

Keep in mind that most women with abnormal cervical screening test results do not have cancer. However, if you have an abnormal test result, it's important to get the follow-up tests and/or treatment that your healthcare provider recommends. Possible next steps and treatments are listed in this section to help you learn more and talk with your healthcare provider

Depending upon your test result, next steps may include:

Pap test: Some women may need to return for another Pap test.

HPV test: An HPV test may be recommended.

Estrogen cream: If you have ASC-US and are near or past menopause, your healthcare provider may prescribe estrogen cream. If the cell changes are caused by low hormone levels, applying estrogen cream will make them go away.

Colposcopy and biopsy: Your healthcare provider will examine your cervix using a colposcope and perform a biopsy. A colposcopy is a procedure to examine your cervix. During this procedure, your doctor inserts a speculum to gently open the vagina and see the cervix. Diluted white vinegar is put on the cervix, causing abnormal areas to turn white. Your doctor then places an instrument called a colposcope close to the vagina. It has a bright light and a magnifying lens and allows your doctor to look closely at your cervix. A colposcopy usually includes a biopsy. A biopsy is done so that the cells or tissues can be checked under a microscope for signs of disease. In addition to removing a sample for further testing, some types of biopsies may be used as treatment, to remove abnormal cervical tissue or lesions.

Types of cervical biopsies include:

- Endocervical curettage: cells are scraped from the lining of the cervical canal

- Punch biopsy: a small piece of cervical tissue is removed

- Cone biopsy (or conization): a cone-shaped sample of cervical tissue is removed

Talk with your doctor to learn what to expect during and after your procedure. Some women have bleeding and/or discharge after a biopsy. Others have pain that feels like menstrual cramps.

Treatments for Cervical Cell Changes

Some abnormal cervical changes need to be removed so they do not turn into cancer. Your doctor will talk with you about which treatment is recommended for you and why. The questions at the end of this section can help you talk with your healthcare provider to learn more.

Common treatment methods include:

- **Cold knife conization** (also called cold knife cone biopsy) is a procedure in which a cone-shaped piece of abnormal tissue is removed from the cervix using a scalpel or laser knife. Some of the tissue is then checked under a microscope for signs of disease, such as cervical cancer. This procedure is done at the hospital and requires general anesthesia.

- **Cryotherapy** is a procedure in which an extremely cold liquid or an instrument called a cryoprobe is used to freeze and destroy abnormal tissue. A cryoprobe is cooled with substances such as liquid nitrogen, liquid nitrous oxide, or compressed argon gas. Also called cryoablation and cryosurgery. This procedure is done in your doctor's office. It takes only a few minutes and usually does not require anesthesia.

- **Laser therapy** is a procedure that uses a laser (narrow beam of intense light) to destroy abnormal tissue. This procedure is done at the hospital and general anesthesia is used.

- **LEEP (loop electrosurgical excision procedure)** is a procedure in which a thin wire loop, through which an electrical current is passed, to remove abnormal tissue. Local anesthesia is used to numb the area. Your doctor usually performs this procedure in the office. It takes only a few minutes, and you will be awake during the procedure.

Section 23.2

Cervical Polyps

What Are Cervical Polyps?

Cervical polyps are elongated growths on the cervix, which is the tubular structure connecting vagina to the uterus. Cervical polyps are usually found in the area where the cervix opens into the vagina. Resembling bulbs on a thin stalk, cervical polyps are usually 1 to 2 centimeters in length and can vary in color from cherry-red to grayish-white. Because certain types of cancer can appear similar to cervical polyps, it is important to have the polyps removed and tested to see if they are cancer.

What Causes Cervical Polyps?

The cause of cervical polyps is not well understood; however, they have been linked to:

- inflammation of the cervix
- abnormal response to high levels of estrogen during the menstrual cycle
- clogged blood vessels in the cervix

Cervical polyps are common in women over the age of 20 who have had children. Young women who are yet to begin their periods generally do not have cervical polyps. Medical professionals usually find a single polyp in women, but in some cases, two to three polyps are also found.

Cervical polyps can be divided into two types:

1. **Ectocervical polyps:** These polyps develop from cells in the outer surface layer of the cervix. They are common in post-menopausal women.

2. **Endocervical polyps:** These polyps develop from the cervical glands in the cervical canal. Most polyps belong to this type and are commonly seen in premenopausal women.

What Are the Symptoms of Cervical Polyps?

Usually there are no noticeable symptoms. However, contact your gynecologist if you experience the following:

- Heavy menstrual periods

- Bleeding after sexual intercourse or douching

- Bleeding in between periods

- Bleeding after menopause

- White or yellow mucus in vaginal discharge

How Are Cervical Polyps Diagnosed?

Cervical polyps cannot be seen or felt by the patient and can be diagnosed by a medical professional during an examination.

How Are Cervical Polyps Treated?

Small polyps do not require surgical removal. This is done only if they are large, infected, or have an unusual appearance. A medical practitioner will remove the polyps in an outpatient procedure. A special instrument known as a polyp forceps is used to surgically remove the polyp. The polyp is grasped with the forceps, twisted and plucked away in a gentle motion, and is then sent for histopathological examination. In most cases, cervical polyps are benign. Rarely, pre-cancerous growth patterns known as neoplastic changes are observed in the polyps, which will warrant treatment depending on the specific type and extent of cancer. After the cervical polyps are removed, the area is dabbed with a solution to stop any bleeding. Surgery with anesthesia may be necessary for removal of large polyps and those that have broad stems.

What Is the Outlook for Women with Cervical Polyps?

In most cases, polyps are not cancerous, and they do not grow back once they are removed surgically.

References

1. "Cervical Polyps," A.D.A.M., Inc., April 5, 2016.

2. "Cervical Polyps," Harvard University, October 2012.

3. "Cervical Polyps—Topic Overview," WebMD, LLC, n.d.

4. Rice, Sandy Calhoun, Nall, Rachel. "What Are Cervical Polyps?" Healthline Media, n.d.

Section 23.3

Cervicitis

What Is Cervicitis?

Cervicitis is an inflammation of the cervix, which is the opening of the uterus that extends into the vagina. Inflammation of the cervix is usually caused by an infection that is contracted during sexual intercourse.

What Are the Symptoms of Cervicitis?

Generally cervicitis does not have any symptoms and can be detected only after sexual intercourse through a Pap smear or biopsy. However, patients may experience symptoms that include:

- Abnormal vaginal discharge that vary in color

- Abnormal vaginal bleeding
  - between periods

- after menopause
- Pain during urination
- Vulvar or vaginal irritation

What Are the Causes and Risk Factors for Cervicitis?

Cervicitis can be caused by:

- Sexually transmitted infections (STIs) such as gonorrhea, chlamydia, herpes virus, trichomoniasis, human papilloma virus (genital warts), etc. STIs are the most common causes of cervicitis.

- An overgrowth of the bacteria normally present in the vaginal cavity

- Allergic reaction to contraceptives and certain feminine hygiene products

- Allergy to latex used in condoms

- Reaction to the chemicals in spermicides

Cervicitis usually occurs in adult women and a few risk factors can increase the chance of having cervicitis, including:

- High-risk sexual behavior (e.g., having sex without a condom)
- Having sex with multiple partners
- Engaging in sexual activity at an early age
- Having had cervicitis before or a history of other sexually transmitted infections

How Is Cervicitis Diagnosed?

The following examinations are done by a healthcare provider to diagnose cervicitis:

- Full pelvic exam
- Pap smear
- Swab to collect vaginal fluid or cells from the cervix for laboratory testing
- Test of any vaginal discharge

- Tests for sexually transmitted diseases such as gonorrhea and chlamydia

The healthcare provider will also take a full medical history from the patient, including asking questions about the use of condoms and other contraceptives as well as questions about the patient's recent sexual history.

How Is Cervicitis Treated?

If cervicitis is diagnosed, it is usually treated with antibiotics that fight bacterial infection. The healthcare provider may also prescribe antifungal or antiviral medications. If antibiotics or other drug protocols do not work, the healthcare provider might suggest surgery. If left untreated, cervicitis can lead to further complications, such as the infection traveling to the uterus, uterine lining and fallopian tubes, pelvic inflammatory disease (PID), and permanent damage to the female reproductive organs.

What Are the Complications of Cervicitis?

Cervicitis can last for a few weeks, months, or even for years. If untreated, cervicitis can cause also pain during intercourse. Having cervicitis can increase the possibility of contracting human immuno-deficiency virus (HIV).

How Can I Avoid Cervicitis?

Cervicitis can be avoided through careful sexual practices, including:

- Limiting the number of sexual partners
- Practicing safe sex, including using condoms consistently
- Avoiding alcohol and drugs when you have sexual intercourse

What Other Precautions Should Be Considered?

If you are diagnosed with cervicitis, then it is vital to inform everyone with whom you have had sex in the last 2–3 months so that they too may be treated for a possible STD. It is also important to finish the course of antibiotics prescribed by your medical practitioner even if the symptoms stop or you feel better. Sexual intercourse should be avoided until treatment is completed.

References

1. "Diseases and Conditions-Cervicitis," MayoClinic, October 24, 2014.

2. "Cervicitis," nyc.gov, n.d.

3. "Cervicitis," Cleveland Clinic, n.d.

4. "Cervicitis," WebMD, n.d.

Chapter 24

Vaginal and Pelvic Infections

Chapter Contents

Section 24.1

Bacterial Vaginosis

This section includes text excerpted from "Bacterial Vaginosis," Office on Women's Health (OWH), U.S. Department of Health and Human Services (HHS), November 19, 2014.

What Is Bacterial Vaginosis (BV)?

Bacterial vaginosis (BV) is an infection in the vagina. BV is caused by changes in the amount of certain types of bacteria in your vagina. BV can develop when your vagina has more harmful bacteria than good bacteria.

BV is common, and any woman can get it. BV is easily treatable with medicine from your doctor or nurse. If left untreated, it can raise your risk for sexually transmitted infections (STIs) and cause problems during pregnancy.

Who Gets BV?

BV is the most common vaginal infection in women ages 15 to 44. But women of any age can get it, even if they have never had sex.

You may be more at risk for BV if you:

- Have a new sex partner.

- Have multiple sex partners.

- Douche.

- Do not use condoms or dental dams.

- Are pregnant. BV is common during pregnancy. About 1 in 4 pregnant women get BV. The risk for BV is higher for pregnant women because of the hormonal changes that happen during pregnancy.

- Are African-American. BV is twice as common in African-American women as in white women.

- Have an intrauterine device (IUD), especially if you also have irregular bleeding.

How Do You Get BV?

Researchers are still studying how women get BV. You can get BV without having sex, but BV can also be caused by vaginal, oral, or anal sex. You can get BV from male or female partners.

What Are the Symptoms of BV?

Many women have no symptoms. If you do have symptoms, they may include:

- Unusual vaginal discharge. The discharge can be white (milky) or gray. It may also be foamy or watery. Some women report a strong fish-like odor, especially after sex.

- Burning when urinating.

- Itching around the outside of the vagina.

- Vaginal irritation.

These symptoms may be similar to vaginal yeast infections and other health problems. Only your doctor or nurse can tell you for sure whether you have BV.

What Is the Difference between BV and a Vaginal Yeast Infection?

BV and vaginal yeast infections are both common causes of vaginal discharge. They have similar symptoms, so it can be hard to know if you have BV or a yeast infection. Only your doctor or nurse can tell you for sure if you have BV.

With BV, your discharge may be white or gray but may also have a fishy smell. Discharge from a yeast infection may also be white or gray but may look like cottage cheese.

How Is BV Diagnosed?

There are tests to find out if you have BV. Your doctor or nurse takes a sample of vaginal discharge. Your doctor or nurse may then look at the sample under a microscope, use an in-office test, or send it to a lab to check for harmful bacteria. Your doctor or nurse may also see signs of BV during an exam.

Before you see a doctor or nurse for a test:

- Don't douche or use vaginal deodorant sprays. They might cover odors that can help your doctor diagnose BV. They can also irritate your vagina.

- Make an appointment for a day when you do not have your period.

How Is BV Treated?

BV is treated with antibiotics prescribed by your doctor.

If you get BV, your male sex partner won't need to be treated. But, BV can be spread to female partners. If your current partner is female, she needs to see her doctor. She may also need treatment.

It is also possible to get BV again.

BV and vaginal yeast infections are treated differently. BV is treated with antibiotics prescribed by your doctor. Yeast infections can be treated with over-the-counter medicines. But you cannot treat BV with over-the-counter yeast infection medicine.

What Can Happen If BV Is Not Treated?

If BV is untreated, possible problems may include:

- **Higher risk of getting STIs, including human immunodeficiency virus (HIV)**. Having BV can raise your risk of getting HIV, genital herpes, chlamydia, pelvic inflammatory disease, and gonorrhea. Women with HIV who get BV are also more likely to pass HIV to a male sexual partner.

- **Pregnancy problems.** BV can lead to premature birth or a low-birth-weight baby (smaller than 5 1/2 pounds at birth). All pregnant women with symptoms of BV should be tested and treated if they have it.

What Should I Do If I Have BV?

BV is easy to treat. If you think you have BV:

- **See a doctor or nurse**. Antibiotics will treat BV.

- **Take all of your medicine**. Even if symptoms go away, you need to finish all of the antibiotic.

- **Tell your sex partner(s) if she is female** so she can be treated.

- **Avoid sexual contact until you finish your treatment.**

- **See your doctor or nurse again if you have symptoms that don't go away** within a few days after finishing the antibiotic.

Is It Safe to Treat Pregnant Women Who Have BV?

Yes. The medicine used to treat BV is safe for pregnant women. All pregnant women with symptoms of BV should be tested and treated if they have it.

If you do have BV, you can be treated safely at any stage of your pregnancy. You will get the same antibiotic given to women who are not pregnant.

How Can I Lower My Risk of BV?

Steps you can take to lower your risk of BV include:

- **Help keep your vaginal bacteria balanced.** Use warm water only to clean the outside of your vagina. You do not need to use soap. Even mild soap can cause infection or irritate your vagina. Always wipe front to back from your vagina to your anus. Keep the area cool by wearing cotton or cotton-lined underpants.

- **Do not douche.** Douching removes some of the normal bacteria in the vagina that protect you from infection. This may raise your risk of BV. It may also make it easier to get BV again after treatment. Doctors do not recommend douching.

- **Practice safe sex.** The best way to prevent the spread of BV through sex is to not have vaginal, oral, or anal sex. If you do have sex, you can lower your risk of getting BV, and any STI, with the following steps. The steps work best when used together. No single step can protect you from BV or every single type of STI. Steps to lower your risk of BV or STIs include:

- **Use condoms.** Condoms are the best way to prevent BV or STIs when you have sex. Make sure to put on the condom before the penis touches the vagina, mouth, or anus. Other methods of birth control, like birth control pills, shots, implants, or diaphragms, will not protect you from STIs.

- **Get tested.** Be sure you and your partner are tested for STIs. Talk to each other about your test results before you have sex.

- **Be monogamous.** Having sex with just one partner can lower your risk for BV or STIs. Be faithful to each other. That means that you only have sex with each other and no one else.

- **Limit your number of sex partners**. Your risk of getting BV and STIs goes up with the number of partners you have.

- **Don't abuse alcohol or drugs, which are linked to sexual risk-taking**. Drinking too much alcohol or using drugs also puts you at risk of sexual assault and possible exposure to STIs.

How Can I Protect Myself If My Female Partner Has BV?

If your partner has BV, you can lower your risk by using protection during sex.

- Use a dental dam every time you have sex. A dental dam is a thin piece of latex that is placed over the vagina before oral sex.

- Cover sex toys with condoms before use. Remove the condom and replace it with a new one before sharing the toy with your partner.

Section 24.2

Pelvic Inflammatory Disease

This section includes text excerpted from "Pelvic Inflammatory Disease," Office on Women's Health (OWH), U.S. Department of Health and Human Services (HHS), March 25, 2014.

Pelvic inflammatory disease (PID) is an infection of a woman's reproductive organs. In 2013, about 88,000 women ages 15–44 in the United States were diagnosed with PID. PID is often caused by a sexually transmitted infection (STI). If left untreated, PID can cause problems getting pregnant, problems during pregnancy, and long-term pelvic pain.

What Is Pelvic Inflammatory Disease (PID)?

PID is an infection of a woman's reproductive organs. The reproductive organs include the uterus (womb), fallopian tubes, ovaries, and cervix.

PID can be caused by many different types of bacteria. Usually PID is caused by bacteria from STIs. Sometimes PID is caused by normal bacteria found in the vagina.

Who Gets PID?

PID affects about 5 percent of women in the United States. Your risk for PID is higher if you:

- Have had an STI.

- Have had PID before.

- Are younger than 25 and have sex. PID is most common in women 15 to 24 years old.

- Have more than one sex partner or have a partner who has multiple sexual partners

- Douche. Douching can push bacteria into the reproductive organs and cause PID. Douching can also hide the signs of PID.

- Recently had an intrauterine device (IUD) inserted. The risk of PID is higher for the first few weeks only after insertion of an IUD, but PID is rare after that. Getting tested for STIs before the IUD is inserted lowers your risk for PID.

How Do You Get PID?

A woman can get PID if bacteria move up from her vagina or cervix and into her reproductive organs. Many different types of bacteria can cause PID. Most often, PID is caused by infection from two common STIs: gonorrhea and chlamydia. The number of women with PID has dropped in recent years. This may be because more women are getting tested regularly for chlamydia and gonorrhea.

You can also get PID without having an STI. Normal bacteria in the vagina can travel into a woman's reproductive organs and can sometimes cause PID. Sometimes the bacteria travel up to a woman's reproductive organs because of douching. Do not douche. No doctor or nurse recommends douching.

What Are the Signs and Symptoms of PID?

Many women do not know they have PID because they do not have any signs or symptoms. When symptoms do happen, they can be mild or more serious.

Signs and symptoms include:

- Pain in the lower abdomen (this is the most common symptom)

- Fever (100.4°F or higher)

- Vaginal discharge that may smell foul

- Painful sex

- Pain when urinating

- Irregular menstrual periods

- Pain in the upper right abdomen (this is rare)

PID can come on fast, with extreme pain and fever, especially if it is caused by gonorrhea.

How Is PID Diagnosed?

To diagnose PID, doctors usually do a physical exam to check for signs of PID and test for STIs. **If you think that you may have PID, see a doctor or nurse as soon as possible.**

If you have pain in your lower abdomen, your doctor or nurse will check for:

- Unusual discharge from your vagina or cervix

- An abscess (collection of pus) near your ovaries or fallopian tubes

- Tenderness or pain in your reproductive organs

Your doctor may do tests to find out whether you have PID or a different problem that looks like PID. These can include:

- Tests for STIs, especially gonorrhea and chlamydia. These infections can cause PID.

- A test for a urinary tract infection or other conditions that can cause pelvic pain

- Ultrasound or another imaging test so your doctor can look at your internal organs for signs of PID

A Pap test is not used to detect PID.

How Is PID Treated?

Your doctor or nurse will give you antibiotics to treat PID. Most of the time, at least two antibiotics are used that work against many different types of bacteria. **You must take all of your antibiotics, even if your symptoms go away.** This helps to make sure the infection is fully cured. See your doctor or nurse again two to three days after starting the antibiotics to make sure they are working.

Your doctor or nurse may suggest going into the hospital to treat your PID if:

- You are very sick.

- You are pregnant.

- Your symptoms do not go away after taking the antibiotics or if you cannot swallow pills. If this is the case, you will need IV antibiotics.

- You have an abscess in a fallopian tube or ovary.

If you still have symptoms or if the abscess does not go away after treatment, you may need surgery. Problems caused by PID, such as chronic pelvic pain and scarring, are often hard to treat. But sometimes they get better after surgery.

What Can Happen If PID Is Not Treated?

Without treatment, PID can lead to serious problems like infertility, ectopic pregnancy, and chronic pelvic pain (pain that does not go away). **If you think you may have PID, see a doctor or nurse as soon as possible.**

Antibiotics will treat PID, but they will not fix any permanent damage done to your internal organs.

Can I Get Pregnant If I Have Had PID?

Maybe. Your chances of getting pregnant are lower if you have had PID more than once. When you have PID, bacteria can get into the fallopian tubes or cause inflammation of the fallopian tubes. This can cause scarring in the tissue that makes up your fallopian tubes.

Scar tissue can block an egg from your ovary from entering or traveling down the fallopian tube to your uterus (womb). The egg needs to be fertilized by a man's sperm and then attach to your uterus for pregnancy to happen. Even having just a little scar tissue can keep you from getting pregnant without fertility treatment.

Scar tissue from PID can also cause a dangerous ectopic pregnancy (a pregnancy outside of the uterus) instead of a normal pregnancy. Ectopic pregnancies are more than six times more common in women who have had PID compared with women who have not had PID. Most of these pregnancies end in miscarriage.

How Can I Prevent PID?

You may not be able to prevent PID. It is not always caused by an STI. Sometimes, normal bacteria in your vagina can travel up to your reproductive organs and cause PID.

But, you can lower your risk of PID by not douching. You can also prevent STIs by not having vaginal, oral, or anal sex.

If you do have sex, lower your risk of getting an STI with the following steps:

- Use condoms.
- Get tested.
- Be monogamous.
- Limit your number of sex partners.
- Do not douche.
- Do not abuse alcohol or drugs.

The steps work best when used together. No single step can protect you from every single type of STI.

Can Women Who Have Sex with Women Get PID?

Yes. It is possible to get PID, or an STI, if you are a woman who has sex only with women.

Talk to your partner about her sexual history before having sex, and ask your doctor about getting tested if you have signs or symptoms of PID.

Section 24.3

Sexually Transmitted Infections

This section includes text excerpted from "Sexually Transmitted Infections," Office on Women's Health (OWH), U.S. Department of Health and Human Services (HHS), March 23, 2017.

Sexually transmitted infections (STIs) are also called sexually transmitted diseases, or STDs. STIs are usually spread by having vaginal, oral, or anal sex. More than 9 million women in the United States are diagnosed with an STI each year. Women often have more serious health problems from STIs than men, including infertility.

What Is a Sexually Transmitted Infection (STI)?

An STI is an infection passed from one person to another person through sexual contact. An infection is when a bacteria, virus, or parasite enters and grows in or on your body. STIs are also called sexually transmitted diseases, or STDs.

Some STIs can be cured and some STIs cannot be cured. For those STIs that cannot be cured, there are medicines to manage the symptoms.

Who Gets STIs?

Nearly 20 million people in the United States get an STI each year. These infections affect women and men of all backgrounds and economic levels. But half of all new infections are among young people 15 to 24 years old.

How Do STIs Affect Women?

Women often have more serious health problems from STIs than men:

- Chlamydia and gonorrhea, left untreated, raise the risk of chronic pelvic pain and life-threatening ectopic pregnancy. Chlamydia and gonorrhea also can cause infertility.

- Untreated syphilis in pregnant women results in infant death up to 40 percent of the time.

- Women have a higher risk than men of getting an STI during unprotected vaginal sex. Unprotected anal sex puts women at even more risk for getting an STI than unprotected vaginal sex.

How Do You Get STIs?

STIs are spread in the following ways:

- Having unprotected (without a condom) vaginal, oral, or anal sex with someone who has an STI. It can be difficult to tell if someone has an STI. STIs can be spread even if there are no signs or symptoms.

- During genital touching. It is possible to get some STIs, such as syphilis and herpes, without having sex.

- Through sexual contact between women who have sex only with other women

- From a pregnant or breastfeeding woman to her baby

Can STIs Cause Health Problems?

Yes. Each STI causes different health problems for women. Certain types of untreated STIs can cause or lead to:

- Problems getting pregnant or permanent infertility

- Problems during pregnancy and health problems for the unborn baby

- Infection in other parts of the body

- Organ damage

- Certain types of cancer, such as cervical cancer

- Death

Having certain types of STIs makes it easier for you to get human immunodeficiency virus (HIV) (another STI) if you come into contact with it.

What Are the Symptoms of STIs?

Many STIs have only mild symptoms or no symptoms at all. When women have symptoms, they may be mistaken for something else, such as a urinary tract infection or yeast infection. Get tested so that you can be treated for the correct infection.

How Do I Get Tested for STIs?

Ask your doctor or nurse about getting tested for STIs. Your doctor or nurse can tell you what test(s) you may need and how they are done. Testing for STIs is also called STI screening.

STI testing can include:

- Pelvic and physical exam. Your doctor looks for signs of infection, such as warts, rashes, or discharge.

- Blood test. A nurse will draw some blood to test for an STI.

- Urine test. You urinate (pee) into a cup. The urine is then tested for an STI.

- Fluid or tissue sample. Your doctor or nurse uses a cotton swab to take fluid or discharge from an infected place on your body. The fluid is looked at under a microscope or sent to a lab for testing.

Find a clinic near you where you can get tested for STIs or get vaccines against hepatitis B and human papillomavirus (HPV).

Does a Pap Test Screen for STIs?

No. Pap testing is mainly used to look for cell changes that could be cancer or precancer. However, your doctor may test you for HPV in addition to doing the Pap test if you are older than 30.

If you want to be tested for STIs, you must ask your doctor or nurse.

Do I Need to Get Tested for STIs?

If you are sexually active, talk to your doctor or nurse about STI testing. Which tests you will need and how often you need to get them will depend on you and your partner's sexual history.

You may feel embarrassed or that your sex life is too personal to share with your doctor or nurse. But being open and honest is the only way your doctor can help take care of you.

Then talk to your doctor or nurse about what tests make sense for you.

How Are STIs Treated?

For some STIs, treatment may involve taking medicine by mouth or getting a shot. For other STIs that can't be cured, like herpes or HIV and acquired immune deficiency syndrome (AIDS), medicines can help reduce the symptoms.

If I Have an STI, Does My Partner Have It Too?

Maybe. If the tests show that you have an STI, your doctor might want your partner to come in for testing. Or the doctor may give you a medicine to take home for your partner.

The STI may have spread to you or your partner from a former sex partner. This is why it is important to get tested after each new sex partner. Also, if you test positive for certain STIs (HIV, syphilis, or gonorrhea), some cities and states require you (or your doctor) to tell any past or current sex partners.

Do Medicines Sold over the Internet Prevent or Treat STIs?

No. Only use medicines prescribed or suggested by your doctor.

Some drugs sold over the Internet claim to prevent or treat STIs. And some of these sites claim their medicines work better than the medicines your doctor prescribes. But in most cases this is not true, and no one knows how safe these products are or even what is in them.

Buying prescription and over-the-counter drugs on the Internet means you may not know exactly what you're getting. An illegal Internet pharmacy may try to sell you unapproved drugs, drugs with the wrong active ingredient, drugs with too much or too little of the active ingredient, or drugs with dangerous ingredients.

How Can I Prevent an STI?

The best way to prevent an STI is to not have vaginal, oral, or anal sex.

If you do have sex, lower your risk of getting an STI with the following steps:

- Get vaccinated.

- Use condoms.

- Get tested.

- Be monogamous.

- Limit your number of sex partners.

- Do not douche.

- Do not abuse alcohol or drugs.

The steps work best when used together. No single step can protect you from every single type of STI.

Section 24.4

Vaginal Yeast Infection

This section includes text excerpted from "Vaginal Yeast Infection," Office on Women's Health (OWH), U.S. Department of Health and Human Services (HHS), January 6, 2015.

A vaginal yeast infection is an infection of the vagina that causes itching and burning of the vulva, the area around the vagina. Three out of four women will have a yeast infection at some point in their life. Yeast infections are easy to treat, but it is important to see your doctor or nurse if you think you have an infection.

Are Some Women More at Risk for Yeast Infections?

Women and girls of all ages can get yeast infections, but they are rare before puberty and after menopause. Your risk for vaginal yeast infections is higher if:

- You are pregnant

- You have diabetes and your blood sugar is not under control

- You use a type of hormonal birth control that has higher doses of estrogen

- You douche or use vaginal sprays

- You recently took antibiotics such as amoxicillin or steroid medicines

- You have a weakened immune system, such as from human immunodeficiency virus (HIV)

What Are the Signs and Symptoms of a Vaginal Yeast Infection?

The most common symptom of a yeast infection is extreme itchiness in and around the vagina. Other signs and symptoms include:

- Burning, redness, and swelling of the vagina and the vulva

- Pain when urinating

- Pain during sex

- Soreness

- A thick, white vaginal discharge that looks like cottage cheese and does not have a bad smell You may only have a few of these symptoms. They may be mild or severe.

Should I Call My Doctor If I Think I Have a Yeast Infection?

Yes. Seeing your doctor is the only way to know for sure if you have a yeast infection. The signs and symptoms of a yeast infection are a lot like symptoms of sexually transmitted infections (STIs) and bacterial vaginosis (BV). If left untreated, STIs and BV can raise your risk of getting other STIs, including HIV, and can lead to problems getting pregnant. BV can also lead to problems during pregnancy, such as premature delivery.

How Are Yeast Infections Treated?

Yeast infections are usually treated with antifungal medicine. See your doctor or nurse to make sure that you have a vaginal yeast infection and not another type of infection. You can then buy antifungal medicine for yeast infections at a store, without a prescription. Antifungal medicines come in the form of creams, tablets, ointments, or suppositories that you insert into your vagina. You can apply treatment in one dose or daily for up to seven days, depending on the brand you choose. Your doctor can also give you a single dose of antifungal medicine taken by mouth, such as fluconazole.

If I Have a Yeast Infection, Does My Sexual Partner Need to Be Treated?

Maybe. It is possible to pass yeast infections to your partner during vaginal, oral, or anal sex.

- **If your partner is a man,** the risk of infection is low. Some men get an itchy rash on their penis. If this happens to your partner, he should see a doctor.
- **If your partner is a woman,** she may be at risk. She should be tested and treated if she has any symptoms.

How Can I Avoid Getting Another Yeast Infection?

You can take steps to lower your risk of getting yeast infections:

- Do not douche. Douching removes some of the normal bacteria in the vagina that protects you from infection.
- Do not use scented feminine products, including bubble bath, sprays, pads, and tampons.
- Change tampons, pads, and pantyliners often.
- Do not wear tight underwear, pantyhose, pants, or jeans. These can increase body heat and moisture in your genital area.
- Wear underwear with a cotton crotch.
- Change out of wet swimsuits and workout clothes as soon as you can.
- After using the bathroom, always wipe from front to back.
- Avoid hot tubs and very hot baths.
- If you have diabetes, be sure your blood sugar is under control.

Chapter 25

Pelvic Floor Disorders

Chapter Contents

Section 25.1

Cystocele

This section includes text excerpted from "Cystocele (Prolapsed Bladder)," National Digestive Diseases, National Institute of Diabetes and Digestive and Kidney Diseases (NIDDK), March 2014.

What Is a Cystocele?

A cystocele, also called a prolapsed or dropped bladder, is the bulging or dropping of the bladder into the vagina. The bladder, located in the pelvis between the pelvic bones, is a hollow, muscular, balloon-shaped organ that expands as it fills with urine. During urination, also called voiding, the bladder empties through the urethra, located at the bottom of the bladder. The urethra is the tube that carries urine outside of the body. The vagina is the tube in a woman's body that runs beside the urethra and connects the womb, or uterus, to the outside of the body.

What Causes a Cystocele?

A cystocele occurs when the muscles and supportive tissues between a woman's bladder and vagina weaken and stretch, letting the bladder sag from its normal position and bulge into the vagina or through the vaginal opening. In a cystocele, the bladder tissue remains covered by the vaginal skin. A cystocele may result from damage to the muscles and tissues that hold the pelvic organs up inside the pelvis. A woman's pelvic organs include the vagina, cervix, uterus, bladder, urethra, and small intestine. Damage to or weakening of the pelvic muscles and supportive tissues may occur after vaginal childbirth and with conditions that repeatedly strain or increase pressure in the pelvic area, such as:

- repetitive straining for bowel movements
- Constipation
- chronic or violent coughing
- heavy lifting
- being overweight or obese

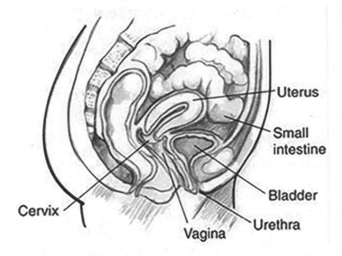

Figure 25.1. *Normal Bladder Position*

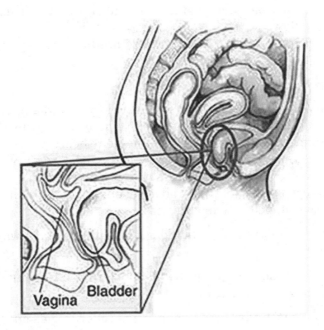

Figure 25.2. *Cystocele*

A woman's chances of developing a cystocele increase with age, possibly because of weakening muscles and supportive tissues from aging. Whether menopause increases a woman's chances of developing a cystocele is unclear.

What are the Symptoms of a Cystocele?

The symptoms of a cystocele may include:

- a vaginal bulge
- the feeling that something is falling out of the vagina
- the sensation of pelvic heaviness or fullness
- difficulty starting a urine stream
- a feeling of incomplete urination
- frequent or urgent urination

Women who have a cystocele may also leak some urine as a result of movements that put pressure on the bladder, called stress urinary incontinence. These movements can include coughing, sneezing, laughing, or physical activity, such as walking. Urinary retention—the inability to empty the bladder completely—may occur with more severe cystoceles if the cystocele creates a kink in the woman's urethra and blocks urine flow.

Women with mild cystoceles often do not have any symptoms.

How Is a Cystocele Diagnosed?

Diagnosing a cystocele requires medical tests and a physical exam of the vagina. Medical tests take place in a healthcare provider's office, an outpatient center, or a hospital. The healthcare provider will ask about symptoms and medical history. A healthcare provider uses a grading system to determine the severity of a woman's cystocele. A cystocele receives one of three grades depending on how far a woman's bladder has dropped into her vagina:

- grade 1—mild, when the bladder drops only a short way into the vagina
- grade 2—moderate, when the bladder drops far enough to reach the opening of the vagina
- grade 3—most advanced, when the bladder bulges out through the opening of the vagina

If a woman has difficulty emptying her bladder, a healthcare provider may measure the amount of urine left in the woman's bladder after she urinates. The remaining urine is called the postvoid residual. A healthcare provider can measure postvoid residual with a bladder ultrasound. A bladder ultrasound uses a device, called a transducer, that bounces safe, painless sound waves off the bladder to create an image and show the amount of remaining urine. A specially trained technician performs the procedure, and a radiologist—a doctor who specializes in medical imaging—interprets the images. A woman does not need anesthesia.

A healthcare provider can also use a catheter—a thin, flexible tube—to measure a woman's postvoid residual. The healthcare provider inserts the catheter through the woman's urethra into her bladder to remove and measure the amount of remaining urine after the woman has urinated. A postvoid residual of 100 mL or more is a sign that the woman is not completely emptying her bladder. A woman receives local anesthesia.

A healthcare provider may use a voiding cystourethrogram—an X-ray exam of the bladder—to diagnose a cystocele as well. A woman gets a voiding cystourethrogram while urinating. The X-ray images show the shape of the woman's bladder and let the healthcare provider see any problems that might block normal urine flow. An X-ray technician performs a voiding cystourethrogram, and a radiologist interprets the images. A woman does not need anesthesia; however, some women may receive sedation. A healthcare provider may order additional tests to rule out problems in other parts of a woman's urinary tract.

How Is a Cystocele Treated?

Cystocele treatment depends on the severity of the cystocele and whether a woman has symptoms. If a woman's cystocele does not bother her, a healthcare provider may recommend only that she avoid heavy lifting or straining, which could worsen her cystocele. If a woman has symptoms that bother her and wants treatment, the healthcare provider may recommend pelvic muscle exercises, a vaginal pessary, or surgery.

Pelvic floor, or Kegel, exercises involve strengthening pelvic floor muscles. Strong pelvic floor muscles more effectively hold pelvic organs in place. A woman does not need special equipment for Kegel exercises.

The exercises involve tightening and relaxing the muscles that support pelvic organs. A healthcare provider can help a woman learn proper technique.

A vaginal pessary is a small, silicone medical device placed in the vagina that supports the vaginal wall and holds the bladder in place. Pessaries come in a number of shapes and sizes. A healthcare provider has many options to choose from to find the most comfortable pessary for a woman.

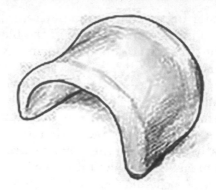

Figure 25.3. *Pessary Device*

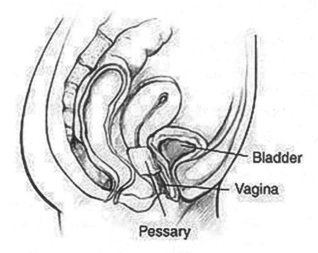

Figure 25.4. *Pessary Inserted in the Vagina*

A healthcare provider may recommend surgery to repair the vaginal wall support and reposition the woman's bladder to its normal position. The most common cystocele repair is an anterior vaginal repair—or anterior colporrhaphy. The surgeon makes an incision in the wall of the woman's vagina and repairs the defect by folding over and sewing together extra supportive tissue between the vagina and bladder. The repair tightens the layers of tissue that separate the organs, creating more support for the bladder. A surgeon who specializes in the urinary tract or female reproductive system performs an anterior vaginal repair in a hospital. The woman receives either regional or general anesthesia. The woman may stay overnight in the hospital, and full recovery may take up to 4 to 6 weeks.

Eating, Diet, and Nutrition

Researchers have not found that eating, diet, and nutrition play a role in causing or preventing a cystocele.

Section 25.2

Rectocele

Pelvic organ prolapse, which is the descent of a pelvic organ toward or through the vaginal opening, is a common condition in women. Rectocele, a type of pelvic organ prolapse, involves the bulging (herniation) of the rectum into the vaginal wall as a result of a weakness in the recto-vaginal septum, which is the connective tissue separating the lower part of the rectum and the vagina.

The condition is more common among older women, and may occur in isolation or together with other pelvic floor disorders, such as a prolapsed bladder (cystocele) or prolapsed small intestine (enterocele). Rectocele is also referred to as posterior prolapse.

Causes

While many factors can cause rectocele, it occurs mostly in conjunction with the weakening of the pelvic floor that can occur with pregnancy, childbirth, and age. It may also be caused by pelvic floor weakness associated with hysterectomy (surgical removal of uterus) or other pelvic surgeries. Other factors that are known to increase the risk of rectocele include chronic constipation, persistent cough, and lifting of heavy weights. These can exert pressure on the pelvic floor and weaken it. According to some studies, assisted delivery using forceps has also been linked to an increased risk of rectocele.

Symptoms

Most cases of posterior prolapse are usually discovered during a routine physical examination and are asymptomatic. Typically, a small pressure or protrusion is felt within the vagina and is accompanied by little or no discomfort. Sometimes, a rectocele may be accompanied by symptoms categorized as either vaginal or rectal. Vaginal symptoms involve the actual protrusion of the prolapsed tissue through the vaginal opening; discomfort or pain during sexual intercourse; and less frequently, vaginal bleeding. On the other hand, rectal symptoms mostly include difficulty having a bowel movement. Rectal symptoms, particularly in moderate to severe cases of posterior prolapse, are usually accompanied by stool being trapped in the rectocele, which can lead to fecal incontinence and rectal discomfort. Stool trapping can lead to excessive straining and frequent urges to defecate, and most women who experience rectal symptoms may resort to splinting—pressing against the vaginal wall with a wad of tissue or fingers to reduce straining and push stool out during a bowel movement.

Diagnosis

A pelvic examination is the first step in diagnosing a rectocele. The patient may be asked to simulate bowel movement by straining or bearing down so the doctor can examine the size and location of the prolapsed tissue. This may be followed up with imaging tests, such as magnetic resonance imaging (MRI) or a special type of X-ray called defecography, which makes a real time visualization of the patient's defecation. Imaging studies such as those provided by a defecogram are being increasingly used for assessing pelvic floor dysfunction and deciding the line of treatment.

Treatment

Most cases of rectocele can be successfully managed with diet and lifestyle changes. Just as laxatives, increased intake of water and dietary fiber also helps ease bowel movement. In recent years, biofeedback has emerged as an effective tool in the management of dysfunctional defecation associated with pelvic floor disorders such as rectocele. This type of therapy aims to restore normal defecation by improving rectal sensory perception.

Rectocele may also be managed with vaginal pessary, one of the oldest and most effective devices for the nonsurgical management of rectocele. Pessaries are designed to provide mechanical support to the collapsed tissues within the walls of the vagina. Pelvic floor strengthening exercises are also particularly useful in the conservative management of rectocele.

Surgical intervention is considered only when symptoms interfere with daily activities and hamper quality of life. Generally, chronic constipation and obstructed defecation are the most common indications for surgical repair of rectocele.

Surgery

A rectocele repair can be performed by a colorectal surgeon or a gynecologist. There are four main approaches for a rectocele surgery:

1. Transanal (through the anus)

2. Transvaginal (through vagina)

3. Transperineal (area between anus and vagina)

4. Transabdominal (through an incision in the abdomen).

While transvaginal reconstruction is the most commonly performed rectocele repair, other approaches can be considered based on the size of the rectocele, severity of symptoms, and presence of other health factors. Surgery, by and large, involves removal of redundant tissue followed by stapling of the prolapsed tissue. Sometimes, a mesh or a prosthetic patch is used to reinforce the repair and strengthen the recto-vaginal septum.

Prophylactic Measures

Activities aimed at strengthening the pelvic floor muscles can go a long way in preventing or worsening a posterior prolapse. Commonly recommended prophylactic measures include:

- Correcting constipation or other metabolic disorders that increase intra-abdominal pressure.

- Avoiding strenuous occupational or recreational activity that could exert pressure on the abdomen and cause potential damage to the pelvic floor.

- Maintaining a healthy body weight.

- Quitting smoking.

- Hormone replacement therapy may be recommended for post-menopausal women to reduce the urogenital atrophy associated with estrogen loss and strengthen the vaginal tissue.

References

1. "Posterior Vaginal Prolapse (Rectocele)," Mayo Clinic, July 25, 2017.

2. Beck, David E., Nechol, Allen L. "Rectocele," National Center for Biotechnology Information (NCBI), June 2010.

3. Lefevre, Roger, Davila, Willy G. "Functional Disorders: Rectocele," National Center for Biotechnology Information (NCBI), May 2008.

Section 25.3

Uterine Prolapse

This section includes text excerpted from documents published by two public domain sources. Text under headings marked 1 are excerpted from "Common Uterine Conditions," Agency for Healthcare Research and Quality (AHRQ), U.S. Department of Health and Human Services (HHS), February 5, 2017; Text under headings marked 2 are excerpted from "Pelvic Floor Disorders: Condition Information," *Eunice Kennedy Shriver* National Institute of Child Health and Human Development (NICHD), December 3, 2012. Reviewed August 2017.

What Is Uterine Prolapse?[1]

If you have uterine prolapse, it means that your uterus has tilted or slipped. Sometimes it slips so far down that it reaches into the vagina. This happens when the ligaments that hold the uterus to the wall of the pelvis become too weak to hold the uterus in its place.

Symptoms of Uterine Prolapse[2]

*   Feel heaviness, fullness, pulling, or aching in the vagina that worsens by the end of the day or when they are having a bowel movement

*   See or feel a "bulge" or "something coming out" of the vagina

- Have a hard time starting to urinate or emptying the bladder completely

- Have frequent urinary tract infections

- Leak urine when they are coughing, laughing, or exercising

- Feel an urgent or frequent need to urinate

- Leak stool or have a hard time controlling gas

- Suffer constipation

- Have a hard time making it to the bathroom in time

Some women with pelvic floor problems do not have symptoms at first. Many women are reluctant to tell their healthcare provider about embarrassing symptoms. In addition, many women think that problems with bladder control are normal and live with their symptoms. However, treatment is available and can help women with pelvic floor problems.

What Can I Do to Reduce or Ease Symptoms?[2]

Researchers are actively studying ways to reduce or ease symptoms, such as:

- **Avoiding foods and drinks that stimulate the bladder or bowel.** Some foods and drinks that can stimulate the bladder and make you need to use the bathroom are caffeinated beverages, citrus fruits and drinks, artificial sweeteners, and alcoholic beverages. Avoiding caffeine and spicy foods may help reduce your chance of having loose stools.

- **Eating a high-fiber diet.** Fiber helps your body to digest food and prevents constipation, making it unnecessary to strain to have a bowel movement. Fiber is found in fruits, vegetables, legumes (such as beans and lentils), and whole grains. Fiber supplements are also available.

- **Losing weight.** For women who are overweight, weight loss may reduce problems with bladder control and pelvic organ prolapse symptoms by relieving pressure on pelvic organs.

- **Bladder training.** This involves using the bathroom on a set schedule to regain bladder control. A woman starts by using the bathroom every 60 or 90 minutes and slowly, over many months, increases that time with a goal of using the bathroom every 2.5 to 3 hours.

Can Uterine Prolapse Be Prevented?[2]

Traditionally, women are taught certain actions that may lower the risk of developing a pelvic floor problem:

- Maintain a healthy weight or lose weight (if overweight). Women who are overweight or obese are more likely to have pelvic floor problems.

- Maintain a high-fiber diet and drink plenty of fluids. This promotes normal bowel function and reduces risk of constipation. Preventing constipation may reduce the risk of some pelvic floor disorders.

- Do not smoke. Smoking can lead to chronic cough, which stresses the pelvic floor.

- Do Kegel exercises regularly to keep pelvic floor muscles toned. To be effective, Kegel exercises must be done correctly and routinely. A healthcare provider can help women who are unsure if they are using the correct muscles.

Some pregnant women wonder if they can prevent pelvic floor problems by having a cesarean delivery rather than a vaginal delivery. The answer is not clear-cut. Women who never become pregnant may develop pelvic floor problems; some women who have multiple pregnancies do not. Undergoing a cesarean delivery presents other significant risks to consider.

If you are pregnant and concerned about future pelvic floor problems, talk to your healthcare provider.

Should I See a Doctor about My Symptoms?[2]

Yes. Do not wait until your symptoms are "really bad" to get help. Without treatment, symptoms can worsen and may affect your self-esteem, your ability to do your job well, your relationships, and many other aspects of daily living. In addition, buying products to deal with the symptoms of bladder or bowel control problems can be costly.

Talk to your healthcare provider if you see or feel a bulge of tissue in your vagina or have other symptoms, including changes in bladder and bowel control.

Diagnosis[2]

A physical exam may be all that is needed to diagnose a PFD. In some cases, a woman's healthcare provider will see or feel a bulge that suggests a prolapse during a routine pelvic exam. In other cases, a woman may see her doctor about symptoms she is experiencing, such as problems with bladder or bowel control. Depending on the findings from the exam or the severity of the symptoms, tests may be performed.

How Is Uterine Prolapse Treated?[1]

Treatment choices depend on how weak the ligaments have become, your age, health, and whether you want to become pregnant.

Options that do not involve an operation include:

- Exercises (called Kegel exercises) can help to strengthen the muscles of the pelvis. How to do Kegel exercises: Tighten your pelvic muscles as if you are trying to hold back urine. Hold the muscles tight for a few seconds and then release them. Repeat this exercise up to 10 times. Repeat the Kegel exercises up to four time each day.

- Taking estrogen to limit further weakening of the muscles and tissues that support the uterus.

- Inserting a pessary—which is a rubber, diaphragm-like device—around the cervix to help prop up the uterus. The pessary does have drawbacks. It may dislodge or cause irritation, it may interfere with intercourse, and it must be removed regularly for cleaning.

- Watchful waiting.

Surgical treatments include:

- Tightening the weakened muscles without taking out the uterus. This is usually done through the vagina, but it also can be done through the abdomen. Although this is a type of surgery, it is not as extensive as a hysterectomy.

- Hysterectomy. Doctors usually recommend this operation if symptoms are bothersome or if the uterus has dropped so far that it is coming through the vagina.

Chapter 26

Vulval Disorders

Chapter Contents

Section 26.1

Vaginitis (Vulvovaginitis)

This section includes text excerpted from "Vaginitis," National
Institutes of Health (NIH), November 15, 2016.

What Is Vaginitis?

Vaginitis, also called vulvovaginitis, is an inflammation or infection
of the vagina. It can also affect the vulva, which is the external part
of a woman's genitals. Vaginitis can cause itching, pain, discharge,
and odor.

Vaginitis is common, especially in women in their reproductive
years. It usually happens when there is a change in the balance of
bacteria or yeast that are normally found in your vagina. There are
different types of vaginitis, and they have different causes, symptoms,
and treatments.

What Are the Different Causes of Vaginitis?

Bacterial vaginosis (BV) is the most common vaginal infection in
women ages 15-44. It happens when there is an imbalance between the
"good" and "harmful" bacteria that are normally found in a woman's
vagina. Many things can change the balance of bacteria, including:

- Taking antibiotics

- Douching

- Using an intrauterine device (IUD)

- Having unprotected sex with a new partner

- Having many sexual partners

Yeast infections (candidiasis) happen when too much candida grows
in the vagina. Candida is the scientific name for yeast. It is a fungus
that lives almost everywhere, including in your body. You may have
too much growing in the vagina because of:

- Antibiotics

- Pregnancy
- Diabetes, especially if it is not well-controlled
- Corticosteroid medicines

Trichomoniasis can also cause vaginitis. Trichomoniasis is a common sexually transmitted disease. It is caused by a parasite.

You can also have vaginitis if you are allergic or sensitive to certain products that you use. Examples include vaginal sprays, douches, spermicides, soaps, detergents, or fabric softeners. They can cause burning, itching, and discharge.

Hormonal changes can also cause vaginal irritation. Examples are when you are pregnant or breastfeeding, or when you have gone through menopause.

Sometimes you can have more than one cause of vaginitis at the same time.

What Are the Symptoms of Vaginitis?

The symptoms of vaginitis depend on which type you have.

With BV, you may not have symptoms. You could have a thin white or gray vaginal discharge. There may be an odor, such as a strong fish-like odor, especially after sex.

Yeast infections produce a thick, white discharge from the vagina that can look like cottage cheese. The discharge can be watery and often has no smell. Yeast infections usually cause the vagina and vulva to become itchy and red.

You may not have symptoms when you have trichomoniasis. If you do have them, they include itching, burning, and soreness of the vagina and vulva. You may have burning during urination. You could also have gray-green discharge, which may smell bad.

How Is the Cause of Vaginitis Diagnosed?

To find out the cause of your symptoms, your healthcare provider may:

- Ask you about your health history
- Do a pelvic exam
- Look for vaginal discharge, noting its color, qualities, and any odor
- Study a sample of your vaginal fluid under a microscope

In some cases, you may need more tests.

What Are the Treatments for Vaginitis?

The treatment depends on which type of vaginitis you have.

BV is treatable with antibiotics. You may get pills to swallow, or cream or gel that you put in your vagina. During treatment, you should use a condom during sex or not have sex at all.

Yeast infections are usually treated with a cream or with medicine that you put inside your vagina. You can buy over-the-counter treatments for yeast infections, but you need to be sure that you do have a yeast infection and not another type of vaginitis. See your healthcare provider if this is the first time you have had symptoms. Even if you have had yeast infections before, it is a good idea to call your healthcare provider before using an over-the-counter treatment.

The treatment for trichomoniasis is usually a single-dose antibiotic. Both you and your partner(s) should be treated, to prevent spreading the infection to others and to keep from getting it again.

If your vaginitis is due to an allergy or sensitivity to a product, you need to figure out which product is causing the problem. It could be a product that you started using recently. Once you figure it out, you should stop using the product.

If the cause of your vaginitis is a hormonal change, your healthcare provider may give you estrogen cream to help with your symptoms.

Can Vaginitis Cause Other Health Problems?

It is important to treat BV and trichomoniasis, because having either of them can increase your risk for getting HIV (human immunodeficiency virus) or another sexually transmitted disease. If you are pregnant, BV or trichomoniasis can increase your risk for preterm labor and preterm birth.

How Can I Prevent Vaginitis?

To help prevent vaginitis:

- Do not douche or use vaginal sprays
- Use a condom when having sex
- Avoid clothes that hold in heat and moisture
- Wear cotton underwear

Section 26.2

Vulvodynia

This section includes text excerpted from "Vulvodynia," *Eunice Kennedy Shriver* National Institute of Child Health and Human Development (NICHD), January 30, 2017.

About Vulvodynia

Vulvodynia is a term used to describe chronic pain (lasting at least 3 months) of the vulva that does not have a clear cause, such as an infection or cancer. The vulva refers to the external female genitalia, including the labia ("lips" or folds of skin at the opening of the vagina), the clitoris, and the vaginal opening. Vulvodynia is usually described as burning, stinging, irritation, or rawness.

Sometimes, vulvodynia is described with more specific terms.

- **Generalized vulvodynia** is pain or discomfort that can be felt in the entire vulvar area.

- **Localized vulvodynia** is felt in only one place on the vulva.

- **Provoked vulvodynia** is pain triggered by an activity or contact with the area, such as having sex, using a tampon, having a gynecological exam, or even wearing tight-fitting pants. Alternatively, spontaneous vulvodynia occurs when the pain is not initiated by any known trigger.

- **Provoked vestibulodynia** is vulvodynia with provoked pain that occurs in the vestibular region of the vulva, or the entry point to the vagina. This condition has formerly been called vulvar vestibulitis syndrome, focal vulvitis, vestibulodynia, or vulvar vestibulitis.

What Are the Symptoms of Vulvodynia?

The main symptom of vulvodynia is pain. The type of pain can be different for each woman.

Vulvodynia can cause burning, stinging, irritation, or rawness of the vulva. Some women may also have itching, aching, soreness, throbbing, or swelling. These symptoms may be caused by pressure on the vulvar area, such as during sex or when inserting a tampon. Symptoms may occur during exercise, after urinating, or even while sitting or resting.

Pain may move around or always be in the same place. It can be constant, or it can come and go.

How Many People Are Affected by or at Risk for Vulvodynia?

The exact number of women with vulvodynia is unknown. Researchers estimate that 9% to 18% of women between the ages of 18 and 64 may experience vulvar pain during their lifetimes.

The evidence suggests that many women either do not seek help at all or go from doctor to doctor seeking a diagnosis and treatment without receiving answers.

What Causes Vulvodynia?

Healthcare providers do not know what causes vulvodynia. It tends to be diagnosed when other causes of vulvar pain, such as infection or skin diseases, are ruled out.

Researchers think that one or more of the following may cause or contribute to vulvodynia:

- Injury to or irritation of the nerves that transmit pain and other sensations from the vulva

- Increased density of the nerve fibers in the vulvar vestibule

- Elevated levels of inflammatory substances in the vulvar tissue

- Abnormal response of vulvar cells to environmental factors

- Altered hormone receptor expression in the vulvar tissue

- Genetic factors such as susceptibility to chronic vestibular inflammation, susceptibility to chronic widespread pain, or inability to combat vulvovaginal infection

- Localized hypersensitivity to *Candida* or other vulvovaginal organisms

- Pelvic floor muscle weakness or spasm

How Do Healthcare Providers Diagnose Vulvodynia?

Vulvodynia tends to be diagnosed only when other causes of vulvar pain, such as infection or skin diseases, have been ruled out.

To diagnose vulvodynia, a healthcare provider will take a detailed medical history, including pain characteristics and any accompanying bowel, bladder, or sexual problems. The provider may recommend that a woman have blood drawn to assess levels of estrogen, progesterone, and testosterone. The provider may also perform a cotton swab test, applying gentle pressure to various vulvar sites and asking the patient to rate the severity of the pain. If any areas of skin appear suspicious, these areas may be further examined with a magnifying instrument or a tissue sample may be taken for biopsy.

Because vulvodynia is often a diagnosis of exclusion, it can be difficult and time-consuming to arrive at an actual diagnosis. The diagnostic process can be especially problematic for women who lack health insurance because they may not have the resources to continue seeking care to exclude the many possible causes of pain. Moreover, some women may be reluctant to discuss their pain or seek treatment.

Researchers sponsored by *Eunice Kennedy Shriver* National Institute of Child Health and Human Development (NICHD) are investigating how to better evaluate and understand vulvar pain. Some have proposed ways to better map the pain to identify nerves that may be involved. Some researchers believe that vulvodynia and vulvar vestibulitis syndrome involve dysfunction in the pathways that process pain.

What Are the Treatments for Vulvodynia?

There are several options to treat the symptoms of vulvodynia. These may include lifestyle changes and therapy, medical treatment, and surgical treatment.

A variety of treatment options may be presented to patients, including:

- Topical medications, such as lidocaine ointment (a local anesthetic) or hormonal creams

- Drug treatment, such as pain relievers, antidepressants, or anticonvulsants

- Biofeedback therapy, intended to help decrease pain sensation

- Physical therapy to strengthen pelvic floor muscles

- Injections of steroids or anesthetics

- Surgery to remove the affected skin and tissue in localized vulvodynia

- Changes in diet (for example, some physicians may suggest a diet low in oxalates, which can form crystals in the body if they aren't filtered out by the kidneys)

- Complementary or alternative therapies (including relaxation, massage, homeopathy, and acupuncture)

Chapter 27

Gynecological Procedures

Chapter Contents

Section 27.1

Common Gynecological Procedures

"Common Gynecological Procedures," © 2018 Omnigraphics.
Reviewed August 2017.

Throughout their lives, women may face one or more gynecological issues that may include certain conditions or illnesses, a pregnancy or the ability to become pregnant, or concerns related to puberty or menopause. Gynecologists and obstetricians employ a range of procedures to test for and treat these issues and conditions. Understanding these procedures is an important aspect of how women can take control of and manage their own healthcare.

Listed below are common gynecological procedures along with a brief description.

Tests and Diagnostic Procedures

Amniocentesis. During a pregnancy, a sample of amniotic fluid (the fluid that surrounds the fetus in the womb) is removed and tested for genetic markers associated with birth defects and other chromosomal abnormalities. Amniocentesis is also used to determine the gender of the fetus.

Cervical Biopsy. Tissue is removed from the cervix to test for cancer, precancerous conditions, and other abnormal conditions.

Chorionic Villus Sampling (CVS). During a pregnancy, a tissue sample from the placenta is removed and tested for chromosomal defects and genetic problems.

Colposcopy. A healthcare professional uses a tubular instrument with a magnifying lens and a light source (called a colposcope) to view the cervix and the vagina to determine if a biopsy is needed.

Endometrial Biopsy. A small sample of tissue is taken from the lining of the uterus, known as the endometrium, for testing and diagnosis of cancer, precancerous conditions, and hormonal imbalances.

Hysteroscopy. A healthcare professional inserts a thin, flexible tube with a light source into the vagina to examine the cervix and uterus.

Loop Electrosurgical Excision Procedure (LEEP). Loop electrosurgical excision procedure (LEEP) is used for both the diagnosis and treatment of abnormal and cancerous growths on the cervix. LEEP uses a wire loop, heated with electric current, as a scalpel to remove a thin layer of cells from the cervix.

Mammogram. A mammogram is an X-ray scan of the breast used to detect cancerous or benign tumors and cysts. A mammogram is a standard diagnostic tool in the case of problems in the breast such as a lump, pain, or discharge from the nipple.

Pelvic Ultrasound. A pelvic ultrasound is a scan that uses sound waves to produce 2D images of structures in the pelvis. A pelvic ultrasound can detect pelvic masses, uterine bleeding, polyps, fibroids, tumors, and other conditions.

Sonohysterography. A sonohysterography is a type of ultrasound exam in which fluid is placed in the uterus to create a more detailed image of the uterus than a standard ultrasound.

Surgical Procedures

Cesarean Section. A cesarean section, or C-section, is a common surgical procedure in which a baby is delivered via an incision in the mother's abdomen and uterus.

Dilation and Curettage (D&C). Dilation and curettage (D&C) is a surgical procedure used to remove abnormal tissues from the uterus. D&C is used to clear out tissues in the uterus in case of a miscarriage, to diagnose and treat uterine bleeding, to remove fibroid tumors, in the detection and treatment of cancer, and in the testing for infertility.

Endometrial Ablation. Endometrial ablation is a procedure carried out to reduce heavy menstrual bleeding by removing the thin layer of tissue lining the uterus known as the endometrium. It is recommended only for women who have decided not to have children in future.

Tubal Ligation. Tubal ligation is a permanent birth control procedure in which a woman's fallopian tubes are either blocked or tied off, preventing sperms from reaching the egg and egg from travelling from ovary to uterus.

Hysterectomy. This is a procedure in which the uterus is surgically removed. Sometimes, one or both the ovaries, the fallopian tubes, and other reproductive organs may be removed along with the uterus in a hysterectomy.

Mastectomy. A mastectomy is the surgical removal of the breast. Mastectomy may be performed in case of any advanced breast cancer.

Myomectomy. A myomectomy is a surgical procedure used to remove uterine fibroids without removing the uterus. Various techniques are employed based on the nature of fibroids in the uterus and the medical history of the women undergoing the procedure. A myomectomy could result in scarring of uterine tissue that could affect fertility.

Oophorectomy. In an oophorectomy, one or both ovaries are surgically removed from a woman's reproductive system.

Trachelectomy. The surgical removal of the cervix without the uterus is known as a trachelectomy. In a radical trachelectomy, the cervix, surrounding tissue, and some pelvic lymph nodes are removed.

References

1. "Gynecological Conditions," The Regents of The University of California, n.d.

2. "Common Gynecologic Procedures," North County Women's Specialists, n.d.

3. "Procedures," University of Rochester Medical Center Rochester, n.d.

4. "Common Gynecologic Procedures," Mission Viejo, n.d.

5. "Gyno Problems," Women's Health Advice, n.d.

6. "Gynecology Tests and Procedures," The Johns Hopkins University, The Johns Hopkins Hospital, and Johns Hopkins Health System, n.d.

7. "Oophorectomy (Ovary Removal Surgery)," Mayo Foundation for Medical Education and Research (MFMER), April 7, 2017.

8. Johnson, Traci C., MD. "Pregnancy and Amniocentesis," WebMD, LLC., June 7, 2017.

Section 27.2

Dilation and Curettage (D&C)

"Dilation and Curettage (D&C),"
© 2018 Omnigraphics. Reviewed August 2017.

What Is Dilation and Curettage (D&C)?

Dilation and curettage, also known as a D&C is a surgical procedure in which abnormal tissues are scraped from the lining (endometrium) of the uterus. It is an outpatient surgery and most women can return home the same day. In dilation and curettage, the cervix is dilated and a spoon-shaped instrument, called a curette, is used to scrape and remove the abnormal tissue. A variation of this procedure is Dilation and Evacuation (D&E) in which the contents of the uterus are removed using suction force.

Why Is D&C Advised?

Dilation and curettage serves diagnostic and therapeutic purposes. It is usually done for:

- Investigating abnormal or excessive uterine bleeding.
- Removal of fibroids (mostly noncancerous connective and muscle tissue growths in the uterus).
- Removal of polyps (growths attached to the inner wall of the uterus).
- Removal of hyperplasia (abnormal growth in the lining of the uterus).
- Examination of potentially cancerous tissue.
- Medical termination of pregnancy, (up to 14 weeks of gestation) also called an abortion.
- Abortion of abnormal fetus (having birth defects).
- Removal of placental and other tissues after miscarriage.

- Removal of remnant placental tissue, postpartum.

- Therapeutic abortion (termination of pregnancy that is dangerous to the mother).

- To determine the cause of infertility.

- Other reasons as seen fit by a doctor.

How Does One Prepare for D&C?

Make arrangements at home to take care of daily activities before you leave for the procedure. Ask someone to drive you home after surgery and arrange for a help when you're recovering. You will be informed as to when you need to stop eating before surgery in order to prevent vomiting during surgery. Inform the hospital about any allergies and medications that you are taking. You will not have to take regular medication on the day of surgery. You will be asked to avoid aspirin because it increases risk of bleeding. If you are allergic to local and general anesthetic agents, iodine, latex or tape, volunteer this information in advance. If you are a smoker, you should quit at least 8 weeks before surgery. Surgery leads to complications and healing time is increased in smokers. Follow instructions given to you by doctors and medical staff. Carry a sanitary napkin to wear when leaving for home.

How Is D&C Performed?

The patient is given sedation for relaxation. D&C is usually done under partial anesthesia, but in certain circumstances, at the request of the patient, she may be fully anesthetized. The patient also will be positioned with both legs harnessed onto stirrups. Prior to surgery, the cervix is dilated with a laminaria stick, which is a thick rod that is inserted in the cervix that absorbs fluid and dilates the cervix so that the uterus can be accessed. Medications are used to numb and soften the cervix to aid dilation. A speculum is then placed into the vagina and clamped into place. Once the cervix has dilated to one and a half inch, the surgeon uses a curette to scrape and clean the abnormal tissue from the uterus. Sometimes tissue samples are sent to the laboratory for analysis. The procedure results in cramps similar to menstrual cramps, which are usually controlled by pain medication.

What Are the Risks and Side Effects of D&C?

- You may experience problems with anesthesia such as nausea or vomiting.
- Abdominal pain or cramping.
- Infection or bleeding.
- Perforation of the uterus or bowel and damage to the cervix.
- Scar tissue may develop in the uterus.
- Foul-smelling discharge.
- Fever or chills.
- Inability to get pregnant after surgery.

Enquire with your medical practitioner about the risks applicable to you and other concerns prior to surgery.

What Happens after the Procedure?

The type of recovery varies along with the kind of procedure applied in your case. You will need to recover from anesthesia and be kept under observation initially. Once your blood pressure, pulse, and breathing have returned to normal you will be taken to recovery and then discharged. Have another person drive you home in case you are discharged on the same day. Sufficient rest will be required if you were anesthetized. After surgery, you will experience spotting or slight vaginal bleeding for a few days. Wear a sanitary napkin. You will also experience cramping. You will be advised not to douche or use tampons and engage in sexual intercourse for a short period of time. Restrictions will be placed on intense physical activity such as lifting heavy objects.

What Is the Follow-Up Required after D&C?

The endometrial lining will rebuild in a few days after surgery and regular menstrual periods will commence in due course of time. If you need pain medication, speak to your doctor. Aspirin could increase chances of bleeding and is not advised. Your cervix is under risk of bacterial infection until it is fully healed. Contact the clinic if you suffer from severe abdominal pain, fever, chills, or foul-smelling discharge.

References

1. "Dilation and Curettage (D and C)," The Johns Hopkins University, n.d.

2. "Dilation and Curettage (D&C)," University of Rochester Medical Center, n.d.

3. "Dilation and Curettage (D and C)," The Cleveland Clinic Foundation, n.d.

4. "Dilation and Curettage (D and C)," Memorial Sloan Kettering Cancer Center, April 3, 2017.

Section 27.3

Hysterectomy

This section includes text excerpted from "Hysterectomy," Office on Women's Health (OWH), U.S. Department of Health and Human Services (HHS), April 28, 2017.

A hysterectomy is a surgery to remove a woman's uterus (also known as the womb). The uterus is where a baby grows when a woman is pregnant. During the surgery the whole uterus is usually removed. Your doctor may also remove your fallopian tubes and ovaries. After a hysterectomy, you no longer have menstrual periods and cannot become pregnant.

What Happens during a Hysterectomy?

Hysterectomy is a surgery to remove a woman's uterus (her womb). The whole uterus is usually removed. Your doctor also may remove your fallopian tubes and ovaries.

Talk to your doctor before your surgery to discuss your options. For example, if both ovaries are removed, you will have symptoms of menopause. Ask your doctor about the risks and benefits of removing your ovaries. You may also be able to try an alternative to hysterectomy, such as medicine or another type of treatment, first.

Why Would I Need a Hysterectomy?

You may need a hysterectomy if you have one of the following:

- **Uterine fibroids.** Uterine fibroids are noncancerous growths in the wall of the uterus. In some women they cause pain or heavy bleeding.

- **Heavy or unusual vaginal bleeding.** Changes in hormone levels, infection, cancer, or fibroids can cause heavy, prolonged bleeding.

- **Uterine prolapse.** This is when the uterus slips from its usual place down into the vagina. This is more common in women who had several vaginal births, but it can also happen after menopause or because of obesity. Prolapse can lead to urinary and bowel problems and pelvic pressure.

- **Endometriosis**. Endometriosis happens when the tissue that normally lines the uterus grows outside of the uterus on the ovaries where it doesn't belong. This can cause severe pain and bleeding between periods.

- **Adenomyosis**. In this condition the tissue that lines the uterus grows inside the walls of the uterus where it doesn't belong. The uterine walls thicken and cause severe pain and heavy bleeding.

- **Cancer (or precancer) of the uterus, ovary, cervix, or endometrium (the lining of the uterus).** Hysterectomy may be the best option if you have cancer in one of these areas. Other treatment options may include chemotherapy and radiation. Your doctor will talk with you about the type of cancer you have and how advanced it is.

Keep in mind that there may be alternative ways to treat your health problem without having a hysterectomy. Hysterectomy is a major surgery. Talk with your doctor about all of your treatment options.

How Common Are Hysterectomies?

Each year in the United States, nearly 500,000 women get hysterectomies. A hysterectomy is the second most common surgery among women in the United States. The most common surgery in women is childbirth by cesarean delivery (C-section).

What Are the Different Types of Hysterectomies?

- A **total hysterectomy** removes all of the uterus, including the cervix. The ovaries and the fallopian tubes may or may not be removed. This is the most common type of hysterectomy.

- A **partial,** also called **subtotal** or **supracervical**, hysterectomy removes just the upper part of the uterus. The cervix is left in place. The ovaries may or may not be removed.

- A **radical hysterectomy** removes all of the uterus, cervix, the tissue on both sides of the cervix, and the upper part of the vagina. A radical hysterectomy is most often used to treat certain types of cancer, such as cervical cancer. The fallopian tubes and the ovaries may or may not be removed.

Will the Doctor Remove My Ovaries during the Hysterectomy?

Whether your ovaries are removed during the hysterectomy may depend on the reason for your hysterectomy.

Ovaries may be removed during hysterectomy to lower the risk for ovarian cancer. However, women who have not yet gone through menopause also lose the protection of estrogen, which helps protect women from conditions such as heart disease and osteoporosis.

Recent studies suggest that removing only the fallopian tubes but keeping the ovaries may help lower the risk for the most common type of ovarian cancer, which is believed to start in the fallopian tubes.

The decision to keep or remove your ovaries is one you can make after talking about the risks and benefits with your doctor.

Will the Hysterectomy Cause Me to Enter Menopause?

All women who have a hysterectomy will stop getting their period. Whether you will have other symptoms of menopause after a hysterectomy depends on whether your doctor removes your ovaries during the surgery.

If you keep your ovaries during the hysterectomy, you should not have other menopausal symptoms right away. But you may have symptoms a few years younger than the average age for menopause (52 years).

If both ovaries are removed during the hysterectomy, you will no longer have periods and you may have other menopausal symptoms right away. Because your hormone levels drop quickly without ovaries, your symptoms may be stronger than with natural menopause. Ask your doctor about ways to manage your symptoms.

How Is a Hysterectomy Performed?

A hysterectomy can be done in several different ways. It will depend on your health history and the reason for your surgery.

Talk to your doctor about the different options:

- **Abdominal hysterectomy**. Your doctor makes a cut, usually in your lower abdomen.
- **Vaginal hysterectomy.** This is done through a small cut in the vagina.
- **Laparoscopic hysterectomy.** A laparoscope is an instrument with a thin, lighted tube and a small camera that allows your doctor to see your pelvic organs. Laparoscopic surgery is when the doctor makes very small cuts to put the laparoscope and surgical tools inside of you. During a laparoscopic hysterectomy the uterus is removed through the small cuts made in either your abdomen or your vagina.
- **Robotic surgery.** Your doctor guides a robotic arm to do the surgery through small cuts in your lower abdomen, like a laparoscopic hysterectomy.

How Long Does It Take to Recover from a Hysterectomy?

Recovering from a hysterectomy takes time. Most women stay in the hospital one to two days after surgery. Some doctors may send you home the same day of your surgery. Some women stay in the hospital longer, often when the hysterectomy is done because of cancer.

Your doctor will likely have you get up and move around as soon as possible after your hysterectomy. This includes going to the bathroom on your own. However, you may have to pee through a thin tube called a catheter for one or two days after your surgery.

The time it takes for you to return to normal activities depends on the type of surgery:

- **Abdominal surgery** can take from four to six weeks to recover.

- **Vaginal, laparoscopic, or robotic surgery** can take from three to four weeks to recover.

You should get plenty of rest and not lift heavy objects for four to six weeks after surgery. At that time, you should be able to take tub baths and resume sexual intercourse. How long it takes for you to recover will depend on your surgery and your health before the surgery. Talk to your doctor.

What Changes Can I Expect after a Hysterectomy?

Hysterectomy is a major surgery, so recovery can take a few weeks. But for most women, the biggest change is a better quality of life. You should have relief from the symptoms that made the surgery necessary.

Other changes that you may experience after a hysterectomy include:

- **Menopause.** You will no longer have periods. If your ovaries are removed during the hysterectomy, you may have other menopause symptoms.

- **Change in sexual feelings**. Some women have vaginal dryness or less interest in sex after a hysterectomy, especially if the ovaries are removed.

- **Increased risk for other health problems**. If both ovaries are removed, this may put you at higher risk for certain conditions such as: bone loss, heart disease, and urinary incontinence (leaking of urine). Talk to your doctor about how to prevent these problems.

- **Sense of loss.** Some women may feel grief or depression over the loss of fertility or the change in their bodies. Talk to your doctor if you have symptoms of depression, including feelings of sadness, a loss of interest in food or things you once enjoyed, or less energy, that last longer than a few weeks after your surgery.

Will My Sex Life Change after a Hysterectomy?

It might. If you had a good sex life before your hysterectomy, you should be able to return to it without any problems after recovery. Many women report a better sex life after hysterectomy because of relief from pain or heavy vaginal bleeding.

Part Four

Sexual and Reproductive Concerns

Chapter 28

Understanding Your Sexuality

The World Health Organization (WHO) defines sexual health as a state of physical, emotional, mental, and social well-being in relation to sexuality; it is not merely the absence of disease, dysfunction, or infirmity. Sexual health requires a positive and respectful approach to sexuality and sexual relationships, as well as the possibility of having pleasurable and safe sexual experiences, free of coercion, discrimination, and violence.

Your Sexuality

As you become a young woman, you may face a lot of changing feelings as your body and your mind—and the people around you!—start developing in whole new ways. You may have lots of changing feelings. Puberty can spark some brand-new urges, and you may start having strong feelings for someone you like. You may start thinking more about your sexuality.

What exactly is sexuality? It's about how your reproductive system works, feeling attractive, and being attracted to someone else. But it's also affected by your values, how you feel about your body, and the messages about bodies and behaviors that you get from the world around you.

This chapter contains text excerpted from the following sources: Text in this chapter begins with excerpts from "Sexual Health," Centers for Disease Control and Prevention (CDC), October 4, 2016; Text beginning with the heading "Your Sexuality" is excerpted from "Your Sexuality," girlshealth.gov, Office on Women's Health (OWH), April 15, 2014.

As you think about your sexuality, a great place to start is knowing that you have the right to feel comfortable, to be treated with respect, and to stay healthy and safe in your relationships.

Dating and Sexual Feelings

Thinking about romance, starting to date, and feeling attraction all can be incredibly cool—and a little intense.

As you start dating, think about what you're looking for. A solid relationship comes from being with someone who supports you, trusts you, and appreciates you for who you are. You want someone who deserves you!

As you start thinking about love and sex, don't forget to focus on feeling good about yourself. Take good care of your body. See a doctor if you are having sex.

When it comes to deciding about kissing and more, remember that so much of what you see on TV and hear in songs is not real or healthy. And remember that there are lots of ways to show affection other than sex. Don't do anything that makes you uncomfortable. You'll probably remember these exciting days for many years, and you want to remember them happily!

Talking with Your Partner about Sex

Anyone you're seriously thinking about having sex with should be someone you can talk to about it. Talk about what kind of birth control you would use to protect yourselves from pregnancy and STDs (sexually transmitted diseases, also called sexually transmitted infections).

Are you worried that you'll sound like you're accusing your partner of having an STD? You can focus instead on protecting your health and respecting each other's feelings.

It's a good idea to talk about all this at a time and in a place where you're comfortable and won't be interrupted. It's a great idea to do this while your clothes are still on!

It's Not Too Late to Stop Having Sex

Some people feel like once they've had sex there's no turning back. That's not true. You don't have to feel bad about yourself if you regret having sex. Everybody makes mistakes—that's just part of learning.

But it doesn't make sense to keep doing something that feels wrong to you.

Could I Be Gay?

If you're having feelings of romantic or physical attraction to other girls, you may wonder if you are gay. It's natural as you develop to wonder about these feelings, and it may take time to figure out whether you are attracted to guys, girls, or both. Keep in mind that being attracted to girls is normal. Also, keep in mind that having a gay or lesbian parent or sibling doesn't mean you are gay.

If you're feeling concerned about your sexual orientation, talk to someone you trust. Also, if you're feeling stressed about telling others you're gay or if you're being bullied about being gay, you can get help. If you feel like you are going to hurt yourself, reach out right away to an adult, a friend, or a counselor. Things can get better.

If you are going to have sex with another girl, keep in mind that women who have sex with women are at risk for many of the same STDs as women who have sex with men. Also, if you are a lesbian, it's a good idea to talk to your doctor about protecting your overall health. Lesbians are more likely to have certain health problems, like obesity, smoking, and depression, so make sure you learn how to stay healthy and strong.

Dating Older Guys

If you date someone even a few years older than you, the chances go up that your partner will want to have sex before you feel ready. Also, if you have sex with a man who is legally an adult and you're underage, he could go to jail. Laws for this are different in each state.

Staying Safe When Dating

You should always feel physically and emotionally safe in a dating relationship. Consider some of the advice below to take good care of yourself.

Remember that you deserve to make your own decisions about sex and not feel rushed or pressured. You don't owe anyone sex, whether they pressure you by being nasty or by being nice! Sometimes in an unhealthy relationship a partner may try to get you pregnant even though you're not ready. Remember that it's your body and your future!

When you go out on a date, take your cell phone and cab money with you. That way you can leave if you start to feel uncomfortable.

Sex you don't agree to is rape, whether it's with a stranger or a date. Rape includes forcing a body part or object into your vagina, rectum (bottom), or mouth. If someone forces you to do anything sexually, tell a trusted adult or call the National Sexual Assault Hotline at 800-656-4673 (800-656-HOPE).

To stay safe in a dating situation, it's a good idea to avoid drugs and alcohol. They make it more likely you'll do something you would never otherwise do, like have unprotected sex. And remember that someone can slip a date rape drug into your drink, so keep it with you at all times.

Protect yourself on the Internet and in text messages. You may think "sexting," or sending sexy photos or messages, is private. But messages can be traced back to you, and you can even get in legal trouble for sending or forwarding them. Whatever you send can get passed around and can stay out there forever. If someone dares you to send this kind of message, think about why they're doing it—and what you have to lose!

Treat your body with the respect it deserves—and make sure others do, too!

What about Masturbation?

You may have heard about or tried masturbation (which basically means giving yourself sexual pleasure). There are lots of opinions about masturbation. From a medical point of view, experts say it's almost always not a problem—unless it's interfering with your responsibilities or your social life. Plus, they say, it can be a way to release tension and learn about your body.

Why Waiting to Have Sex Makes Sense

You may hear so many messages suggesting that it's a good idea to have sex, from songs on the radio. You may also feel curious about sex or have a strong attraction to someone.

Deciding to have sex is a big deal, though, so think it through. You could wind up with an unplanned pregnancy. You could also catch an STD.

Having sex before you're ready can seriously hurt your relationship—and your feelings. Few people regret waiting to have sex, but many wish they hadn't started early.

Keep in mind that even if you've already had sex, you can still choose to stop.

Unplanned Pregnancy

Three out of 10 young women in the United States get pregnant before they turn 20. And most teen pregnancies are not planned.

Getting pregnant before you're ready can be a huge shock. The emotional stress and money worries of raising a baby can be a lot even for an older couple. Imagine what your life would be like if you had to get up with a baby in the night and take care of it every day!

Abstinence is the safest way to prevent the challenges that come with pregnancy. Check out some of these facts about teen pregnancy:

- Teen mothers are less likely to finish high school.

- Teen moms are more likely to be—and stay—single parents.

- Babies born to teen moms face greater health risks.

- Teen moms face health risks, too, including possibly being obese later in life.

- Teen moms are at a higher risk of being poor.

- Kids of teen moms are more likely to have problems in school and with the police.

If you do get pregnant, remember that you need to take care of yourself. Be sure to see a doctor.

Sexually Transmitted Diseases (STDs)

STDs are a huge problem among young people.

Consider some reasons that abstinence makes sense in staying safe from STDs:

- One in 4 teen girls has an STD.

- Condoms decrease the risk of STDs, but they are not 100% effective. This is especially true for STDs that can spread just by skin-to-skin contact, such as herpes, which has no cure.

- Having an STD increases your chances of getting HIV, too, and there is no cure for HIV.

- Some STDs have no symptoms, so you can't know if your partner is infected. A partner with no symptoms can still give the STD to you, though.

- Some STDs have no symptoms, so you can't know if you have them, but they can cause serious health problems. These problems include trouble getting pregnant when you are ready to have a baby.

What If I Don't Have "Real" Sex?

Different people may have different definitions of abstinence. Some think it means not having sexual intercourse, but others think it means avoiding other sexual acts, too. Experts say complete abstinence—not having vaginal, oral, and anal sex—is safest. Consider these facts:

- Even if you don't have intercourse but semen (cum) gets in your vagina, there's a chance you could get an STD or get pregnant.

- You can get some STDs from oral sex.

- It's easier to get some STDs from anal sex than from vaginal sex.

Avoiding intimate sexual contact, including skin-to-skin genital contact, is the only sure way to prevent all STDs and pregnancy. If you are having sexual contact, though, it's super-smart to use a condom.

Also keep in mind that acts like oral sex are intimate acts. Try to think about whether you want to do something intimate before you do it. Think about having respect for yourself and having the respect of your partner.

Ways to Stick to Abstinence

It's not always easy to abstain from sex. It can help to make a plan ahead of time and get support from people you trust. You also might keep in mind the reasons you made the choice to be abstinent.

Don't be afraid to take a stand with your partner. If you are close enough with someone to consider having sex, you should be close enough to talk about the decision. If you and your partner can't agree, then you might think about whether you'd be better off with someone whose beliefs are closer to your own.

Your own body may tell you to give up on abstinence. Remember that your body is not in charge! Remind yourself of the possible physical, emotional, and financial costs of having sex before you're really ready.

Consider these tips for staying abstinent:

- **Get involved.** Some people find it helps to get involved in activities that let them focus on something other than sex, like volunteering or joining a sports team.

- **Get together.** When you hang out with your date, it can help to hang out in a group. Also, try not to spend a lot of time in secluded places with no one else around or at someone's house when no adults are home.

- **Get out.** Always take a cell phone and cab or bus money in case you want to get out of an uncomfortable situation.

- **Practice.** Think about how to say "no" ahead of time, so you don't have to come up with replies on the spot.

- **Stay sober.** Drugs and alcohol can make you more likely to do something you otherwise never would.

Deciding about Sex

What Is Sex?

Here are some key points about sex and "fooling around":

- When people say "sex," they usually mean sexual intercourse, or a man putting his penis in a woman's vagina.

- There are other types of sexual contact, like touching a partner's genitals. These also are very personal acts and are worth thinking about in a serious way.

- It's possible to get pregnant if a guy ejaculates ("comes") on the outside of your vagina.

- You can get some STDs from giving or receiving oral sex or from genital-to-genital contact that isn't intercourse. Using a condom can help protect you.

- Above all, don't do anything sexual that doesn't feel right to you!

Ways to Decide If You're Ready for Sex

If you are deciding about sex, you've got a lot to think about. And it makes sense to do your thinking in advance—not when you're swept up in the excitement of the moment.

Think about your values, deepest feelings, and future goals. Remember that having sex with someone is no guarantee that you'll stay together. Not even having a baby together guarantees that. And as much as you care what the other person thinks, it's what you think that really matters!

For young women, not having sex—abstinence—makes good sense. That's partly because your chances of staying safe from unplanned pregnancy and HIV and other STDs are better if you wait. It's also partly because being older can help you handle the strong emotional aspects of sex. Just because your body seems ready doesn't mean that you are!

Questions to Ask Yourself about Sex

Here are some questions you can ask yourself to help decide about sex:

- Do you really feel ready to have sex and not just excited about the idea?

- Do you really trust and feel safe with your partner?

- Are you feeling pressure—from friends, your partner, or even yourself—or is this something that's really right for you?

- Are you doing this because you think everyone else is?

- Do you feel really nervous—not just a little worried but really concerned or scared?

- Can you talk to your partner about preventing pregnancy and STDs?

- Do you know what to do help prevent pregnancy and STDs?

- Do you know what you would do if you got pregnant?

- How would you feel if other people found out you had sex?

Remember, you're in charge of your body and your life!

Birth Control

Birth control (also called contraception) may seem confusing and overwhelming. If you think you're ready to have sex, though, you need to be ready to protect your body and your future. It may be tempting to have sex without birth control, but that can cause serious problems.

Remember, if you feel close enough with someone to have sex, you should feel close enough to discuss birth control—even if it makes you feel a little uncomfortable.

There are lots of possible questions about birth control. It's a good idea to talk with your doctor or nurse, before you have sex.

What Do I Need to Know about Birth Control?

The more you know about birth control, the more you can take charge of protecting yourself. Here are some key points:

- Not having sex—abstinence—is the only sure way to prevent pregnancy or a STD.

- All types of birth control can fail. Some fail more than others, and some work very well. For example, the intrauterine device (IUD) works almost 100% of the time.

- Whatever type of birth control you choose, use it right and every time to be safest.

- If you're not sure how to use your birth control, ask a doctor or nurse. It's worth a little embarrassment to avoid serious problems.

- Male latex condoms (or synthetic ones) are the best protection against STDs. And even they don't fully protect against all STDs.

- It's important to use condoms and another birth control method for both STD protection and pregnancy prevention.

How Does Birth Control Work?

During vaginal sex, the man's penis goes into the woman's vagina, which leads to her reproductive organs, including her uterus, or womb. When the man ejaculates ("comes"), his penis spurts semen, which contains millions of sperm. The sperm swim up into the woman's uterus and fallopian tubes. If a sperm joins with an egg from the woman,

349

she will become pregnant. There's also a chance a woman can get pregnant if her partner's sperm gets on the outside of her vagina and then swims inside.

Most birth control methods work either by preventing the egg from being released or by stopping the sperm from getting to the egg.

Do I Need to See a Doctor to Get Birth Control?

Only condoms, contraceptive sponges, spermicides, and some kinds of emergency contraception are sold in stores like supermarkets and drugstores. All other kinds of birth control require a visit to a health-care professional. Some people get contraception at a family planning clinic, where services are confidential (kept private) and often cost less or are free.

In the United States, most insurance companies have to pay for the whole cost of an appointment to talk to your doctor about birth control and for most types of birth control your doctor prescribes.

If you are having sex, you should see a healthcare professional regularly to protect your health even if you aren't going for birth control.

Why Do Youngsters Sometimes Not Use Birth Control?

There are a number of reasons youngsters sometimes don't use birth control. Check out some common ones and why they don't make good sense.

- **Some young women think they are not likely to get pregnant.** Unfortunately, 4 out of 5 pregnancies among girls 19 and younger are not planned.

- **You might be afraid of what your partner will think.** Anyone worth sharing sex with should be willing to talk about staying safe.

- **Some people think that using a birth control method now will not allow them to get pregnant when they are ready to have a baby.** The truth is that nearly all kinds of birth control stop working right away when you stop using them. And condoms can actually protect your ability to have a baby later by helping to prevent STDs that can hurt your reproductive system.

Whatever the possible reasons to avoid birth control, there are so many more reasons to use it. Women who get pregnant face a huge number of challenges, including possibly having their partner leave them and taking care of a baby's many needs.

What If I Need Birth Control in an Emergency?

Emergency contraception (EC) is birth control used to prevent pregnancy after unprotected sex. Women sometimes seek emergency contraception if they didn't use birth control, if their birth control failed (like if the condom broke), or if they were forced to have sex.

Mainly, emergency contraception works by preventing your body from releasing an egg.

Here's some important information about emergency contraception:

- **Emergency contraception sometimes is called the "morning-after pill."** It really shouldn't be, though. You actually should take it as soon as possible after unprotected sex.

- **Emergency contraception is only for emergencies.** It is not meant as a regular means of birth control.

- **You can get emergency contraception in a hospital emergency room, a family planning clinic, and many drugstores.**

- **There's a chance you can still get pregnant if you use emergency contraception.** If more than seven days pass after you expect to get your period, you should take a pregnancy test.

- **Don't use emergency contraception if you are already pregnant.** If you are already pregnant, EC will not stop or harm your pregnancy.

- **Emergency contraception does not protect against sexually transmitted diseases.**

- **Emergency contraception may not work as well if you are obese.**

There are different types of emergency contraception:

- Plan B One-Step pill and similar generic versions, such as Next Choice One Dose

- You should take Plan B One-Step or generic versions as soon as possible within three days (72 hours) after unprotected sex.

- You do not need a prescription from a doctor or proof of your age to buy these.

- These are on the drugstore shelf. If you don't see them, ask the pharmacist for help.

- Levonorgestrel tablets (two-pill generic Next Choice and LNG tablets 0.75 mg)

- You take the first pill as soon as possible within 3 days (72 hours) after unprotected sex.

- You take the second pill 12 hours later.

- If you are under 17, you need a prescription for these pills.

- Even if you are over 17, you need to ask for them because they are kept behind the pharmacy counter.

- ella

- You take ella as soon as possible within five days (120 hours) after unprotected sex.

- You need a prescription for ella.

What Causes Pregnancy?

Here are some basic facts of (making) life:

Pregnancy happens when a male's sperm joins with (fertilizes) a female's egg.

For you to get pregnant, sperm has to get into your vagina. Sperm can get into your vagina a few different ways.

- **Sperm is in the fluid (sometimes called "ejaculate" or "cum") that spurts out when a guy ejaculates ("comes").** The main way sperm get into the vagina is when a guy ejaculates during sexual intercourse.

- **Sperm also sometimes can get into the vagina in pre-ejaculate ("pre-cum").** This is a little bit of fluid that leaks out during sex before a guy ejaculates. A guy wouldn't know that pre-ejaculate was leaking out. That means you could get pregnant even if he pulls his penis out before he ejaculates.

- **Sperm can get into your vagina even if you're not having sexual intercourse.** This can happen if sperm get on the outside of your vagina and swim inside.

For you to get pregnant, one of your eggs has to be in the right place at the right time. Keep in mind that:

- It's hard to know exactly when an egg is released, which means that avoiding sex at certain times of the month is not a very reliable way to avoid pregnancy.

- You can get pregnant if you don't have regular periods.

- You can even get pregnant during your period!

What Doesn't Cause Pregnancy?

Kissing, hugging, and rubbing clothed bodies don't cause pregnancy. The only time pregnancy can happen is when sperm can get to an egg.

Of course, touching, and other kinds of fooling around are pretty personal, and they definitely can affect your feelings and relationships even if they can't cause pregnancy. Plus, it can be hard to stop before having sex if you're in the heat of the moment. It's a good idea to think in advance about what you want and don't want to do sexually.

You may have heard lots of rumors about ways to have sex to avoid pregnancy. Make sure you have reliable info. For example, you should know that:

- A plastic bag or wrap does not work in place of a condom.

- Jumping up and down after sex does not stop sperm from getting to an egg.

- Using certain positions during sex does not prevent pregnancy.

Understanding the Human Papillomavirus (HPV) Vaccine

HPV, or human papillomavirus, is often passed through sexual contact. Some types of HPV cause genital warts, cervical cancer, and other cancers. A safe and effective vaccine can help protect you against a few types of HPV.

Here are some key points about the HPV vaccine:

- **The HPV vaccine works best if you get it before you are ever exposed to the virus.** That's why it's important to get the vaccine before you ever have sex. Experts recommend that you get it at age 11 or 12. You can even get the vaccine as young as 9.

- **If you missed getting the vaccine when you were 11 or 12, you can still get it.** The vaccine is given as a series of three shots over the course of several months. You need all three shots.

- **The vaccine was tested on tens of thousands of people.** The U.S. Food and Drug Administration (FDA) says it is safe.

- **The vaccine won't protect you against all types of HPV.** It also won't protect against other sexually transmitted diseases or STDs. So even if you get the vaccine, use a latex condom every time you have sex to help stay safe.

- **The vaccine comes under two brand names.** Cervarix helps protect against cervical cancer. Gardasil helps protect against cervical cancer and some types of genital warts.

- **Ask your healthcare professional which one is right for you.**

Chapter 29

Female Sexual Dysfunction

Chapter Contents

Section 29.1

Dyspareunia (Painful Intercourse)

What Is Dyspareunia?

Dyspareunia refers to the pain a woman experiences during or after vaginal intercourse. This condition can affect many aspects of a woman's life, including her relationship with her partner, her physical health, and her emotional wellbeing. Painful sex is a problem that affects women of all ages; however, 25 percent to 45 percent of postmenopausal women find intercourse painful. Dyspareunia can be caused by a range of factors, from physical problems to psychological concerns, most of which can be treated.

Causes of Dyspareunia

There are two main classifications of dyspareunia based on where the pain occurs:

1. Superficial pain (entry pain)

2. Deep dyspareunia (deep pain)

Superficial pain occurs when penetration is attempted and deep dyspareunia is experienced at the top of the vagina while thrusting.

Physical Causes

- **Entry pain** occurs during penetration of the penis into the vagina, and can be caused by a number of factors, including:

  - **Insufficient Lubrication**—Insufficient or lack of lubrication can often be attributed to insufficient foreplay. When a woman is relaxed and sufficiently aroused, the glands around her vagina secrete fluids that reduce friction and allows for penetration without pain. Also, a drop in estrogen levels after menopause and few medications such as antidepressant sedatives, certain birth control pills, and antihistamines also reduce lubrication, causing pain.

- **Vaginismus (spasms)**—When the vaginal muscles spasm, there could be a feeling of tightness that makes entry point penetration extremely difficult and painful.

- **Inflammation or Infection**—Skin problems such as eczema, lichen planus and lichen sclerosus, vulvar vestibulitis (inflammation around the vaginal opening), vaginal yeast infections, urinary tract infections, and sexually transmitted diseases (which may include genital warts, sores, etc.), and other sexually transmitted infections can cause pain during penetration. Allergic reactions to clothing, spermicides, or douches can also make intercourse painful.

- **Injury or Trauma**—Trauma to the genitals or to an area of the body nearby can also be a factor that contributes to pain. Such trauma includes surgery, female circumcision, injury to vulva or the genital area, a cut (episiotomy) in the perineum (area of skin between the vagina and the anus), or a tear from childbirth.

- **Atrophic vaginitis**—This condition refers to a thinning of the vaginal lining that usually occurs in postmenopausal women.

- **Vulvodynia**—Another common condition in premenopausal women that causes discomfort or pain in the vulvar area for no obvious reason. The pain is usually experienced only when the area is touched. Tense pelvic floor muscles also contribute to painful intercourse.

- **Menopause**—When a woman goes through menopause, the normal moisture and thickness of the vaginal lining could be lost, making it thin and dry, which further leads to pain during intercourse.

- **Other Causes**—Congenital abnormalities of the genitals can be an underlying cause of pain during intercourse as well as an ectopic pregnancy, which occurs when an egg develops outside of the uterus. Intercourse can be painful soon after a surgery, childbirth, or while breastfeeding.

- **Deep Pain** occurs when the penis is thrust deeply into the vagina. This abnormal pain can be caused due to several factors. Some of them include:

- Certain illnesses and conditions such as endometriosis
- Irritable bowel syndrome
- Hemorrhoids and ovarian cysts
- Cervix infections
- Retroverted uterus, a condition in which the uterus is tipped toward the back
- Uterine fibroids
- Uterine prolapse or when the uterus slips or sags into the vagina
- Adenomyosis, a condition in which the lining of the uterus grows into the uterine wall
- Interstitial cystitis or painful bladder syndrome

Psychological Causes

Depression, fears about physical appearance, fear about a relationship, anxiety, stress, history of sexual or physical abuse, etc. are all psychological factors that may be responsible for painful intercourse.

Symptoms of Dyspareunia

Most cases of dyspareunia are diagnosed if patient experiences the following symptoms:

- Pain while inserting a tampon
- Pain when the penis penetrates the vagina
- Deep pain while thrusting
- An irritation or burning sensation during intercourse
- Pain immediately after intercourse in the genital area
- Sudden onset of new pain

In most diagnoses, the patient regularly experiences pain during penetration or when inserting a tampon. In some cases, fear of pain over a protracted period of time may indicate the existence of the condition.

To diagnose dyspareunia, a doctor will take a full medical history and complete a physical exam to rule out any other diseases or conditions. The doctor will also likely apply gentle pressure to different areas of the genitals to determine the location, intensity, and possible cause of the pain.

Treatment of Dyspareunia

Treatment of dyspareunia generally focuses on the underlying cause of the pain. Physicians may also prescribe medications that treat nerve and muscular pain, including antidepressants, anticonvulsants, or topical anesthetics to rule out any other causes. In the case of vaginal dryness associated with menopause, estrogen therapy may be recommended. If pain is occurring immediately after childbirth and/or during breastfeeding, it is recommended to avoid intercourse for the first six weeks after delivery.

Pain can also be reduced through desensitization therapy. This usually involves vaginal relaxation exercises and pelvic floor exercises as recommended by the physician.

When sexual pain cannot be traced to any particular reason, sex therapy and counseling are recommended. With internal conflicts, guilt, or memories of bad experiences possibly contributing to painful intercourse, resolving such issues can prove effective in treating the condition. Having open communication with your partner can also help address pain during the intercourse. Changing positions, engaging in longer foreplay, and introducing lubricants can effectively address vaginal dryness as well as the pain associated with deep thrusting.

References

1. "Painful sex (dyspareunia)," Jean Hailes for Women's Health, July 24, 2017.

2. "Painful intercourse (dyspareunia)," Mayo Clinic, January 24, 2015.

3. "Painful Sexual Intercourse (Dyspareunia)," Harvard Health Publications, December 2013.

4. "Sexual Health: Female Pain during Sex," Cleveland Clinic, n.d.

5. "Painful Sex: What You Need to Know," Healthy Women, n.d.

6. Gordon, Stephanie. "When Sex Hurts," Healthy Women, n.d.

Section 29.2

Hypoactive Sexual Desire Disorder

"Hypoactive Sexual Desire Disorder,"
© 2018 Omnigraphics. Reviewed August 2017.

Hypoactive sexual desire disorder (HSDD) is a condition characterized by a sustained lack of interest in sex. Considered one of the most common sexual disorders that affect women of all ages—research suggests that 1 out of 10 women have experienced this condition. HSDD can affect various aspects of a woman's life, including her relationship with her partner, her quality of life, and her emotional well-being. HSDD can be caused by a range of factors such as beliefs, lifestyle, current relationship, intimacy with her partner, and her physical and emotional well-being. HSDD is a treatable condition.

Causes

Causes of HSDD include:

Physical Causes

- Conditions such as cancer, arthritis, heart disease, neurological diseases, and diabetes
- Certain medications such as antidepressants, antipsychotics, birth control pills, beta-blockers, and opioids
- A substantial decrease of estrogen and testosterone hormone levels
- Menopause and hormonal changes during and after pregnancy

Psychological and Emotional Causes

- Psychological factors such as depression, mental health issues, anxiety, and a low self-esteem
- A history of sexual or physical abuse

- Stress caused by the demands of work and family life

- Feelings of anger, distrust, or fear regarding a partner or spouse

- Lack of an emotional bond with a partner or spouse

Diagnosis

No diagnostic test exists for HSDD. Instead, physicians must take into account the level of distress experienced by the patient, her medical and personal history, the health of her relationship with her partner, and other factors. The doctor may also use a diagnostic tool, the Decreased Sexual Desire Screener (DSDS), a simple questionnaire intended to help screen for the condition. Finally, to determine if there is a physical cause, a doctor will conduct a physical examination of the pelvic and genital areas and a complete medical history.

Treatment

When HSDD is due to an underlying medical condition, physicians will focus on treating that condition. For example, he or she may prescribe estrogen in pill or cream form for women with low levels of the hormone. If the condition is the result of a drug side effect, patients may be given an alternative or told to stop the medication all together. In some cases, doctors may prescribe Flibanserin (Addyi), a drug approved by the U.S. Food and Drug Administration (FDA) to enhance female sexual desire. Flibanserin works by altering the chemistry of certain neurotransmitters in the brain that control sexual desire.

For non-physical causes, individual and couples' counseling is recommended. Psychotherapy can help treat previously undiagnosed mental health issues, such as depression, and can help women overcome serious emotional issues, such as memories of previous sexual trauma. Sex therapists can help patients understand their own sexuality and how to best communicate their sexual needs to their partner. Couples therapy is recommended when the underlying cause can be traced to issues in a patient's relationship with her partner or spouse. Learning how to communicate, resolve conflicts, and build trust can help partners achieve a healthier and more positive sexual relationship.

References

1. "Conditions: HSDD," Sex Health Matters, n.d.

2. "Female Sexual Health," International Society for Sexual Medicine (ISSM), n.d.

3. Kingsberg, Sheryl A. "Hypoactive Sexual Desire Disorder: Understanding the Impact on Midlife Women," The North American Menopause Society (NAMS), March 2011.

4. Lynn B Hook, Debra. "What Is Hypoactive Sexual Desire Disorder?" Everyday Health, April 27, 2010.

Section 29.3

Female Orgasmic Disorder

"Female Orgasmic Disorder," © 2018 Omnigraphics.
Reviewed August 2017.

Female orgasmic disorder (FOD) is a condition in which a woman either cannot reach orgasm or has difficulty achieving an orgasm when sexually aroused. In cases of FOD, a woman either has no orgasm at all or has an orgasm of significantly less intensity during most or all sexual encounters. FOD is divided into two categories:

1. Primary FOD. The patient has never had an orgasm.

2. Secondary FOD. The patient has experienced orgasms in the past but has stopped having them.

Researchers have estimated that 16–28 percent of women in the United States suffer from FOD, making it the second most common sexual dysfunction. FOD can refer to both a general failure to achieve orgasm or to difficulty in achieving orgasm in relationship to specific types of stimulation, situations, and partners.

Symptoms

Symptoms include difficulty in climaxing during a sexual interaction, reduced intensity of an orgasm, or complete failure to have an orgasm despite being fully aroused. This is usually accompanied with anxiety, conflicts in relationships, or shame. Women who experience FOD can see sex as a mundane activity rather than a pleasurable one, leading to an increasing disinterest in sex and a decline in the frequency of intercourse. Women may also experience resentment and conflict with their partner as a result of FOD.

Causes

Both physical and mental health issues contribute to orgasmic dysfunction. Apart from this, sociocultural factors and relationship issues can also play a role. Below are some of the causes of FOD:

Physical Causes

- Diabetes
- Spinal cord injuries
- Pelvic disorders
- Traumatic pelvic injuries
- Cardiovascular disease
- Vulvodynia
- Conditions that affect nerve supply to the pelvis
- Multiple sclerosis
- Hormone disorders
- Chronic illnesses that inhibit sexual desire
- Certain prescription drugs such as antipsychotics, cancer treatment drugs, and some medicines given for heart disease
- Antidepressants such as Fluoxetine (Prozac), Paroxetine (Paxil), and Sertraline (Zoloft)

Mental and Sociocultural Causes

- History of sexual abuse and rape
- Negative attitude toward sex learned in childhood
- Anxiety regarding achieving an orgasm
- Shameful thoughts brought on by cultural and religious messages that reinforce negative views of female sexuality and pleasure

Relationship Issues

- Lack of sufficient stimulation by the partner

- Boredom

- Inexperience or lack of knowledge regarding sexual intercourse

- Lack of emotional connection with the partner

- Feeling resentful, angry, or fearful about the partner

- Shyness about discussing what preferred types of sexual stimulation

Diagnosis and Treatment

A woman exhibiting symptoms for a period of at least 6 months may have to be diagnosed with FOD. For a diagnosis, a physician will take a medical history and complete a physical examination with the goal of understanding the underlying cause of the condition and if it co-occurs with other sexual dysfunction (such as pain during sex).

If the condition is due to a treatable physical condition, the healthcare provider may prescribe medications or other protocols to address the problem. If the cause is a side effect of prescription medication being taken by the patient, the provider will recommend alternatives or discontinuing the drug all together if possible.

When FOD happens due to psychological issues such as a history of sexual abuse, undiagnosed anxiety or depression, or a fear of sex associated with childhood, then treatment may involve psychotherapy or cognitive behavioral therapy (CBT). In some cases, desensitization can bring a gradual end to FOD and relieve sexual anxiety. Therapists may also find it necessary to explain the importance of nonsexual touch.

Sex therapy is a common approach to cases of FOD that do not have a physical cause. The therapist may spend time teaching the patient the process of arousal and climaxing as well as what types of stimulation works best for that individual. Therapist will often focus on clitoral stimulation, which most women require for climax, and how it can be incorporated into sexual activity with the partner. Or the therapist may recommend teach the woman to masturbate in order to better understand how she becomes sexually aroused.

When relationship issues are the cause of the problem, couples therapy can be recommended. Learning how to communicate, resolve conflicts, and build trust can help partners achieve a healthier and more positive sexual relationship. Studies have shown that women have a higher rate of achieving orgasm if they are in an emotionally healthy and loving relationship.

Prevention

The following are some of the ways to prevent this disorder:

- Understand that every person is responsible for their own sexual fulfilment.

- Spend some time on finding out what sexual technique and type of stimulation suit you the best.

- Be relaxed. Anxiety and pressure to have an orgasm can themselves prove to be detrimental to your desire to have one.

- Work towards a healthy and loving relationship with your partner.

- Focus on developing verbal and nonverbal communication skills to guide your partner during intercourse.

- Work on overcoming embarrassments to talk openly about sex with your partner.

- Develop a healthy attitude towards sex.

References

1. "Orgasmic Dysfunction," Health Medicine Network, April 5, 2012.

2. "What Is Female Orgasmic Disorder (FOD)?" International Society for Sexual Medicine (ISSM), n.d.

3. "Orgasmic Disorder," GoodTherapy.org, August 17, 2015.

4. "Orgasmic Disorder," Psychology Today, March 30, 2017.

Chapter 30

Birth Control

Chapter Contents

Section 30.1

Birth Control Methods and Effectiveness

This section includes text excerpted from "Birth Control
Methods," Office on Women's Health (OWH), U.S. Department
of Health and Human Services (HHS), April 24, 2017.

Birth control (contraception) is any method, medicine, or device
used to prevent pregnancy. Women can choose from many different
types of birth control. Some work better than others at preventing
pregnancy. The type of birth control you use depends on your health,
your desire to have children now or in the future, and your need to
prevent sexually transmitted infections. Your doctor can help you
decide which type is best for you right now.

What Is the Best Method of Birth Control?

There is no "best" method of birth control for every woman. The
birth control method that is right for you and your partner depends
on many things, and may change over time.

Before choosing a birth control method, talk to your doctor or nurse
about:

- whether you want to get pregnant soon, in a few years, or never

- how well each method works to prevent pregnancy

- possible side effects

- how often you have sex

- the number of sex partners you have

- your overall health

- how comfortable you are with using the method (For example,
  can you remember to take a pill every day? Will you have to ask
  your partner to put on a condom each time?)

Keep in mind that even the most effective birth control methods
can fail. But your chances of getting pregnant are lower if you use a
more effective method.

What Are the Different Types of Birth Control?

Women can choose from many different types of birth control methods. These include, in order of most effective to least effective at preventing pregnancy:

- **Female and male sterilization** (female tubal ligation or occlusion, male vasectomy)—Birth control that prevents pregnancy for the rest of your life through surgery or a medical procedure.

- **Long-acting reversible contraceptives or "LARC" methods** (intrauterine devices, hormonal implants)—Birth control your doctor inserts one time and you do not have to remember to use birth control every day or month. LARCs last for 3 to 10 years, depending on the method.

- **Short-acting hormonal methods** (pill, mini pills, patch, shot, vaginal ring)—Birth control your doctor prescribes that you remember to take every day or month. The shot requires you to get a shot from your doctor every 3 months.

- **Barrier methods** (condoms, diaphragms, sponge, cervical cap)—Birth control you use each time you have sex.

- **Natural rhythm methods**—Not using a type of birth control but instead avoiding sex and/or using birth control only on the days when you are most fertile (most likely to get pregnant). An ovulation home test kit or a fertility monitor can help you find your most fertile days.

Table 30.1. Types of Birth Control

Method	Number of Pregnancies Per 100 Women Within Their First Year of Typical Use	Side Effects and Risks*	How Often You Have to Take or Use
Abstinence (no sexual contact)	Unknown (0 for perfect use)	No medical side effects	No action required, but it does take willpower. You may want to have a back-up birth control method, such as condoms.
Permanent sterilization surgery for women (tubal ligation, "getting your tubes tied")	Less than 1	• Possible pain during recovery (up to 2 weeks) • Bleeding or other complications from surgery • Less common risk includes ectopic (tubal) pregnancy	No action required after surgery
Permanent sterilization implant for women (Essure®)	Less than 1	• Pain during the insertion of Essure; some pain during recovery • Cramping, vaginal bleeding, back pain during recovery • Implant may move out of place • Less common but serious risk includes ectopic (tubal) pregnancy	No action required after surgery

Table 30.1. Continued

Method	Number of Pregnancies Per 100 Women Within Their First Year of Typical Use	Side Effects and Risks*	How Often You Have to Take or Use
Implantable rod (Implanon®, Nexplanon®)	Less than 1	• Headache • Irregular periods • Weight gain • Sore breasts • Less common risk includes difficulty in removing the implant	No action required for up to 3 years before removing or replacing
Copper intrauterine device (IUD) (ParaGard®)	Less than 1	• Cramps for a few days after insertion • Missed periods, bleeding between periods, heavier periods • Less common but serious risks include pelvic inflammatory disease and the IUD being expelled from the uterus or going through the wall of the uterus.	No action required for up to 10 years before removing or replacing
Hormonal intrauterine devices (IUDs) (Liletta, Mirena®, and Skyla®)	Less than 1	• Irregular periods, lighter or missed periods • Ovarian cysts • Less common but serious risks include pelvic inflammatory disease and the IUD being expelled from the uterus or going through the wall of the uterus.	No action required for 3 to 5 years, depending on the brand, before removing or replacing

Table 30.1. Continued

Method	Number of Pregnancies Per 100 Women Within Their First Year of Typical Use	Side Effects and Risks*	How Often You Have to Take or Use
Shot/injection (Depo-Provera®)	6	• Bleeding between periods, missed periods • Weight gain • Changes in mood • Sore breasts • Headaches • Bone loss with long-term use (bone loss may be reversible once you stop using this type of birth control)	Get a new shot every 3 months
Oral contraceptives, combination hormones ("the pill")	9	• Headache • Upset stomach • Sore breasts • Changes in your period • Changes in mood • Weight gain • High blood pressure • Less common but serious risks include blood clots, stroke and heart attack; the risk is higher in smokers and women older than 35	Take at the same time every day

Table 30.1. Continued

Method	Number of Pregnancies Per 100 Women Within Their First Year of Typical Use	Side Effects and Risks*	How Often You Have to Take or Use
Oral contraceptives, progestin-only pill ("mini-pill")	9	• Spotting or bleeding between periods • Weight gain • Sore breasts • Headache • Nausea	Take at the same time every day
Skin patch (Xulane®)	9 May be less effective in women weighing 198 pounds or more	• Skin irritation • Upset stomach • Changes in your period • Changes in mood • Sore breasts • Headache • Weight gain • High blood pressure • Less common but serious risks include blood clots, stroke and heart attack; the risk is higher in smokers and women older than 35	Wear for 21 days, remove for 7 days, replace with a new patch

Table 30.1. Continued

Method	Number of Pregnancies Per 100 Women Within Their First Year of Typical Use	Side Effects and Risks*	How Often You Have to Take or Use
Vaginal ring (NuvaRing®)	9	• Headache • Upset stomach • Sore breasts • Vaginal irritation and discharge • Changes in your period • High blood pressure • Less common but serious risks include blood clots, stroke and heart attack; the risk is higher in smokers and women older than 35	Wear for 21 days, remove for 7 days, replace with a new ring
Diaphragm with spermicide (Koromex®, Ortho-Diaphragm®)	12 If you gain or lose than 15 pounds, or have a baby, have your doctor check you to make sure the diaphragm still fits.	• Irritation • Allergic reactions • Urinary tract infection (UTI) • Vaginal infections • Rarely, toxic shock if left in for more than 24 hours • Using a spermicide often might increase your risk of getting HIV	Insert each time you have sex

Table 30.1. Continued

Method	Number of Pregnancies Per 100 Women Within Their First Year of Typical Use	Side Effects and Risks*	How Often You Have to Take or Use
Sponge with spermicide (Today Sponge®)	12 (among women who have never given birth before) or 24 (among women who have given birth)	• Irritation • Allergic reactions • Rarely, toxic shock if left in for more than 24 hours • Using a spermicide often might increase your risk of getting HIV	Insert each time you have sex
Cervical cap with spermicide (FemCap®)	23	• Vaginal irritation or odor • Urinary tract infections (UTIs) • Allergic reactions • Rarely, toxic shock if left in for more than 48 hours • Using a spermicide often might increase your risk of getting HIV	Insert each time you have sex
Female condom	21	• Irritation • Condom may tear or slip out • Allergic reaction	Use each time you have sex
Natural family planning (rhythm method)	24	• Can be hard to know the days you are most fertile (when you need to avoid having sex or use back-up birth control)	Depending on method used, takes planning each month
Spermicide alone	28 Works best if used along with a barrier method, such as a diaphragm	• Irritation • Allergic reactions • Urinary tract infection • Frequent use of a spermicide might increase your risk of getting HIV	Use each time you have sex

* These are not all of the possible side effects and risks. Talk to your doctor or nurse for more information.

Which Types of Birth Control Can I Get without a Prescription?

You can buy these types of birth control over-the-counter at a drugstore or supermarket:

- Male condoms

- Female condoms

- Sponges

- Spermicides

- Emergency contraception (EC) pills. Plan B One-Step® and its generic versions are available in drugstores and some supermarkets to anyone, without a prescription. However you should not use EC as your regular birth control because it does not work as well as regular birth control. EC is meant to be used only when your regular birth control does not work for some unexpected reason.

Which Types of Birth Control Do I Have to See My Doctor to Get?

You need a prescription for these types of birth control:

- Oral contraceptives: the pill and the mini-pill (in some states, birth control pills are now available without a prescription, through the pharmacy)

- Patch

- Vaginal ring

- Diaphragms (your doctor or nurse needs to fit one to the shape of your vagina)

- Shot/injection (you get the shot at your doctor's office or family planning clinic)

- Cervical cap

- Implantable rod (inserted by a doctor in the office or clinic)

- IUD (inserted by a doctor in the office or clinic)

You will need surgery or a medical procedure for:

- Female sterilization (tubal ligation)

- Male sterilization (vasectomy)
- Tubal implant (Essure®)

How Can I Get Free or Low-Cost Birth Control?

Under the Affordable Care Act (ACA) [the healthcare law], most insurance plans cover U.S. Food and Drug Administration (FDA)-approved prescription birth control for women, such as the pill, IUDs, and female sterilization, at no additional cost to you. This also includes birth control counseling.

- If you have insurance, check with your insurance provider to find out what is included in your plan.

- If you have Medicaid, your insurance covers birth control. This includes birth control prescriptions and visits to your doctor related to birth control. Programs vary between states, so check with your state's Medicaid program (www.medicaid.gov/medicaid/by-state/by-state.html) to learn what your benefits are.

- If you don't have insurance, don't panic. Family planning (reproductive health) clinics may provide some birth control methods for free or at low cost.

How Does Birth Control Work?

Birth control works to prevent pregnancy in different ways, depending upon the type of birth control you choose:

- **Female or male sterilization surgery** prevents the sperm from reaching the egg by cutting or damaging the tubes that carry sperm (in men) or eggs (in women).

- **Long-acting reversible contraceptives or "LARC" methods** (intrauterine devices, hormonal implants) prevent your ovaries from releasing eggs, prevent sperm from getting to the egg, or make implantation of the egg in the uterus (womb) unlikely.

- **Short-acting hormonal methods,** such as the pill, mini-pill, patch, shot, and vaginal ring, prevent your ovaries from releasing eggs or prevent sperm from getting to the egg.

- **Barrier methods,** such as condoms, diaphragms, sponge, cervical cap, prevent sperm from getting to the egg.

- **Natural rhythm methods** involve avoiding sex or using other forms of birth control on the days when you are most fertile (most likely to get pregnant).

Which Types of Birth Control Help Prevent Sexually Transmitted Infections (STIs)?

Only two types can protect you from STIs, including human immunodeficiency virus (HIV): male condoms and female condoms.

While condoms are the best way to prevent STIs if you have sex, they are not the most effective type of birth control. If you have sex, the best way to prevent both STIs and pregnancy is to use what is called "dual protection." Dual protection means you use a condom to prevent STIs each time you have sex, and at the same time, you use a more effective form of birth control, such as an intrauterine device (IUD), implant, or shot.

Are Birth Control Pills Safe?

Yes, hormonal birth control methods, such as the pill, are safe for most women. Today's birth control pills have lower doses of hormones than in the past. This has lowered the risk of side effects and serious health problems.

Today's birth control pills can have health benefits for some women, such as a lower risk of some kinds of cancer. Also, different brands and types of birth control pills (and other forms of hormonal birth control) can increase your risk for some health problems and side effects. Side effects can include weight gain, headaches, irregular bleeding, breast tenderness, and mood changes.

Talk to your doctor about whether hormonal birth control is right for you.

Does Birth Control Raise My Risk for Health Problems?

It can, depending on your health and the type of birth control you use. Talk to your doctor to find the birth control method that is right for you.

Different forms of birth control have different health risks and side effects. Some birth control methods that increase your risk for health problems include:

- **Hormonal birth control.** Combination birth control pills (birth control with both estrogen and progesterone) and some other forms of hormonal birth control, such as the vaginal ring or skin patch, may raise your risk for blood clots and high blood pressure. Blood clots and high blood pressure can cause a heart attack or stroke. A blood clot in the legs can also go to your lungs, causing serious damage or even death. These are serious side effects of hormonal birth control, but they are rare.

- **Spermicides (used alone or with the cervical cap, diaphragm or sponge).** Spermicides that have nonoxynol-9 can irritate the vagina. This can raise your risk for getting HIV. Use spermicides with nonoxynol-9 only if you are in a monogamous relationship (you have sex only with each other) with a man you know is HIV-negative. Also, medicines for vaginal yeast infections may make spermicides less effective.

- **IUDs.** IUDs can slightly raise your risk of an ectopic pregnancy. Ectopic pregnancies happen when a fertilized egg implants somewhere outside of the uterus (womb), usually in one of the fallopian tubes. An ectopic pregnancy is a serious medical problem that should be treated as soon as possible. IUDs also have a very rare but serious risk of infection or puncture of the uterus.

What Do I Do If I Miss a Day Taking the Pill?

Follow the instructions that came with your birth control about using back-up birth control (such as a condom and spermicide). You also can follow these recommendations from the Centers for Disease Control and Prevention (CDC).

If you are late or miss a day taking your pill:

- Take the late or missed pill as soon as possible.

- Continue taking the rest of your pills at your normal time, even if it means taking two pills on the same day.

- You do not need other forms of birth control, such as a condom, unless you need to protect against STIs.

If you miss two or more days in a row:

- Take only the most recent missed pill as soon as possible.

- Continue taking the rest of your pills at your normal time, even if it means taking two pills on the same day.

- Use back-up birth control, such as a condom and spermicide, or do not have sex until you have taken a pill for seven days in a row.

- If you missed pills during days in the last week of active pills (days 15–21 for 28-day pill packs), start a new pack the next day. If you are not able to start a new pack right away, use back-up birth control or avoid sex until hormone pills from a new pack have been taken for 7 days in a row.

- Consider emergency contraception if you missed pills during the first week and had sex.

Talk to your doctor if you continue to miss taking your birth control pill or find it hard to take the pill at the same time each day. You may want to consider a different type of birth control, such as an IUD, an implant, shot, ring, or patch that you don't have to remember to take every day.

Section 30.2

Emergency Contraception

This section includes text excerpted from "Emergency Contraception," Office on Women's Health (OWH), U.S. Department of Health and Human Services (HHS), February 6, 2017.

Emergency contraception can help keep you from getting pregnant if you had sex without using birth control or if your birth control method did not work. There are two types of U.S. Food and Drug Administration (FDA) approved emergency contraceptive pills (ECP's). Some ECPs can work when taken within five days of unprotected sex or when your birth control does not work correctly. Some ECPs are available without a prescription.

What Is Emergency Contraception?

Emergency contraception is a method of birth control you can use if you had sex without using birth control or if your birth control method did not work correctly. You must use emergency contraception as soon as possible after unprotected sex.

Emergency contraception pills are different from the abortion pill. If you are already pregnant, emergency contraception pills do not stop or harm your pregnancy. Emergency contraception has also been called the "morning-after pill," but you do not need to wait until the morning after unprotected sex to take it.

Emergency contraception is not meant to be used for regular birth control. Talk to your doctor or nurse about regular birth control to help prevent pregnancy. Nearly half of all pregnancies in the United States are unplanned.

What Types of Emergency Contraception Pills Are Available?

In the United States, there are two types of FDA-approved ECPs available for emergency contraception:

- **ella®** (ulipristal acetate)

- **Plan B One-Step®** (LNG-only)—Plan B One-Step® has several generic versions. Some common generic versions include After-Pill™, My Way®, Next Choice One Dose™, and Take Action™.

How Do Emergency Contraception Pills Prevent Pregnancy?

Research shows that emergency contraception pills work mostly by preventing or delaying ovulation (the release of an egg from the ovary). Less commonly, emergency contraception may prevent fertilization of the egg by the sperm if ovulation has already happened. If a fertilized egg has already implanted in your uterus (you are pregnant), emergency contraception pills will not stop or harm your pregnancy.

When Should I Think about Using Emergency Contraception?

Consider using emergency contraception if you had sex and:

- You didn't use birth control

- You think your birth control didn't work

Consider asking your doctor for a prescription for emergency contraception pills, or having some type of emergency contraception pill already at home or with you in case you need it.

381

How Do I Get Emergency Contraception?

It depends on the type of emergency contraception you need.

- **Plan B One-Step®** and similar generic versions are available in stores without a prescription to anyone, of any age. If you do not see it on the shelf, ask the pharmacist for help.

- **Levonorgestrel tablets** (two-pill generic Next Choice® and LNG tablets 0.75 mg) are available to people aged 17 and older without a prescription. These brands are sold from behind the pharmacy counter.

- **ella®** is available only by prescription from your doctor, nurse, or family planning clinic.

How Quickly Should I Use Emergency Contraception after Unprotected Sex?

Emergency contraception works best when you use it as soon as possible after unprotected sex. If you are unable to take it right away, emergency contraception can still work to prevent pregnancy if taken up to three to five days after unprotected sex. How long after depends on which type of emergency contraception you use.

- Take Plan B One-Step® or a generic version as soon as possible within three days (or 72 hours) after unprotected sex.

- For the two-dose version (Next Choice®, LNG tablets 0.75 mg), take one pill as soon as possible within 3 days and the second pill 12 hours later.

- Take ella® (ulipristal acetate) as soon as possible within five days (or 120 hours) after unprotected sex.

Does Emergency Contraception Have Side Effects?

Yes, but the side effects are rarely serious. Side effects differ for each woman and may include:

- Headache
- Abdominal pain
- Tiredness (fatigue)

- Dizziness

- Nausea

- Breast pain

The side effects are usually mild and do not last long. Your next period may come early or late, and you may have spotting (light bleeding that happens between menstrual periods).

Does Body Weight Affect How Well Emergency Contraception Works for Women?

Maybe. Research from the Centers for Disease Control and Prevention (CDC) shows that ECPs may not prevent pregnancy as often for obese women (with a body mass index, or BMI, of 30 or greater) as for women who are not obese.

If your BMI is greater than 30, talk to your doctor or nurse about your risk and your options for emergency contraception.

How Can I Get Free or Low-Cost Emergency Contraception?

Under the Affordable Care Act (the healthcare law), most insurance plans cover FDA-approved prescriptions for emergency contraception and birth control at no cost to you. This includes Plan B One-Step® and ella®. Since you can buy Plan B One-Step® or the generic version in a store, without a prescription, call your insurance company to find out if your plan covers over-the-counter emergency contraception. You may need to get a prescription from your doctor if you want your insurance plan to pay for it.

- If you have insurance, check with your insurance provider to find out what's included in your plan.

- If you have Medicaid, your insurance may cover emergency contraception. Coverage varies between states, so check with your state's Medicaid program to learn about your benefits.

- If you don't have insurance, find a family planning clinic in your area. They may provide emergency contraception for free or at low cost.

Can I Get Emergency Contraception Pills before I Need Them?

Yes. Your doctor can give you a prescription to fill so you can have emergency contraception at home to use when you need it. Or, you can buy some types of emergency contraception pills from a store at any time.

Can I Use Emergency Contraception as My Regular Form of Birth Control?

No. Do not use Plan B One-Step® (or a generic version) or ella® as your regular birth control. Most other types of FDA-approved birth control, when used correctly, are much better at preventing pregnancy than emergency contraception pills and usually cost less. Also, while emergency contraception pills are safe for emergency use, they have not been tested as regular birth control and are not approved by the FDA for this purpose.

Women who are sexually active will need to use birth control to prevent pregnancy. What type of regular birth control you can use right away depends on the type of emergency contraception you take.

- If you take **ella®**, do not use hormonal birth control (the pill, patch, vaginal ring, or intrauterine device) for at least five days after you take ella. Using them together may cause ella® not to work. Instead, use a condom, diaphragm, sponge, or cervical cap until you get your next period.10

- If you take **Plan B One-Step®** (or a generic version), you can start right away or continue using a regular form of birth control.

Will Emergency Contraception Pills Affect My next Period?

Maybe. After you take an emergency contraception pill, your next period may come sooner or later than normal. Most women will get their period within a week of the expected date. Your period also may be heavier, lighter, spotty, and more or less painful than is normal for you.

If you do not get your period more than one week after expected or if you think you might be pregnant after taking emergency contraception pills, take a pregnancy test to find out for sure.

Chapter 31

Abortion

Chapter Contents

Section 31.1

Medical Abortion Procedures

The term "abortion" means any medical treatment intended to remove the embryo or fetus and placenta from the uterus. Also called induced termination of pregnancy, abortion can be performed with medication or surgery. A medical abortion is a non-surgical treatment that uses pharmaceutical abortifacients (medicines that induce abortion) to terminate pregnancy. Generally, a medical abortion is performed up to about 9 weeks of gestation. The procedure is done by a licensed abortion provider and can be performed in an outpatient setting. For the most part, the method chosen to induce abortion depends on the stage of pregnancy, patient needs, and policies of the healthcare facility where the treatment is sought.

Medical Abortion Regimens

Three of the most widely used protocols for drug-induced abortion include:

1. **Mifepristone**: Also known as "Mifeprex" or "RU-486," Mifepristone is a synthetic steroid that works by blocking progesterone, the hormone responsible for sustaining pregnancy. It causes the uterine lining to shed and initiates uterine contractions. Mifepristone can be used alone or in conjunction with other medicines to induce abortion.

2. **Misoprostol**: A hormone-like substance that can induce uterine contractions and cervical effacement (thinning of the cervix in preparation for labor), this drug is commonly used for second trimester (13–27 weeks) abortions. Sold under the brand name Cytotec, misoprostol is more effective when used in combination with other abortion-inducing drugs, such as methotrexate or mifepristone. The route of administration of

misoprostol may be oral, sublingual (under the tongue), buccal (between gum and cheek), or intravaginal (inside the vagina).

3. **Methotrexate (MTX)**: Also used to treat some cancers as part of chemotherapy, this works by interfering with cell division and preventing implantation of embryo to the uterine wall. It is particularly effective in terminating early pregnancies and is usually used in conjunction with Misoprostol.

A typical treatment schedule involves:

- Laboratory tests, pelvic examination, and sometimes, an ultrasound to determine the stage of pregnancy.

- Mifepristone or a combination of abortifacient drugs is administered orally at the clinic or at home to end the pregnancy.

- Two to four days later Misoprostol is administered orally or as a vaginal suppository.

- A follow up visit to the clinic after a week and a second ultrasound scan to determine if the abortion is complete.

How It Works

Cramping and vaginal bleeding caused by uterine contractions are the first signs of a medical abortion. These symptoms are more severe than the cramps normally associated with menstruation and usually start within a few hours of administering Misoprostol. It is also normal to pass small to large blood clots in the first few days. Vaginal bleeding usually lasts 2–3 weeks following a medical abortion, after which it tapers off and eventually stops. Some women may also notice the passage of tissue (products of conception) together with the vaginal discharge. Most pregnancies end within 24 hours after taking Misoprostol. In some cases, however, these symptoms may be delayed by a few days. Most women may require heating pads and analgesics for pain relief.

If It Fails

About three percent of medical abortions may fail and the pregnancy may continue. A second dose of Misoprostol or surgical intervention (aspiration or dilation and curettage [D&C]) may be required to terminate the pregnancy. Misoprostol has been linked to birth defects when given in early pregnancy. Therefore, a failed medical abortion is almost always followed up with surgical abortion.

Side Effects

While some women have little or no medication side effects, others may experience pelvic pain, nausea, vomiting, diarrhea, headache, dizziness, fever, or chills. Medical abortion is fairly safe as there is minimal risk of bleeding and infection, and studies have shown no significant long-term risks associated with medical abortion. If heavy bleeding, fever, and abdominal pain persist beyond 24 hours after taking medication, a woman should contact her healthcare provider or go to a hospital emergency room immediately.

Contraindications for Medical Abortion

Medical abortions are not recommended for women with ectopic pregnancy, hemorrhagic disorders, chronic renal disease, or seizures. Further, abortion medications have to be used with caution in women with a history of heart disease, severe anemia, and chronic asthma. It is also important to provide your healthcare professional with information regarding any previous allergy to abortion medication. Certain prescription and nonprescription medications such as steroids, herbal supplements, and vitamins may interact with abortion medication and cause side effects. If an intrauterine device (IUD) is being used, it has to be removed before administering abortion medications.

References

1. "Medication Guide," U.S. Food and Drug Administration (FDA), March 2016.

2. "Clinical Care for Women Undergoing Abortion," National Center for Biotechnology Information (NCBI), 2012.

3. "Medical Abortion Using Mifepristone and Misoprostol," Michigan.Gov, n.d.

Section 31.2

Surgical Abortion Procedures

Surgical abortion is an invasive procedure to end a pregnancy and involves surgically removing the fetus and placenta from the uterus. There are different procedures by which a surgical abortion can be performed and the choice depends, by and large, on the stage of pregnancy and any other health issues that may require consideration.

Surgical abortion may use any one of the following protocols:

- Vacuum aspiration
- Dilation and Curettage (D&C)
- Dilation and Evacuation (D&E)
- Dilation and Extraction (D&X)

Vacuum Aspiration

Also known as suction aspiration, this is the quickest, simplest, and safest procedure for surgical abortion, and is commonly performed when the gestation period is less than 12 weeks. Most vacuum aspirations are performed under local anesthesia and require not more than 10–15 minutes. The procedure is done in an outpatient setting: either in a hospital or an abortion clinic. As with any abortion procedure, confirming the pregnancy with laboratory tests and ultrasound scan is the first step prior to a vacuum aspiration. A vacuum aspiration can be used either as a stand-alone procedure for ending early pregnancies or in combination with dilation and evacuation for more advanced pregnancies.

The procedure involves two steps:

Dilation: The cervix (opening of the uterus) is dilated by administering oral or intravaginal medication. Sometimes, laminaria (a type of seaweed) is used to enlarge the cervix. A cannula or a small rod (dilator) is inserted into the dilated or stretched cervix.

Aspiration: A suction apparatus attached to the cannula is moved around the inner walls of the uterus to remove fetal tissues and other products of pregnancy from the uterus. The suction may be produced by an electric or manual pump.

Aftercare

Analgesics or sedatives are administered to relieve cramping and pain from uterine contractions associated with the procedure. Prophylactic antibiotics are prescribed to prevent infection.

Complications

Vacuum aspirations are relatively safer than a dilation and curettage (D&C) procedure. However, abortions for pregnancies earlier than six weeks sometimes run the risk of retaining products of conception following the procedure. A second aspiration procedure or a D&C becomes necessary under such circumstances. Other complications, although rare, include hemorrhage, infection, and cervical trauma.

Dilatation and Curettage (D&C)

This type of abortion is performed during the second trimester (gestation period of 14–23 weeks). The procedure involves two steps: Dilation of the cervical canal followed by evacuation of the uterus to expel the products of conception (fetus, placenta, and membranes). Preparation for the procedure begins with routine blood tests and an ultrasound scan to assess the stage of pregnancy and location of the fetus attaching to the uterine wall. The dilation of the cervix may take a few hours or up to a day depending on the type of cervical dilator used. Medication, such as Misoprostol, can dilate the cervix in a couple of hours. On the other hand, the commonly used medical seaweed (laminaria) needs to be inserted in the vagina and left overnight before the procedure can be performed. After the cervix is sufficiently dilated, a cannula or suction tube is inserted into the cervix to aspirate the fetus and tissues associated with pregnancy. A surgical instrument called the curette is inserted into the uterus. The scoop-shaped curette is used to empty the uterus by scraping the lining of the uterus, hence the name curettage.

Risks and Complications

While abortions in general—both medical and surgical—are relatively safe and do not involve any serious complications, the chances for complications are slightly higher for surgical abortions. Infection, although rare, can be serious and may need hospitalization. Indications of an infection include fever, abdominal pain, and vaginal discharge.

Other potential complications include:

- Trauma to uterine lining or cervical tears.

- Hemorrhage resulting in a serious blood loss requiring blood transfusion or hospitalization.

- Adverse reaction to medications including anesthetics, antibiotics, or medication administered for dilation.

Dilation and Evacuation (D&E)

This procedure is usually performed to terminate late second trimester pregnancies and the preoperative protocol is essentially the same as for a D&C. The cervix is dilated using medication, such as Misoprostol, or a laminaria stick. Pain medication and sedatives are administered before the procedure that can be done under local anesthesia (in an abortion clinic) or under general anesthesia (in a hospital). The protocol for D&E procedure is the same as for D&C in that it combines vacuum aspiration and curettage, but also uses surgical instruments, such as forceps, to remove the fetus and other tissues associated with pregnancy. The surgeon uses an ultrasound to guide the procedure.

Complications

Complications following a D&E are primarily the same as with any surgical procedure and include infection, bleeding, or adverse reaction to medication. While early abortions using D&E procedures may be relatively risk free, those involving later stages may carry potential risks. This is primarily due to the larger fetus size and the thinning of the uterine walls. Some of these complications include trauma to the uterus and cervix, uterine perforations, and, sometimes, injury to other pelvic organs such as the bladder or bowel. D&E is also associated with the risk of intrauterine adhesions caused by the buildup of scar tissue between the uterine walls as a result of trauma or infection following D&E. These complications, if severe, may be associated with adverse outcomes for future pregnancies, which include infertility, miscarriage, and ectopic pregnancy. Having multiple abortions may also elevate the risk for incompetent cervix (weakened cervix), which in turn may cause preterm birth.

Dilation and Extraction (D&X)

Also called partial birth abortion in nonmedical parlance, this procedure is performed for third trimester abortions, and it involves partially delivering the fetus, followed by in utero fetal dismemberment and extraction of the fetus from the uterus. As in other surgical abortion procedures, dilation of the cervix is the first step and may occur over a sequence of days. Instruments may be used to manipulate the fetus to a footling breech (a presentation in which the feet of the fetus are the first to exit the uterus). After this, the fetus, excluding the head, is extracted. The final step in the procedure involves intrauterine cranial evacuation of the fetus using medical instruments. This causes decompression (collapse) of the skull. Vaginal delivery of the fetus completes the procedure.

Indications for D&X

While elective abortions performed using D&X procedures are rare and most are done for serious medical reasons involving either the mother or the fetus, this is, by and large, the only safe method for terminating late-term pregnancies. Also, standard abortion procedures, such as D&E are not generally performed for advanced gestational age as they are associated with a greater risk of maternal trauma.

Late-term abortions using D&X may have legal implications in some states, particularly when they are based on fetal viability (ability of fetus to survive outside the womb). Under such circumstances D&X procedures may be restricted to a certain gestation period prior to viability, most often around 22 weeks.

Risks and Complications

Procedural risks and complications involved in D&X procedures are primarily the same as for childbirth and includes heavy bleeding, uterine infection, and high blood pressure. Trauma to the cervix and uterus from use of surgical instruments may have long-term effects on reproductive health and future pregnancy. Another factor that complicates late abortions is embolism. This can often be fatal and is caused by the sudden entry of amniotic fluid, blood clots, or fetal tissues into maternal circulation.

References

1. Jacobson, John D., MD. "Abortion-Surgical," A.D.A.M., Inc., October 4, 2016.

2. "Surgical Abortion Procedures," American Pregnancy Association, January 26, 2017.

3. "Clinical Care for Women Undergoing Abortion," National Institutes of Health (NIH), n.d.

Chapter 32

Infertility and Infertility Treatment Options

What Is Infertility?

In general, infertility is defined as not being able to get pregnant (conceive) after one year (or longer) of unprotected sex. Because fertility in women is known to decline steadily with age, some providers evaluate and treat women aged 35 years or older after 6 months of unprotected sex. Women with infertility should consider making an appointment with a reproductive endocrinologist—a doctor who specializes in managing infertility. Reproductive endocrinologists may also be able to help women with recurrent pregnancy loss, defined as having two or more spontaneous miscarriages.

Pregnancy is the result of a process that has many steps.

To get pregnant:

- a woman's body must release an egg from one of her ovaries (ovulation).

- a man's sperm must join with the egg along the way (fertilize).

- the fertilized egg must go through a fallopian tube toward the uterus (womb).

This chapter includes text excerpted from "Infertility FAQs," Centers for Disease Control and Prevention (CDC), March 30, 2017.

- the fertilized egg must attach to the inside of the uterus (implantation).

Infertility may result from a problem with any or several of these steps.

Impaired fecundity is a condition related to infertility and refers to women who have difficulty getting pregnant or carrying a pregnancy to term.

Is Infertility a Common Problem?

Yes. About 6 percent of married women aged 15 to 44 years in the United States are unable to get pregnant after one year of trying (infertility). Also, about 12 percent of women aged 15 to 44 years in the United States have difficulty getting pregnant or carrying a pregnancy to term, regardless of marital status (impaired fecundity).

Is Infertility Just a Woman's Problem?

No, infertility is not always a woman's problem. Both women and men can contribute to infertility.

Many couples struggle with infertility and seek help to become pregnant, but it is often thought of as only a woman's condition. However, in about 35 percent of couples with infertility, a male factor is identified along with a female factor. In about 8 percent of couples with infertility, a male factor is the only identifiable cause.

Almost 9 percent of men aged 25 to 44 years in the United States reported that they or their partner saw a doctor for advice, testing, or treatment for infertility during their lifetime.

What Causes Infertility in Women?

Women need functioning ovaries, fallopian tubes, and a uterus to get pregnant. Conditions affecting any one of these organs can contribute to female infertility. Some of these conditions are listed below and can be evaluated using a number of different tests.

Disruption of Ovarian Function

A woman's menstrual cycle is, on average, 28 days long. Day 1 is defined as the first day of "full flow." Regular predictable periods that occur every 24 to 32 days likely reflect ovulation. A woman with irregular periods is likely not ovulating.

Ovulation can be predicted by using an ovulation predictor kit and can be confirmed by a blood test to check the woman's progesterone level on day 21 of her menstrual cycle. Although several tests exist to evaluate a woman's ovarian function, no single test is a perfect predictor of fertility. The most commonly used markers of ovarian function include follicle stimulating hormone (FSH) value on day 3 to 5 of the menstrual cycle, antimüllerian hormone value (AMH), and antral follicle count (AFC) using a transvaginal ultrasound.

Disruptions in ovarian function may be caused by several conditions and warrants an evaluation by a doctor.

When a woman doesn't ovulate during a menstrual cycle, it's called anovulation. Potential causes of anovulation include the following:

- **Polycystic ovary syndrome (PCOS)**. PCOS is a condition that causes women to not ovulate, or to ovulate irregularly. Some women with PCOS have elevated levels of testosterone, which can cause acne and excess hair growth. PCOS is the most common cause of female infertility.

- **Diminished ovarian reserve (DOR)**. Women are born with all of the eggs that they will ever have, and a woman's egg count decreases over time. Diminished ovarian reserve is a condition in which there are fewer eggs remaining in the ovaries than normal. The number of eggs a woman has declines naturally as a woman ages. It may also occur due to congenital, medical, surgical, or unexplained causes. Women with diminished ovarian reserve may be able to conceive naturally, but will produce fewer eggs in response to fertility treatments.

- **Functional hypothalamic amenorrhea (FHA)**. FHA is a condition caused by excessive exercise, stress, or low body weight. It is sometimes associated with eating disorders such as anorexia.

- **Improper function of the hypothalamus and pituitary glands**. The hypothalamus and pituitary glands in the brain produce hormones that maintain normal ovarian function. Production of too much of the hormone prolactin by the pituitary gland (often as the result of a benign pituitary gland tumor), or improper function of the hypothalamus or pituitary gland, may cause a woman not to ovulate.

- **Premature ovarian insufficiency (POI)**. POI, sometimes referred to as premature menopause, occurs when a woman's ovaries fail before she is 40 years of age. Although certain exposures, such as chemotherapy or pelvic radiation therapy, and certain medical conditions may cause POI, the cause is often unexplained. About 5–10 percent of women with POI conceive naturally and have a normal pregnancy.

- **Menopause**. Menopause is an age-appropriate decline in ovarian function that usually occurs around age 50. By definition, a woman in menopause has not had a period in one year. She may experience hot flashes, mood changes, difficulty sleeping, and other symptoms as well.

Fallopian Tube Obstruction

Risk factors for blocked fallopian tubes (tubal occlusion) can include a history of pelvic infection, history of ruptured appendicitis, history of gonorrhea or chlamydia, known endometriosis, or a history of abdominal surgery.

Tubal evaluation may be performed using an X-ray that is called a hysterosalpingogram (HSG), or by chromopertubation (CP) in the operating room at time of laparoscopy, a surgical procedure in which a small incision is made and a viewing tube called a laparoscope is inserted.

- **Hysterosalpingogram (HSG)** is an X-ray of the uterus and fallopian tubes. A radiologist injects dye into the uterus through the cervix and simultaneously takes X-ray pictures to see if the dye moves freely through fallopian tubes. This helps evaluate tubal caliber (diameter) and patency.

- **Chromopertubation** is similar to an HSG but is done in the operating room at the time of a laparoscopy. Blue-colored dye is passed through the cervix into the uterus and spillage and tubal caliber (shape) is evaluated.

Abnormal Uterine Contour

Depending on a woman's symptoms, the uterus may be evaluated by transvaginal ultrasound to look for fibroids or other anatomic abnormalities. If suspicion exists that the fibroids may be entering the endometrial cavity, a sonohysterogram (SHG) or hysteroscopy (HSC) may be performed to further evaluate the uterine environment.

What Increases a Woman's Risk of Infertility?

Female fertility is known to decline with:

- Age. More women are waiting until their 30s and 40s to have children. In fact, about 20 percent of women in the United

States now have their first child after age 35. About one-third of couples in which the woman is older than 35 years have fertility problems. Aging not only decreases a woman's chances of having a baby, but also increases her chances of miscarriage and of having a child with a genetic abnormality.

- Aging decreases a woman's chances of having a baby in the following ways:

    - She has a smaller number of eggs left.

    - Her eggs are not as healthy.

    - She is more likely to have health conditions that can cause fertility problems.

    - She is more likely to have a miscarriage.

- Smoking.

- Excessive alcohol use.

- Extreme weight gain or loss.

- Excessive physical or emotional stress that results in amenorrhea (absent periods).

How Long Should Couples Try to Get Pregnant before Seeing a Doctor?

Most experts suggest at least one year for women younger than age 35. However, for women aged 35 years or older, couples should see a healthcare provider after 6 months of trying unsuccessfully. A woman's chances of having a baby decrease rapidly every year after the age of 30.

Some health problems also increase the risk of infertility. So, couples with the following signs or symptoms should not delay seeing their healthcare provider when they are trying to become pregnant:

- Irregular periods or no menstrual periods

- Very painful periods

- Endometriosis

- Pelvic inflammatory disease

- More than one miscarriage

- Suspected male factor (i.e., history of testicular trauma, hernia surgery, chemotherapy, or infertility with another partner)

It is a good idea for any woman and her partner to talk to a health-care provider before trying to get pregnant. They can help you get your body ready for a healthy baby, and can also answer questions on fertility and give tips on conceiving.

How Will Doctors Find Out If a Woman and Her Partner Have Fertility Problems?

Doctors will begin by collecting a medical and sexual history from both partners. The initial evaluation usually includes a semen analysis, a tubal evaluation, and ovarian reserve testing.

How Do Doctors Treat Infertility?

Infertility can be treated with medicine, surgery, intrauterine insemination, or assisted reproductive technology.

Often, medication and intrauterine insemination are used at the same time. Doctors recommend specific treatments for infertility on the basis of:

- The factors contributing to the infertility.

- The duration of the infertility.

- The age of the female.

- The couple's treatment preference after counseling about success rates, risks, and benefits of each treatment option.

What Medicines Are Used to Treat Infertility in Women?

Some common medicines used to treat infertility in women include:

- Clomiphene citrate (Clomid®*) is a medicine that causes ovulation by acting on the pituitary gland. It is often used in women who have polycystic ovary syndrome (PCOS) or other problems with ovulation. It is also used in women with normal ovulation to increase the number of mature eggs produced. This medicine is taken by mouth.

- Letrozole (Femara ®*) is a medication that is frequently used off-label to cause ovulation. It works by temporarily lowering a woman's progesterone level, which causes the brain to naturally make more FSH. It is often used to induce ovulation in women with PCOS, and in women with normal ovulation to increase the number of mature eggs produced in the ovaries.

- Human menopausal gonadotropin or hMG (Menopur®*; Repronex®*; Pergonal®*) is a medication often used for women who don't ovulate because of problems with their pituitary gland—hMG acts directly on the ovaries to stimulate development of mature eggs. It is an injectable medicine.

- Follicle-stimulating hormone or FSH (Gonal-F®*; Follistim®*) is a medication that works much like hMG. It stimulates development of mature eggs within the ovaries. It is an injectable medication.

- Gonadotropin-releasing hormone (GnRH) analogs and GnRH antagonists are medications that act on the pituitary gland to prevent a woman from ovulating. They are used during in vitro fertilization cycles, or to help prepare a woman's uterus for an embryo transfer. These medications are usually injected or given with a nasal spray.

- Metformin (Glucophage®*) is a medicine doctors use for women who have insulin resistance or diabetes and PCOS. This drug helps lower the high levels of male hormones in women with these conditions. This helps the body to ovulate. Sometimes clomiphene citrate or FSH is combined with metformin. This medicine is taken by mouth.

- Bromocriptine (Parlodel®*) and Cabergoline (Dostinex ®*) are medications used for women with ovulation problems because of high levels of prolactin.

Note: Use of trade names and commercial sources is for identification only and does not imply endorsement by the U.S. Department of Health and Human Services (HHS).

Many fertility drugs increase a woman's chance of having twins, triplets, or other multiples. Women who are pregnant with multiple fetuses may have more problems during pregnancy. Multiple fetuses have a higher risk of being born prematurely (too early). Premature babies are at a higher risk of health and developmental problems.

What Is Intrauterine Insemination (IUI)?

Intrauterine insemination (IUI) is an infertility treatment that is often called artificial insemination. In this procedure, specially prepared sperm are inserted into the woman's uterus. Sometimes the woman is also treated with medicines that stimulate ovulation before IUI.

IUI is often used to treat:

• Mild male factor infertility.

• Couples with unexplained infertility.

What Is Assisted Reproductive Technology (ART)?

Assisted reproductive technology (ART) includes all fertility treatments in which both eggs and embryos are handled outside of the body. In general, ART procedures involve removing mature eggs from a woman's ovaries using a needle, combining the eggs with sperm in the laboratory, and returning the embryos to the woman's body or donating them to another woman. The main type of ART is in vitro fertilization (IVF).

How Often Is Assisted Reproductive Technology (ART) Successful?

Success rates vary and depend on many factors, including the clinic performing the procedure, the infertility diagnosis, and the age of the woman undergoing the procedure. This last factor—the woman's age—is especially important.

The Centers for Disease Control and Prevention (CDC) collects success rates on ART for some fertility clinics. According to the CDC's 2014 ART Success Rates, the average percentage of fresh, non donor ART cycles that led to a live birth were:

• 37 percent in women younger than 35 years of age

• 30 percent in women aged 35 to 37 years

• 20 percent in women aged 38 to 40 years

• 10 percent in women aged 41 to 42 years

• 4 percent in women aged 43 to 44 years

• 1 percent in women older than 44 years of age

Success rates also vary from clinic to clinic and with different infertility diagnoses.

ART can be expensive and time-consuming, but it has allowed many couples to have children that otherwise would not have been conceived. The most common complication of ART is a multiple pregnancy. This is a problem that can be prevented or minimized by limiting the number of embryos that are transferred back to the uterus. For example, transfer of a single embryo, rather than multiple embryos, greatly reduces the chances of a multiple pregnancy and its risks such as preterm birth.

What Are the Different Types of Assisted Reproductive Technology (ART)?

- In vitro fertilization (IVF), meaning fertilization outside of the body, is the most effective and the most common form of ART.

- Intracytoplasmic sperm injection (ICSI) is a type of IVF that is often used for couples with male factor infertility. With ICSI, a single sperm is injected into a mature egg. The alternative to ICSI is "conventional" fertilization where the egg and many sperm are placed in a petri dish together and the sperm fertilizes an egg on its own.

Older ART methods that are rarely used in the United States today include:

- **Zygote intrafallopian transfer (ZIFT)** or tubal embryo transfer. This is similar to IVF. Fertilization occurs in the laboratory. Then the very young embryo is transferred to the fallopian tube instead of the uterus.

- **Gamete intrafallopian transfer (GIFT)**, involves transferring eggs and sperm into the woman's fallopian tube. Fertilization occurs in the woman's body.

ART procedures sometimes involve the use of donor eggs (eggs from another woman), donor sperm, or previously frozen embryos. Donor eggs are sometimes used for women who cannot produce eggs. Also, donor eggs or donor sperm are sometimes used when the woman or man has a genetic disease that can be passed on to the baby. An infertile woman or couple may also use donor embryos. These are embryos that were either created by couples in infertility treatment or were created from donor sperm and donor eggs. The donated embryo

403

is transferred to the uterus. The child will not be genetically related to either parent.

Gestational Carrier

Women with ovaries but no uterus may be able to use a gestational carrier. This may also be an option for women who shouldn't become pregnant because of a serious health problem. In this case, a woman uses her own egg. It is fertilized by her partner's sperm and the embryo is placed inside the carrier's uterus.

Chapter 33

Having a Healthy Pregnancy

Chapter Contents

Section 33.1

Preconception and Prenatal Care

This section includes text excerpted from "Planning for Pregnancy," Centers for Disease Control and Prevention (CDC), February 13, 2017.

If you are trying to have a baby or are just thinking about it, it is not too early to start getting ready for pregnancy. Preconception health and healthcare focus on things you can do before and between pregnancies to increase the chances of having a healthy baby. For some women, getting their body ready for pregnancy takes a few months. For other women, it might take longer. Whether this is your first, second, or sixth baby, the following are important steps to help you get ready for the healthiest pregnancy possible.

Make a Plan and Take Action

Whether or not you've written them down, you've probably thought about your goals for having or not having children, and how to achieve those goals. For example, when you didn't want to have a baby, you used effective birth control methods to achieve your goals. Now that you're thinking about getting pregnant, it's really important to take steps to achieve your goal—getting pregnant and having a healthy baby!

See Your Doctor

Before getting pregnant, talk to your doctor about preconception healthcare. Your doctor will want to discuss your health history and any medical conditions you currently have that could affect a pregnancy. He or she also will discuss any previous pregnancy problems, medicines that you currently are taking, vaccinations that you might need, and steps you can take before pregnancy to prevent certain birth defects.

If your doctor has not talked with you about this type of care—ask about it! Take a list of talking points so you don't forget anything!

406

Be sure to talk to your doctor about:

Medical Conditions

If you currently have any medical conditions, be sure they are under control and being treated. Some of these conditions include: sexually transmitted diseases (STDs), diabetes, thyroid disease, phenylketon-uria (PKU), seizure disorders, high blood pressure, arthritis, eating disorders, and chronic diseases.

Lifestyle and Behaviors

Talk with your doctor or another health professional if you smoke, drink alcohol, or use "street" drugs; live in a stressful or abusive environment; or work with or live around toxic substances. Healthcare professionals can help you with counseling, treatment, and other support services.

Medications

Taking certain medicines during pregnancy can cause serious birth defects. These include some prescription and over-the-counter medications and dietary or herbal supplements. If you are planning a pregnancy, you should discuss the need for any medication with your doctor before becoming pregnant and make sure you are taking only those medications that are necessary

Vaccinations (Shots)

Some vaccinations are recommended before you become pregnant, during pregnancy, or right after delivery. Having the right vaccinations at the right time can help keep you healthy and help keep your baby from getting very sick or having lifelong health problems.

Take 400 Micrograms of Folic Acid Every Day

Folic acid is a B vitamin. If a woman has enough folic acid in her body at least 1 month before and during pregnancy, it can help prevent major birth defects of the baby's brain and spine.

Stop Drinking Alcohol, Smoking, and Using Street Drugs

Smoking, drinking alcohol, and using street drugs can cause many problems during pregnancy for a woman and her baby, such as premature birth, birth defects, and infant death.

If you are trying to get pregnant and cannot stop drinking, smoking, or using drugs—get help! Contact your doctor or local treatment center.

Avoid Toxic Substances and Environmental Contaminants

Avoid toxic substances and other environmental contaminants harmful materials at work or at home, such as synthetic chemicals, metals, fertilizer, bug spray, and cat or rodent feces. These substances can hurt the reproductive systems of men and women. They can make it more difficult to get pregnant. Exposure to even small amounts during pregnancy, infancy, childhood, or puberty can lead to diseases. Learn how to protect yourself and your loved ones from toxic substances at work and at home.

Reach and Maintain a Healthy Weight

People who are overweight or obese have a higher risk for many serious conditions, including complications during pregnancy, heart disease, type 2 diabetes, and certain cancers (endometrial, breast, and colon). People who are underweight are also at risk for serious health problems.

The key to achieving and maintaining a healthy weight isn't about short-term dietary changes. It's about a lifestyle that includes healthy eating and regular physical activity.

If you are underweight, overweight, or obese, talk with your doctor about ways to reach and maintain a healthy weight before you get pregnant.

Get Help for Violence

Violence can lead to injury and death among women at any stage of life, including during pregnancy. The number of violent deaths experienced by women tells only part of the story. Many more survive violence and are left with lifelong physical and emotional scars.

If someone is violent toward you or you are violent toward your loved ones—get help. Violence destroys relationships and families.

Learn Your Family History

Collecting your family's health history can be important for your child's health. You might not realize that your sister's heart defect or your cousin's sickle cell disease could affect your child, but sharing this family history information with your doctor can be important.

Based on your family history, your doctor might refer you for genetic counseling. Other reasons people go for genetic counseling include having had several miscarriages, infant deaths, or trouble getting pregnant (infertility), or a genetic condition or birth defect that occurred during a previous pregnancy.

Get Mentally Healthy

Mental health is how we think, feel, and act as we cope with life. To be at your best, you need to feel good about your life and value yourself. Everyone feels worried, anxious, sad, or stressed sometimes. However, if these feelings do not go away and they interfere with your daily life, get help. Talk with your doctor or another health professional about your feelings and treatment options.

Have a Healthy Pregnancy!

Once you are pregnant, be sure to keep up all of your new healthy habits and see your doctor regularly throughout pregnancy for prenatal care.

Section 33.2

Pregnancy and Medicines

This section includes text excerpted from "Medicine and Pregnancy,"
U.S. Food and Drug Administration (FDA), May 19, 2017.

Are you pregnant and taking medicines? You are not alone. Many women need to take medicines when they are pregnant. There are about six million pregnancies in the United States each year, and 50 percent of pregnant women say that they take at least one medicine. Some women take medicines for health problems, like diabetes, morning sickness or high blood pressure that can start or get worse when a woman is pregnant. Others take medicines before they realize they are pregnant.

Pregnancy can be an exciting time. However, this time can also make you feel uneasy if you are not sure how your medicines will affect your baby. Not all medicines are safe to take when you are pregnant. Even headache or pain medicine may not be safe during certain times in your pregnancy.

Here are four tips to help you talk to your healthcare provider about how prescription and over-the-counter medicines might affect you and your baby.

Ask Questions

Always talk to your healthcare provider before you take any medicines, herbs, or vitamins. Don't stop taking your medicines until your healthcare provider says that it is OK.

Use these questions to help you talk to your doctor, nurse, or pharmacist:

- Will I need to change my medicines if I want to get pregnant? Before you get pregnant, work with your healthcare provider to make a plan to help you safely use your medicines.

- How might this medicine affect my baby? Ask about the benefits and risks for you and your baby.

- What medicines and herbs should I avoid? Some drugs can harm your baby during different stages of your pregnancy. At these times, your healthcare provider may have you take something else.

- Will I need to take more or less of my medicine? Your heart and kidneys work harder when you are pregnant. This makes medicines pass through your body faster than usual.

- Can I keep taking this medicine when I start breastfeeding? Some drugs can get into your breast milk and affect your baby.

- What kind of vitamins should I take? Ask about special vitamins for pregnant women called prenatal vitamins.

Prenatal Vitamins

Some dietary supplements may have too much or too little of the vitamins that you need. Talk to your healthcare provider about what kind of prenatal vitamins you should take.

What is folic acid? Folic acid helps to prevent birth defects of the baby's brain or spine. Ask about how much folic acid you should take before you become pregnant and through the first part of your pregnancy.

Read the Label

Check the drug label and other information you get with your medicine to learn about the possible risks for women who are pregnant or breastfeeding. The labeling tells you what is known about how the drugs might affect pregnant women. Your healthcare provider can help you decide if you should take the medicine.

New Prescription Drug Information

The prescription drug labels are changing. The new labels will replace the old A, B, C, D, and X categories with more helpful information about a medicine's risks. The labels will also have more information on whether the medicine gets into breast milk and how it can possibly affect the baby.

Be Smart Online

Ask your doctor, nurse, or pharmacist about the information you get online. Some websites say that drugs are safe to take during pregnancy, but you should check with your healthcare provider first. Every woman's body is different. It may not be safe for you.

- Do not trust that a product is safe just because it says 'natural'.

- Check with your healthcare provider before you use a product that you heard about in a chat room or group.

Section 33.3

Nutrition and Fitness during Pregnancy

This section includes text excerpted from "Health Tips for Pregnant Women," National Institute of Diabetes and Digestive and Kidney Diseases (NIDDK), June 2016.

This section gives you tips on how to eat better and be more active while you are pregnant and after your baby is born. Use the ideas and tips in this publication to improve your eating pattern and be more physically active.

These tips can also be useful if you are not pregnant but are thinking about having a baby! By making changes now, you can get used to new eating and activity habits and be a healthy example for your family for a lifetime.

Healthy Weight

Why Is Gaining a Healthy Amount of Weight during Pregnancy Important?

Gaining the right amount of weight during pregnancy helps your baby grow to a healthy size. But gaining too much or too little weight may lead to serious health problems for you and your baby.

Too much weight gain raises your chances for diabetes and high blood pressure during pregnancy and after. If you are overweight when you get pregnant, your chances for health problems may be even higher. It also makes it more likely that you will have a hard delivery and need a cesarean section (C-section).

Gaining a healthy amount of weight helps you have an easier pregnancy and delivery. It may also help make it easier for you to get back to your normal weight after delivery. Research shows that a healthy weight gain can also lower the chances that you or your child will have obesity and weight-related problems later in life.

How Much Weight Should I Gain during My Pregnancy?

How much weight you should gain depends on how much you weighed before pregnancy.

Weight Gain during Pregnancy

General weight-gain advice below refers to weight before pregnancy and is for women having only one baby.

Table 33.1. Weight Gain during Pregnancy

If You Area	You Should Gain About
underweight (BMI* less than 18.5)	28 to 40 pounds
normal weight (BMI of 18.5 to 24.9)	25 to 35 pounds
overweight (BMI of 25 to 29.9)	15 to 25 pounds
obese (BMI of 30+)	11 to 20 pounds

The body mass index (BMI) measures your weight in relation to your height.

It is important to gain weight very slowly. The old myth that you are "eating for two" is not true. During the first 3 months, your baby is only the size of a walnut and does not need very many extra calories. The following rate of weight gain is advised:

- 1 to 4 pounds total in the first 3 months
- 2 to 4 pounds each month from 4 months until delivery

Talk to your healthcare provider about how much weight you should gain. Work with him or her to set goals for your weight gain. Take into account your age, weight, and health. Track your weight at home or at your provider visits using charts from the Institute of Medicine.

Do not try to lose weight if you are pregnant. Healthy food is needed to help your baby grow. Some women may lose a small amount of weight at the start of pregnancy. Speak to your healthcare provider if this happens to you.

Healthy Eating

How Much Should I Eat?

Eating healthy foods and the right amount of calories helps you and your baby gain the proper amount of weight.

How much food you need depends on things like your weight before pregnancy, your age, and how fast you gain weight. In the first 3 months of pregnancy, most women do not need extra calories. You also may not need extra calories during the final weeks of pregnancy.

Check with your doctor about this. If you are not gaining the right amount of weight, your doctor may advise you to eat more calories. If you are gaining too much weight, you may need to cut down on calories.

Each woman's needs are different. Your needs depend on if you were underweight, overweight, or obese before you became pregnant, or if you are having more than one baby.

What Kinds of Foods Should I Eat?

A healthy eating plan for pregnancy includes nutrient-rich foods. *Dietary guidelines* advise eating these foods each day:

- fruits and veggies (provide vitamins and fiber)

- whole grains, like oatmeal, whole-wheat bread, and brown rice (provide fiber, B vitamins, and other needed nutrients)

- fat-free or low-fat milk and milk products or nondairy soy, almond, rice, or other drinks with added calcium and vitamin D

- protein from healthy sources, like beans and peas, eggs, lean meats, seafood (8 to 12 ounces per week), and unsalted nuts and seeds

A healthy eating plan also limits salt, solid fats (like butter, lard, and shortening), and sugar-sweetened drinks and foods.

What If I Am a Vegetarian?

A vegetarian eating plan during pregnancy can be healthy. Talk to your healthcare provider to make sure you are getting calcium, iron, protein, vitamin B12, vitamin D, and other needed nutrients. He or she may ask you to meet with a registered dietitian (a nutrition expert who has a degree in diet and nutrition approved by the Academy of Nutrition and Dietetics, has passed a national exam, and is licensed to practice in your state) who can help you plan meals. Your doctor may also tell you to take vitamins and minerals that will help you meet your needs.

Do I Have Any Special Nutrition Needs Now That I Am Pregnant?

Yes. During pregnancy, you need more vitamins and minerals, like folate, iron, and calcium.

Getting the right amount of folate is very important. Folate, a B vitamin also known as folic acid, may help prevent birth defects. Before pregnancy, you need 400 mcg per day. During pregnancy and when breastfeeding, you need 600 mcg per day from foods or vitamins. Foods high in folate include orange juice, strawberries, spinach, broccoli, beans, and fortified breads and breakfast cereals.

Most healthcare providers tell women who are pregnant to take a prenatal vitamin every day and eat a healthy diet. Ask your doctor about what you should take.

What Other New Eating Habits May Helps My Weight Gain?

Pregnancy can create some new food and eating concerns. Meet the needs of your body and be more comfortable with these tips:

- **Eat breakfast every day**. If you feel sick to your stomach in the morning, try dry whole-wheat toast or whole-grain crackers when you first wake up. Eat them even before you get out of bed. Eat the rest of your breakfast (fruit, oatmeal, whole-grain cereal, low-fat milk or yogurt, or other foods) later in the morning.

- **Eat high-fiber foods**. Eating high-fiber foods, drinking plenty of water, and getting daily physical activity may help prevent constipation. Try to eat whole-grain cereals, vegetables, fruits, and beans.

- **If you have heartburn, eat small meals more often**. Try to eat slowly and avoid spicy and fatty foods (such as hot peppers or fried chicken). Have drinks between meals instead of with meals. Do not lie down soon after eating.

What Foods Should I Avoid?

There are certain foods and drinks that can harm your baby if you have them while you are pregnant. Here is a list of items you should avoid:

- **Alcohol**. Do not drink alcohol like wine or beer. Enjoy decaf coffee or tea, nonsugar-sweetened drinks, or water with a dash of juice. Avoid diet drinks and drinks with caffeine.

- **Fish that may have high levels of mercury** (a substance that can buildup in fish and harm an unborn baby). You should eat 8 to 12 ounces of seafood per week, but limit white (albacore) tuna to 6 ounces per week. Do not eat tilefish, shark, swordfish, and king mackerel.

- **Anything that is not food**. Some pregnant women may crave something that is not food, such as laundry starch or clay. This may mean that you are not getting the right amount of a nutrient. Talk to your doctor if you crave something that is not food. He or she can help you get the right amount of nutrients.

Physical Activity

Should I Be Physically Active during My Pregnancy?

Almost all women can and should be physically active during pregnancy. Regular physical activity may:

- help you and your baby gain the right amounts of weight
- reduce backaches, leg cramps, and bloating
- reduce your risk for gestational diabetes (diabetes that develops when a woman is pregnant)

If you were physically active before you became pregnant, you may not need to change your exercise habits. Talk with your healthcare provider about how to change your workouts during pregnancy.

It can be hard to be physically active if you do not have child care for your other children, have not worked out before, or do not know what to do. Keep reading for tips about how you can work around these things and be physically active.

How Much Physical Activity Do I Need?

Most women need the same amount of physical activity as before they became pregnant. Aim for at least 30 minutes of aerobic activity per day on most days of the week. Aerobic activities use large muscle groups (back, chest, and legs) to increase heart rate and breathing.

The aerobic activity should last at least 10 minutes at a time and should be of moderate intensity. This means it makes you breathe harder but does not overwork or overheat you.

If you have health issues like obesity, high blood pressure, diabetes, or anemia (too few healthy red blood cells), ask your healthcare provider about a level of activity that is safe for you.

How Can I Stay Active While Pregnant?

Even if you have not been active before, you can be active during your pregnancy by using the tips below:

Go for a walk around the block, in a local park, or in a shopping mall with a family member or friend. If you already have children, take them with you and make it a family outing.

Get up and move around at least once an hour if you sit in a chair most of the day. When watching TV, get up and move around during commercials. Even a simple activity like walking in place can help.

How Can I Stay Safe While Being Active?

For your health and safety, and for your baby's, you should not do some physical activities while pregnant. Some of these are listed below. Talk to your healthcare provider about other physical activities that you should not do.

Make a plan to be active while pregnant. List the activities you would like to do, such as walking or taking a prenatal yoga class. Think of the days and times you could do each activity on your list, like first thing in the morning, during lunch break from work, after dinner, or on Saturday afternoon. Look at your calendar or planner to find the days and times that work best, and commit to those plans.

Table 33.2. Safety Do's and Don'ts

Follow These Safety Tips While Being Active	
Do...	Don't...
Choose moderate activities that are not likely to injure you, such as walking or aqua aerobics.	Avoid brisk exercise outside during very hot weather.
Drink fluids before, during, and after being physically active.	Don't use steam rooms, hot tubs, and saunas.
Wear comfortable clothing that fits well and supports and protects your breasts.	After the end of week 12 of your pregnancy, avoid exercises that call for you to lie flat on your back.
top exercising if you feel dizzy, short of breath, tired, or sick to your stomach.	

Lifespan Tip Sheet for Pregnancy

- Talk to your healthcare provider about how much weight you should gain during your pregnancy. Track your progress on a weight-gain graph.

- Eat foods rich in folate, iron, calcium, and protein. Ask your healthcare provider about prenatal supplements (vitamins you may take while pregnant).

- Eat breakfast every day.

- Eat foods high in fiber and drink plenty of water to avoid constipation.

- Cut back on "junk" foods and soft drinks.

- Avoid alcohol, raw or undercooked fish, fish high in mercury, undercooked meat and poultry, and soft cheeses.

- Be physically active on most, or all, days of the week during your pregnancy. If you have health issues, talk to your healthcare provider before you begin.

- After pregnancy, slowly get back to your routine of regular, moderate-intensity physical activity.

- Return to a healthy weight slowly.

Chapter 34

The Birth of Your Baby

Chapter Contents

Section 34.1

Labor and Delivery Basics

This section includes text excerpted from "Labor and Delivery,"
Eunice Kennedy Shriver National Institute of Child Health and
Human Development (NICHD), December 17, 2014.

Labor and delivery describe the process of childbirth. With regular
contractions of the uterus and changes of the cervix (the opening of
the uterus), a woman's body prepares for childbirth, the baby is born,
and the placenta follows.

Preterm labor and delivery, also called premature labor and birth,
share many features with regular labor and delivery. But they also
have specific features all their own. For this reason, preterm labor and
birth are addressed in a separate topic.

What Are Labor and Delivery?

Labor and delivery are the process by which a baby is born. Early labor
prepares the body for delivery. This is a period of hours or days when
the uterus regularly contracts and the cervix gradually thins out (called
effacing) and opens (called dilation) to allow the baby to pass through.

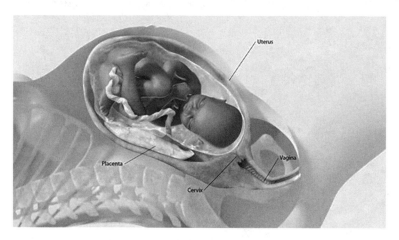

Figure 34.1. *Fetus*

Once the cervix has opened completely, pushing begins. If the baby and placenta come out through the vagina, this is known as a vaginal delivery.

When Does Labor Usually Start?

The due date is 40 weeks after the first day of the last menstrual period, although sometimes it is determined by an ultrasound. For most women, labor occurs sometime between week 37 and week 42 of pregnancy. Labor that occurs before 37 weeks of pregnancy is considered premature, or preterm labor. Labor that occurs at 37 or 38 weeks is now considered early term because babies born at that gestational age are still immature.

Just as pregnancy is different for every woman, the start of labor, the signs of labor, and the length of time it takes to go through labor will vary from woman to woman and even from pregnancy to pregnancy.

Signs of Labor

Some signs that labor may be close (although, in fact, it still might be weeks away) can include:

- "Lightening." This term describes when the fetus "drops," or moves lower in the uterus. Not all fetuses drop before birth. Lightening gets its name from the feeling of lightness or relief that some women experience when the fetus moves away from the rib cage to the pelvic area. This allows some women to breathe easier and more deeply and to get relief from heartburn.

- Increase in vaginal discharge. Called "show" or "the bloody show," the discharge can be clear, pink, or slightly bloody. This occurs as the cervix begins to open (dilate) and can happen several days before labor or just as labor begins.

If a woman experiences any of the following signs of labor at any point in pregnancy, she should contact her healthcare provider:

- Contractions every 10 minutes or more often

- Change in color of vaginal discharge

- Pain or pressure around the front of the pelvis or the rectum

- Low, dull backache

- Vaginal spotting or bleeding

- Abdominal cramps, with or without diarrhea

Sometimes, if the health of the mother or the fetus is at risk, a woman's healthcare provider will recommend inducing labor, using medically supervised methods, such as medication, to bring on labor.

Unless earlier delivery is medically necessary, waiting until at least 39 weeks before delivering gives mother and baby the best chance for healthy outcomes. During the last few weeks of pregnancy, the fetus's lungs, brain, and liver are still developing.

What Are the Stages of Labor?

Stage One

The first stage of labor happens in two phases: early labor and active labor.

During early labor:

- The cervix starts to open or dilate.

- Strong and regular contractions last 30 to 60 seconds and come every 5 to 20 minutes.

- The woman may have a bloody show.

A woman may experience this phase for a few hours or days, especially if she is giving birth for the first time.

During active labor:

- Contractions become stronger, longer, and more painful.

- Contractions come closer together.

- The woman may not have much time to relax between contractions.

- The woman may feel pressure in her lower back.

- The cervix fully dilates to 10 centimeters.

Stage Two

During this stage, the cervix is fully dilated and ready for delivery. The woman will begin to push (or is sometimes told to "bear down") to allow the baby to move through the birth canal.

During stage 2:

- The woman may feel pressure on her rectum as the baby's head moves through the vagina.
- She may feel the urge to push, as if having a bowel movement.
- The baby's head starts to show (called "crowning").
- The healthcare provider guides the baby out of the vagina.
- Once the baby comes out, the healthcare provider cuts the umbilical cord, which connected mother and fetus during pregnancy.

This stage can last between 20 minutes and several hours. It usually lasts longer for first-time mothers.

Stage Three

During this stage, the placenta is delivered. The placenta is the organ that gave the fetus food and oxygen through the umbilical cord during the pregnancy.

During stage 3:

- Contractions begin 5 to 10 minutes after the baby is delivered.
- The woman may have chills or feel shaky.

It may take 5 to 30 minutes for the placenta to exit the vagina.

What Are the Options for Pain Relief during Labor and Delivery?

The amount of pain felt during labor and delivery is different for every woman. The level of pain can depend on many factors, including the size and position of the baby and the strength of contractions. Some women learn breathing and relaxation techniques to help them cope with the pain. These techniques can be used along with one or more pain-relieving drugs.

A woman should discuss the many aspects of labor with her healthcare provider well before labor begins to ensure that she understands all of the options, risks, and benefits of pain relief during labor and delivery. It might also be helpful to put all the decisions in writing to clarify the options chosen.

Types of Pain-Relieving Medications

Pain-relief drugs fall into two categories: analgesics and anesthetics. There are different forms of each.

Analgesics

Analgesics relieve pain without causing total loss of feeling or muscle movement. These drugs do not always stop pain completely, but they reduce it.

- **Systemic analgesics** affect the whole nervous system rather than a single area. They ease pain but do not cause the patient to go to sleep. Systemic analgesics are often used in early labor. They are not given right before delivery because they may slow the baby's breathing and reflexes. They are given in two ways:

  - Injected into a muscle or vein

  - Inhaled or breathed in with a mixture of oxygen. The woman holds a mask to her face, meaning she decides how much or how little analgesic is needed for pain relief.

- **Regional analgesics** relieve pain in one region of the body. In the United States, regional analgesia is the most common way to relieve pain during labor. Several types of regional analgesia can be given during labor:

  - Epidural analgesia, also called an epidural block or an epidural, causes loss of feeling in the lower body while the patient stays awake. The drug starts working about 10 to 20 minutes after it is given. A healthcare provider injects the drug near the spinal cord. A small tube (catheter) is placed through the needle. The needle is then withdrawn, but the tube stays in place. Small amounts of the drug can then be given through the catheter throughout labor without the need for another injection.

  - A spinal block is an injection of a much smaller amount of the drug into the sac of spinal fluid around the spine. The drug starts working right away, but it only lasts for 1 to 2 hours. Usually a spinal block is given only once during labor, to help with pain during delivery.

  - A combined spinal-epidural block, also called a "walking epidural," gives the benefits of an epidural block and a spinal block. The spinal part relieves pain immediately. The epidural part allows drugs to be given throughout labor. Some women may be able to walk around after a combined spinal-epidural block.

Anesthetics

Anesthetics block all feeling, including pain.

- **General anesthesia** causes the patient to go to sleep. The patient does not feel pain while asleep.

- **Local anesthesia** removes all feeling, including pain, from a small part of the body while the patient stays awake. It does not lessen the pain of contractions. Healthcare providers often use it when performing an episiotomy, a surgical cut made in the region between the vagina and anus to widen the vaginal opening for delivery, or when repairing vaginal tears that happen during birth.

What Is Natural Childbirth?

Natural childbirth can refer to many different ways of giving birth without using pain medication, either in the home or at the hospital or birthing center.

Natural Forms of Pain Relief

Women who choose natural childbirth can use a number of natural ways to ease pain. These include:

- Emotional support
- Relaxation techniques
- A soothing atmosphere
- Moving and changing positions frequently
- Using a birthing ball
- Using soothing phrases and mental images
- Placing a heating pad or ice pack on the back or stomach
- Massage
- Taking a bath or shower
- Hypnosis
- Using soothing scents (aromatherapy)

- Acupuncture or acupressure

- Applying small doses of electrical stimulation to nerve fibers to activate the body's own pain-relieving substances (called transcutaneous electrical nerve stimulation, or TENS)

- Injecting sterile water into the lower back, which can relieve the intense discomfort and pain in the lower back known as back labor

A woman should discuss the many aspects of labor with her healthcare provider well before labor begins to ensure that she understands all of the options, risks, and benefits of pain relief during labor and delivery. It might also be helpful to put all the decisions in writing to clarify the options chosen.

What Is a Cesarean Section (C-Section)?

A cesarean section (C-section), short for cesarean section, is also called cesarean birth. Cesarean birth is the delivery of a baby through surgical cuts in a woman's abdomen and uterus. The uterus is then closed with stitches that later dissolve. Stitches or staples also close the skin on the belly.

When Is Cesarean Delivery Needed?

Cesarean delivery may be necessary in the following circumstances:

- **A pregnancy with two or more fetuses (multiple pregnancy).** A cesarean delivery may be needed if labor has started too early (preterm labor), if the fetuses are not in good positions in the uterus for natural delivery, or if there are other problems.

- **Labor is not progressing.** Contractions may not open the cervix enough for the baby to move into the vagina.

- **The infant's health is in danger.** The umbilical cord, which connects the fetus to the uterus, may become pinched, or the fetus may have an abnormal heart rate. In these cases, a C-section allows the baby to be delivered quickly to address and resolve the baby's health problems.

- **Problems with the placenta**. Sometimes the placenta is not formed or working correctly, is in the wrong place in the uterus, or is implanted too deeply or firmly in the uterine wall. This can cause problems, such as depriving the fetus of needed oxygen and nutrients or vaginal bleeding.

- **The baby is too large.** Women with gestational diabetes, especially if their blood sugar levels are not well controlled, are at increased risk for having large infants. And larger infants are at risk for complications during delivery. These include shoulder dystocia, when the infant's head is delivered through the vagina but the shoulders are stuck.

- **The baby is breech, or in a breech presentation,** meaning the baby is coming out feet first instead of head first.

- **The mother has an infection,** such as human immunodeficiency virus (HIV) or herpes, that could be passed to the baby during vaginal birth. Cesarean delivery could help prevent transmission of the virus to the infant.

- **The mother has a medical condition.** A C-section enables the healthcare provider to better manage the mother's health issues.

Women who have a cesarean delivery may be given pain medication with an epidural block, a spinal block, or general anesthesia. An epidural block numbs the lower part of the body through an injection in the spine. A spinal block also numbs the lower part of the body but through an injection directly into the spinal fluid. Women who receive general anesthesia, often used for emergency cesarean deliveries, will not be awake during the surgery.

What Are the Risks of a C-Section?

Cesarean birth is a type of surgery, meaning it has risks and possible complications for both mother and infant.

Possible risks from a C-section (which are also associated with vaginal birth) include:

- Infection

- Blood loss

- Blood clots in the legs, pelvic organs, or lungs

- Injury to surrounding structures, such as the bowel or bladder

- Reaction to medication or anesthesia used

A woman who has a C-section also may have to stay in the hospital longer. The more C-sections a woman has, the greater her risk for certain medical problems and problems with future pregnancies, such as uterine rupture and problems with the placenta.

427

Can a C-Section Be Requested?

Some women may want to have a cesarean birth even if vaginal delivery is an option. Women should discuss this option in detail with their healthcare provider before making a final decision about a C-section. As is true for vaginal births, unless there is a medical necessity, delivery should not occur before 39 weeks of pregnancy (called full term).

What Is Induction of Labor?

Labor induction is the use of medications or other methods to cause, or induce, labor. This practice is used to make contractions start.

When Would a Provider Induce Labor?

Induction is usually limited to situations when there is a problem with the pregnancy, or when a baby is overdue. Several weeks before labor begins, the cervix begins to soften (called "ripening"), thin out, and open to prepare for delivery. If the cervix is not ready, especially if labor has not started 2 weeks or more after your due date, your healthcare provider may recommend labor induction.

A healthcare provider may also recommend labor induction if there is a health risk to mother or fetus. Healthcare providers use a scoring system, called the Bishop score, to determine how ready the cervix is for labor. The scoring system ranges from 0 to 13. A score of less than 6 means the cervix may need a procedure to prepare it for labor.

Preparing the Cervix for Labor

If the cervix is not ready for labor, a healthcare provider may suggest one of the following to ripen the cervix:

- **Stripping the membranes.** Your healthcare provider can disconnect the thin tissue of the amniotic sac containing the fetus from the wall of the uterus. Stripping the membranes causes the body to release prostaglandins, which soften the cervix and cause contractions.

- **Giving prostaglandins**. This drug may be inserted into the vagina or given by mouth. The body naturally makes these chemicals to ripen the cervix.

- **Inserting a catheter.** A small tube with an inflatable balloon on the end can be placed in the cervix to widen it.

How Is Labor Induced?

Once the cervix is ripe, a healthcare provider may recommend one of the following techniques to start contractions or make them stronger:

- **Amniotomy.** A healthcare provider uses a tool to make a small hole in the amniotic sac, causing it to rupture (or the water to break) and contractions to start.

- **Giving oxytocin (also called Pitocin).** Oxytocin is a hormone the body naturally makes that causes contractions. It is given to start labor or to speed up labor that has already begun.

Can Induction Be Requested?

In most cases, induction is limited to situations when there is a problem with the pregnancy, or when a baby is overdue. But sometimes labor induction is requested for reasons other than a problem with the pregnancy.

A woman might want labor induction for several reasons, including:

- Physical discomfort at the end of pregnancy

- Concern with getting to the hospital in time

- Ensuring her own healthcare provider or midwife can be at the delivery

- Ensuring her spouse or partner can be at the delivery

- Scheduling issues with work or child care

It is best not to induce labor before 39 weeks of pregnancy (full term) unless there is a medical reason. Preterm infants (born before 37 weeks) and early term infants (born in the 37th and 38th weeks of pregnancy) are at increased risk of illness and even death.

What Is Vaginal Birth after Cesarean (VBAC)?

Vaginal birth after cesarean (VBAC) refers to successful vaginal delivery of a baby after a woman has delivered a baby by C-section in a previous pregnancy.

In the past, pregnant women who had a prior cesarean delivery would automatically have another C-section. But research shows that, for many women who had prior C-sections, attempting to give birth vaginally—called a trial of labor after cesarean delivery trial of labor after cesarean (TOLAC)—should be considered.

When Is VBAC Appropriate?

VBAC may be a safe and appropriate choice for some women, including those:

- Whose prior cesarean incision was across the uterus toward its base (called a low-transverse incision), the most common type of incision. Note that the incision on the uterus is different than the incision on the skin.

- With two previous low-transverse cesarean incisions

- Who are carrying twins

- With an unknown type of uterine incision

Benefits of VBAC include:

- No abdominal surgery

- A lowered risk of hemorrhage and infection, compared with a C-section

- Faster recovery

- Possibly avoiding the risks of many cesareans, such as hysterectomy, bowel and bladder injury, infection, and abnormal placenta conditions

- Greater likelihood of being able to have more children in the future

Eunice Kennedy Shriver National Institute of Child Health and Human Development (NICHD) research has shown that among appropriate candidates, about 75 percent of VBAC attempts are successful. A National Institutes of Health (NIH) Consensus Development Conference on Vaginal Birth After Cesarean evaluated data on VBAC and issued a statement determining that it is a reasonable option for many women.

But it is still possible that a woman will have to have a cesarean after having a trial of labor. Most risks associated with TOLAC are similar to those associated with choosing a repeat cesarean. They include:

- Uterine rupture

- Maternal hemorrhage and infection

- Blood clots

- Possible need for a hysterectomy

A woman considering VBAC should discuss the issue with her healthcare provider.

What Are Some Common Complications during Labor and Delivery?

Labor and delivery are different for everyone. Complications some-times happen. Possible complications include (but are not limited to):

- **Labor that does not progress.** Sometimes the cervix does not dilate in a timely manner to ready the body for delivery. If labor is not progressing, a healthcare provider may give the woman medications to speed up labor, or the woman may need a cesar-ean delivery.

- **Abnormal heart rate of the baby.** Many times an abnormal heart rate during labor does not mean there is a problem. A healthcare provider will likely ask the woman to switch posi-tions to help the infant get more blood flow. In certain instances or if test results show there is a problem, delivery might have to happen right away. When this happens, the woman is more likely to need a cesarean delivery, or the healthcare provider will need to do an episiotomy (a surgical cut between the vagina and anus) to widen the vaginal opening for delivery.

- **Perinatal asphyxia.** This condition occurs when the baby does not get enough oxygen in the uterus, during labor and delivery, or just after birth.

- **Shoulder dystocia.** In this situation, the infant's head has come out of the vagina but one of the shoulders becomes stuck.

- **Excessive bleeding.** If delivery results in tears to the uterus or if the uterus does not contract to deliver the placenta, heavy bleeding can result. Worldwide, such bleeding is a leading cause of maternal death.

Section 34.2

Premature Labor and Birth

This section includes text excerpted from "Preterm Labor and Birth—
Condition Information," *Eunice Kennedy Shriver* National Institute
of Child Health and Human Development (NICHD), March 16, 2014.

In general, a normal human pregnancy lasts about 40 weeks, or
just more than 9 months, from the start of the last menstrual period to
childbirth. Labor that begins before 37 weeks is called preterm labor
(or premature labor). A birth that occurs before 37 weeks is considered
a preterm birth.

Preterm birth is the most common cause of infant death and is the leading cause of long-term disability related to the nervous system in children.

What Is Preterm Labor?

In general, a normal human pregnancy is about 40 weeks long (9.2
months). Healthcare providers now define "full-term" birth as birth
that occurs between 39 weeks and 40 weeks and 6 days of pregnancy.
Infants born during this time are considered full-term infants.

Infants born in the 37th and 38th weeks of pregnancy—previously
called term but now referred to as "early term"—face more health risks
than do those born at 39 or 40 weeks.

Deliveries before 37 weeks of pregnancy are considered "preterm"
or premature:

- Labor that begins before 37 weeks of pregnancy is preterm or
  premature labor.

- A birth that occurs before 37 weeks of pregnancy is a preterm or
  premature birth.

- An infant born before 37 weeks in the womb is a preterm or premature infant. (These infants are commonly called "preemies" as
  a reference to being born prematurely.)

"Late preterm" refers to 34 weeks through 36 weeks of pregnancy.
Infants born during this time are considered late-preterm infants, but
they face many of the same health challenges as preterm infants. More

than 70 percent of preterm infants are born during the late-preterm time frame.

Preterm birth is the most common cause of infant death and is the leading cause of long-term disability in children. Many organs, including the brain, lungs, and liver, are still developing in the final weeks of pregnancy. The earlier the delivery, the higher the risk of serious disability or death.

Infants born prematurely are at risk for cerebral palsy (a group of nervous system disorders that affect control of movement and posture and limit activity), developmental delays, and vision and hearing problems.

Late-preterm infants typically have better health outcomes than those born earlier, but they are still three times more likely to die in the first year of life than are full-term infants. Preterm births can also take a heavy emotional and economic toll on families.

What Are the Symptoms of Preterm Labor?

Preterm labor is any labor that occurs from 20 weeks through 36 weeks of pregnancy. Here are the symptoms:

- Contractions (tightening of stomach muscles, or birth pains) every 10 minutes or more often
- Change in vaginal discharge (leaking fluid or bleeding from the vagina)
- Feeling of pressure in the pelvis (hip) area
- Low, dull backache
- Cramps that feel like menstrual cramps
- Abdominal cramps with or without diarrhea

It is normal for pregnant women to have some uterine contractions throughout the day. It is not normal to have frequent uterine contractions, such as six or more in one hour. Frequent uterine contractions, or tightenings, may cause the cervix to begin to open.

If a woman thinks that she might be having preterm labor, she should call her doctor or go to the hospital to be evaluated.

How Many People Are Affected by Preterm Labor and Birth?

According to the Centers for Disease Control and Prevention (CDC), in 2014, preterm birth affected about 1 of every 10 infants born in the United States. The rate of preterm births peaked in 2006 at nearly 13 percent, which was more than one-third higher than rates during the early 1980s. But in the past 5 years, the rates of preterm births have been falling. Between 2009 and 2010 (the latest year for which data are available), the rate declined to less than 12 percent of births.

Going into preterm labor does not always mean that a pregnant woman will deliver the baby prematurely. Up to one-half of women who experience preterm labor eventually deliver at 37 weeks of pregnancy or later.

In some cases, intervention from a healthcare provider is needed to stop preterm labor. In other cases, the labor may stop on its own. A woman who thinks she is experiencing preterm labor should contact a healthcare provider immediately.

How Many Women Are at Risk for Preterm Labor and Delivery?

Any pregnant woman could experience preterm labor and delivery. But there are some factors that increase a woman's risk of going into labor or giving birth prematurely.

What Causes Preterm Labor and Birth?

The causes of preterm labor and premature birth are numerous, complex, and only partly understood. Medical, psychosocial, and biological factors may all play a role in preterm labor and birth.

There are three main situations in which preterm labor and premature birth may occur:

- **Spontaneous preterm labor and birth.** This term refers to unintentional, unplanned delivery before the 37th week of pregnancy. This type of preterm birth can result from a number of causes, such as infection or inflammation, although the cause of spontaneous preterm labor and delivery is usually not known. A history of delivering preterm is one of the strongest predictors for subsequent preterm births.

- **Medically indicated preterm birth.** If a serious medical condition—such as preeclampsia—exists, the healthcare provider might recommend a preterm delivery. In these cases, healthcare providers often take steps to keep the baby in the womb as long as possible to allow for additional growth and development, while also monitoring the mother and fetus for health issues.

Providers also use additional interventions, such as steroids, to help improve outcomes for the baby.

- **Nonmedically indicated (elective) preterm delivery.** Some late-preterm births result from inducing labor or having a cesarean delivery even though there is not a medical reason to do so, even though this practice is not recommended. Research indicates that even babies born at 37 or 38 weeks of pregnancy are at higher risk for poor health outcomes than are babies born at 39 weeks of pregnancy or later. Therefore, unless there are medical problems, healthcare providers should wait until at least 39 weeks of pregnancy to induce labor or perform a cesarean delivery to prevent possible health problems.

What Are the Risk Factors for Preterm Labor and Birth?

There are several risk factors for preterm labor and premature birth, including ones that researchers have not yet identified. Some of these risk factors are "modifiable," meaning they can be changed to help reduce the risk. Other factors cannot be changed.

Healthcare providers consider the following factors to put women at high risk for preterm labor or birth:

- Women who have delivered preterm before, or who have experienced preterm labor before, are considered to be at high risk for preterm labor and birth.

- Being pregnant with twins, triplets, or more (called "multiple gestations") or the use of assisted reproductive technology is associated with a higher risk of preterm labor and birth. One study showed that more than 50 percent of twin births occurred preterm, compared with only 10 percent of births of single infants.

- Women with certain abnormalities of the reproductive organs are at greater risk for preterm labor and birth than are women who do not have these abnormalities. For instance, women who have a short cervix (the lower part of the uterus) or whose cervix shortens in the second trimester (fourth through sixth months) of pregnancy instead of the third trimester are at high risk for preterm delivery.

Certain medical conditions, including some that occur only during pregnancy, also place a woman at higher risk for preterm labor and delivery. Some of these conditions include:

- Urinary tract infections
- Sexually transmitted infections
- Certain vaginal infections, such as bacterial vaginosis and trichomoniasis
- High blood pressure
- Bleeding from the vagina
- Certain developmental abnormalities in the fetus
- Pregnancy resulting from in vitro fertilization
- Being underweight or obese before pregnancy
- Short time period between pregnancies (less than 6 months between a birth and the beginning of the next pregnancy)
- Placenta previa, a condition in which the placenta grows in the lowest part of the uterus and covers all or part of the opening to the cervix
- Being at risk for rupture of the uterus (when the wall of the uterus rips open). Rupture of the uterus is more likely if you have had a prior cesarean delivery or have had a uterine fibroid removed.
- Diabetes (high blood sugar) and gestational diabetes (which occurs only during pregnancy)
- Blood clotting problems

Other factors that may increase risk for preterm labor and premature birth include:

- Ethnicity. Preterm labor and birth occur more often among certain racial and ethnic groups. Infants of African American mothers are 50 percent more likely to be born preterm than are infants of white mothers.
- Age of the mother.
  - Women younger than age 18 are more likely to have a preterm delivery.
  - Women older than age 35 are also at risk of having preterm infants because they are more likely to have other conditions (such as high blood pressure and diabetes) that can cause complications requiring preterm delivery.

- Certain lifestyle and environmental factors, including:
  - Late or no healthcare during pregnancy
  - Smoking
  - Drinking alcohol
  - Using illegal drugs
  - Domestic violence, including physical, sexual, or emotional abuse
  - Lack of social support
  - Stress
  - Long working hours with long periods of standing
  - Exposure to certain environmental pollutants

Is It Possible to Predict Which Women Are More Likely to Have Preterm Labor and Birth?

There is no definitive way to predict preterm labor or premature birth. By identifying which women are at increased risk, healthcare providers may be able to provide early interventions, treatments, and close monitoring of these pregnancies to prevent preterm delivery or to improve health outcomes.

However, in some situations, healthcare providers know that a preterm delivery is very likely.

Shortened Cervix

As a preparation for birth, the cervix (the lower part of the uterus) naturally shortens late in pregnancy. However, in some women, the cervix shortens prematurely, around the fourth or fifth month of pregnancy, increasing the risk for preterm delivery.

In some cases, a healthcare provider may recommend measuring a pregnant woman's cervical length, especially if she previously had preterm labor or a preterm birth. Ultrasound scans may be used to measure cervical length and identify women with a shortened cervix.

"Incompetent" Cervix

The cervix normally remains closed during pregnancy. In some cases, the cervix starts to open early, before a fetus is ready to be born.

437

Healthcare providers may refer to a cervix that begins to open as an "incompetent" cervix. The process of cervical opening is painless and unnoticeable, without labor contractions or cramping.

Approximately 5 to 10 out of 1,000 pregnant women are diagnosed as having an incompetent cervix.

To try to prevent preterm birth, a doctor may place a stitch around the cervix to keep it closed. This procedure is called cervical cerclage.

How Do Healthcare Providers Diagnose Preterm Labor?

If a woman is concerned that she could be showing signs of preterm labor, she should call her healthcare provider or go to the hospital to be evaluated. In particular, a woman should call if she has more than six contractions in an hour or if fluid or blood is leaking from the vagina.

Physical Exam

If a woman is experiencing signs of labor, the healthcare provider may perform a pelvic exam to see if:

- The membranes have ruptured

- The cervix is beginning to get thinner (efface)

- The cervix is beginning to open (dilate)

Any of these situations could mean the woman is in preterm labor. Providers may also do an ultrasound exam and use a monitor to electronically record contractions and the fetal heart rate.

Fetal Fibronectin (fFN) Test

This test is used to detect whether the protein fetal fibronectin is being produced. fFN is like a biological "glue" between the uterine lining and the membrane that surrounds the fetus.

Normally fFN is detectable in the pregnant woman's secretions from the vagina and cervix early in the pregnancy (up to 22 weeks, or about 5 months) and again toward the end of the pregnancy (1 to 3 weeks before labor begins). It is usually not present between 24 and 34 weeks of pregnancy (5½ to 8½ months). If fFN is detected during this time, it may be a sign that the woman may be at risk of preterm labor and birth.

In most cases, the fFN test is performed on women who are showing signs of preterm labor. Testing for fFN can predict with about 50 percent accuracy which pregnant women showing signs of preterm labor are likely to have a preterm delivery. It is typically used for its negative predictive value, meaning that if it is negative, it is unlikely that a woman will deliver within the next 7 days.

What Treatments Are Used to Prevent Preterm Labor and Birth?

Treatment options for preventing preterm labor or birth are somewhat limited, in part because the cause of preterm labor or birth is often unknown.

- Hormone treatment
- Cerclage
- Bed rest

Women should discuss all of their treatment options—including the risks and benefits—with their healthcare providers. If possible, these discussions should occur during regular prenatal care visits, before there is any urgency, to allow for a complete discussion of all the issues.

What Treatments Can Reduce the Chances of Preterm Labor and Birth?

If a pregnant woman is showing signs of preterm labor, her doctor will often try treatments to stop labor and prolong the pregnancy until the fetus is more fully developed. Treatments include therapies to try to stop labor (tocolytics) and medications administered before birth to improve outcomes for the infant if born preterm (antenatal steroids to improve the respiratory outcomes and neuroprotective medications such as magnesium sulfate).

Medications to Delay Labor

Drugs called tocolytics can be given to many women with symptoms of preterm labor. These drugs can slow or stop contractions of the uterus and may prevent labor for 2 to 7 days. One common treatment for delaying labor is magnesium sulfate, given to the pregnant woman intravenously through a needle inserted in an arm vein.

Medications to Speed Development of the Fetus

Tocolytics may provide the extra time for treatment with corticosteroids to speed up development of the fetus's lungs and some other organs or for the pregnant woman to get to a hospital that offers specialized care for preterm infants. Corticosteroids can be particularly effective if the pregnancy is between 24 and 34 weeks (between 5½ and 7¾ months) and the woman's healthcare provider suspects that the birth may occur within the next week. Intravenously delivered magnesium sulfate may also reduce the risk of cerebral palsy if the child is born early.

What Methods Do Not Work to Prevent Preterm Labor?

Researchers have found that some methods for trying to stop preterm labor are not as effective as once thought. These include:

- Home uterine monitors

- Routine screening of all asymptomatic women for bacterial vaginosis *(Trichomonas vaginalis)* infection. Routine screening and treatment with antibiotics did not reduce preterm birth; in fact, the latter increased the risk of preterm birth.

Section 34.3

Maternal Health Benefits of Breastfeeding

This section includes text excerpted from "Making the Decision to Breastfeed," Office on Women's Health (OWH), U.S. Department of Health and Human Services (HHS), May 3, 2017.

When you breastfeed, you give your baby a healthy start that lasts a lifetime. Breastmilk is the perfect food for your baby. Breastfeeding saves lives, money, and time.

What Health Benefits Does Breastfeeding Give My Baby?

The cells, hormones, and antibodies in breast milk help protect babies from illness. This protection is unique and changes every day to meet your baby's growing needs.

Research shows that breastfed babies have lower risks of:

- Asthma

- Leukemia (during childhood)

- Obesity (during childhood)

- Ear infections

- Eczema (atopic dermatitis)

- Diarrhea and vomiting

- Lower respiratory infections

- Necrotizing enterocolitis, a disease that affects the gastrointestinal tract in premature babies, or babies born before 37 weeks of pregnancy

- Sudden infant death syndrome (SIDS)

- Type 2 diabetes

What Is Colostrum and How Does It Help My Baby?

Your breast milk helps your baby grow healthy and strong from day one.

- **Your first milk is liquid gold.** Called liquid gold for its deep yellow color, colostrum is the thick first milk that you make during pregnancy and just after birth. This milk is very rich in nutrients and includes antibodies to protect your baby from infections.

Colostrum also helps your newborn's digestive system to grow and function. Your baby gets only a small amount of colostrum at each feeding, because the stomach of a newborn infant is tiny and can hold only a small amount.

- **Your milk changes as your baby grows**. Colostrum changes into mature milk by the third to fifth day after birth. This mature milk has just the right amount of fat, sugar, water, and protein to help your baby continue to grow. It looks thinner than colostrum, but it has the nutrients and antibodies your baby needs for healthy growth.

What Are the Health Benefits of Breastfeeding for Mothers?

Breastfeeding helps a mother's health and healing following childbirth. Breastfeeding leads to a lower risk of these health problems in mothers:

- Type 2 diabetes

- Certain types of breast cancer

- Ovarian cancer

How Does Breastfeeding Compare to Formula Feeding?

- **Formula can be harder for your baby to digest.** For most babies, especially premature babies (babies born before 37 weeks of pregnancy), breast milk substitutes like formula are harder to digest than breast milk. Formula is made from cow's milk, and it often takes time for babies' stomachs to adjust to digesting it.

- **Your breast milk changes to meet your baby's needs.** As your baby gets older, your breast milk adjusts to meet your baby's changing needs. Researchers think that a baby's saliva transfers chemicals to a mother's body through breastfeeding. These chemicals help a mother's body create breast milk that meets the baby's changing needs.

- **Life can be easier for you when you breastfeed.** Breastfeeding may seem like it takes a little more effort than formula feeding at first. But breastfeeding can make your life easier once you and your baby settle into a good routine. When you breastfeed, there are no bottles and nipples to sterilize. You do not have to buy, measure, and mix formula. And there are no bottles to warm in the middle of the night! When you breastfeed, you can satisfy your baby's hunger right away.

- **Not breastfeeding costs money.** Formula and feeding supplies can cost well over $1,500 each year. As your baby gets older he or she will eat more formula. But breast milk changes with the baby's needs, and babies usually need the same amount of breast milk as they get older. Breastfed babies may also be sick less often, which can help keep your baby's health costs lower.

- **Breastfeeding keeps mother and baby close**. Physical contact is important to newborns. It helps them feel more secure, warm, and comforted. Mothers also benefit from this closeness. The skin-to-skin contact boosts your oxytocin levels. Oxytocin is a hormone that helps breast milk flow and can calm the mother.

Sometimes, formula feeding can save lives:

- Very rarely, babies are born unable to tolerate milk of any kind. These babies must have an infant formula that is hypoaller-genic, dairy free, or lactose free. A wide selection of specialist baby formulas now on the market include soy formula, hydro-lyzed formula, lactose-free formula, and hypoallergenic formula.

- Your baby may need formula if you have a health problem that won't allow you to breastfeed and you do not have access to donor breast milk.

Can Breastfeeding Help Me Lose Weight?

Besides giving your baby nourishment and helping to keep your baby from becoming sick, breastfeeding may help you lose weight. Many women who breastfed their babies said it helped them get back to their prepregnancy weight more quickly, but experts are still looking at the effects of breastfeeding on weight loss.

How Does Breastfeeding Benefit Society?

Society benefits overall when mothers breastfeed.

- **Breastfeeding saves lives.** Research shows that if 90 percent of families breastfed exclusively for six months, nearly 1,000 deaths among infants could be prevented each year.

- **Breastfeeding saves money.** Medical costs may be lower for fully breastfed infants than never-breastfed infants. Breastfed infants usually need fewer sick care visits, prescriptions, and hospitalizations.

- **Breastfeeding also helps make a more productive work-force.** Mothers who breastfeed may miss less work to care for sick infants than mothers who feed their infants formula. Employer medical costs may also be lower.

- **Breastfeeding is better for the environment.** Formula cans and bottle supplies create more trash and plastic waste. Your milk is a renewable resource that comes packaged and warmed.

How Does Breastfeeding Help in an Emergency?

During an emergency, such as a natural disaster, breastfeeding can save your baby's life:

- Breastfeeding protects your baby from the risks of an unclean water supply.

- Breastfeeding can help protect your baby against respiratory illnesses and diarrhea.

- Your milk is always at the right temperature for your baby. It helps to keep your baby's body temperature from dropping too low.

- Your milk is always available without needing other supplies.

Chapter 35

Recovering from Birth and Managing Postpartum Depression

When you are pregnant or after you have a baby, you may be depressed and not know it. Some normal changes during and after pregnancy can cause symptoms similar to those of depression. Your doctor can figure out if your symptoms are caused by depression or something else.

What Is Depression?

Depression is more than just feeling "blue" or "down in the dumps" for a few days. It's a serious illness that involves the brain. With depression, sad, anxious, or "empty" feelings don't go away and interfere with day-to-day life and routines. These feelings can be mild to severe. The good news is that most people with depression get better with treatment.

How Common Is Depression during and after Pregnancy?

Depression is a common problem during and after pregnancy. About 13 percent of pregnant women and new mothers have depression.

This chapter includes text excerpted from "Depression during and after Pregnancy," Office on Women's Health (OWH), U.S. Department of Health and Human Services (HHS), June 12, 2017.

How Do I Know If I Have Depression?

When you are pregnant or after you have a baby, you may be depressed and not know it. Some normal changes during and after pregnancy can cause symptoms similar to those of depression. But if you have any of the following symptoms of depression for more than 2 weeks, call your doctor:

- Feeling restless or moody

- Feeling sad, hopeless, and overwhelmed

- Crying a lot

- Having no energy or motivation

- Eating too little or too much

- Sleeping too little or too much

- Having trouble focusing or making decisions

- Having memory problems

- Feeling worthless and guilty

- Losing interest or pleasure in activities you used to enjoy

- Withdrawing from friends and family

- Having headaches, aches and pains, or stomach problems that don't go away

Your doctor can figure out if your symptoms are caused by depression or something else.

What Causes Depression? What about Postpartum Depression?

There is no single cause. Rather, depression likely results from a combination of factors:

- Depression is a mental illness that tends to run in families. Women with a family history of depression are more likely to have depression.

- Changes in brain chemistry or structure are believed to play a big role in depression.

- Stressful life events, such as death of a loved one, caring for an aging family member, abuse, and poverty, can trigger depression.

- Hormonal factors unique to women may contribute to depression in some women. We know that hormones directly affect the brain chemistry that controls emotions and mood. We also know that women are at greater risk of depression at certain times in their lives, such as puberty, during and after pregnancy, and during perimenopause. Some women also have depressive symptoms right before their period.

Depression after childbirth is called postpartum depression. Hormonal changes may trigger symptoms of postpartum depression. When you are pregnant, levels of the female hormones estrogen and progesterone increase greatly. In the first 24 hours after childbirth, hormone levels quickly return to normal. Researchers think the big change in hormone levels may lead to depression. This is much like the way smaller hormone changes can affect a woman's moods before she gets her period.

Levels of thyroid hormones may also drop after giving birth. The thyroid is a small gland in the neck that helps regulate how your body uses and stores energy from food. Low levels of thyroid hormones can cause symptoms of depression. A simple blood test can tell if this condition is causing your symptoms. If so, your doctor can prescribe thyroid medicine.

Other factors may play a role in postpartum depression. You may feel:

- Tired after delivery

- Tired from a lack of sleep or broken sleep

- Overwhelmed with a new baby

- Doubts about your ability to be a good mother

- Stress from changes in work and home routines

- An unrealistic need to be a perfect mom

- Loss of who you were before having the baby

- Less attractive

- A lack of free time

Are Some Women More at Risk for Depression during and after Pregnancy?

Certain factors may increase your risk of depression during and after pregnancy:

- A personal history of depression or another mental illness
- A family history of depression or another mental illness
- A lack of support from family and friends
- Anxiety or negative feelings about the pregnancy
- Problems with a previous pregnancy or birth
- Marriage or money problems
- Stressful life events
- Young age
- Substance abuse

Women who are depressed during pregnancy have a greater risk of depression after giving birth. The U.S. Preventive Services Task Force (USPSTF) recommends screening for depression during and after pregnancy, regardless of a woman's risk factors for depression.

What Is the Difference between "Baby Blues," Postpartum Depression, and Postpartum Psychosis?

Many women have the baby blues in the days after childbirth. If you have the baby blues, you may:

- Have mood swings
- Feel sad, anxious, or overwhelmed
- Have crying spells
- Lose your appetite
- Have trouble sleeping

The baby blues most often go away within a few days or a week. The symptoms are not severe and do not need treatment.

The symptoms of postpartum depression last longer and are more severe. Postpartum depression can begin anytime within the first year after childbirth. If you have postpartum depression, you may have any of the symptoms of depression listed above. Symptoms may also include:

- Thoughts of hurting the baby
- Thoughts of hurting yourself
- Not having any interest in the baby

Postpartum depression needs to be treated by a doctor.

Postpartum psychosis is rare. It occurs in about 1 to 4 out of every 1,000 births. It usually begins in the first 2 weeks after childbirth. Women who have bipolar disorder or another mental health problem called schizoaffective disorder have a higher risk for postpartum psychosis. Symptoms may include:

- Seeing things that aren't there
- Feeling confused
- Having rapid mood swings
- Trying to hurt yourself or your baby

What Should I Do If I Have Symptoms of Depression during or after Pregnancy?

Call your doctor if:

- Your baby blues don't go away after 2 weeks
- Symptoms of depression get more and more intense
- Symptoms of depression begin any time after delivery, even many months later
- It is hard for you to perform tasks at work or at home
- You cannot care for yourself or your baby
- You have thoughts of harming yourself or your baby

Your doctor can ask you questions to test for depression. Your doctor can also refer you to a mental health professional who specializes in treating depression.

Some women don't tell anyone about their symptoms. They feel embarrassed, ashamed, or guilty about feeling depressed when they are supposed to be happy. They worry they will be viewed as unfit parents.

Any woman may become depressed during pregnancy or after having a baby. It doesn't mean you are a bad or "not together" mom. You and your baby do not have to suffer. There is help.

Here are some other helpful tips:

- Rest as much as you can. Sleep when the baby is sleeping.

- Don't try to do too much or try to be perfect.

- Ask your partner, family, and friends for help.

- Make time to go out, visit friends, or spend time alone with your partner.

- Discuss your feelings with your partner, family, and friends.

- Talk with other mothers so you can learn from their experiences.

- Join a support group. Ask your doctor about groups in your area.

- Don't make any major life changes during pregnancy or right after giving birth. Major changes can cause unneeded stress. Sometimes big changes can't be avoided. When that happens, try to arrange support and help in your new situation ahead of time.

How Is Depression Treated?

The two common types of treatment for depression are:

- **Talk therapy**. This involves talking to a therapist, psychologist, or social worker to learn to change how depression makes you think, feel, and act.

- **Medicine.** Your doctor can prescribe an antidepressant medicine. These medicines can help relieve symptoms of depression.

These treatment methods can be used alone or together. If you are depressed, your depression can affect your baby. Getting treatment is important for you and your baby. Talk with your doctor about the benefits and risks of taking medicine to treat depression when you are pregnant or breastfeeding.

What Can Happen If Depression Is Not Treated?

Untreated depression can hurt you and your baby. Some women with depression have a hard time caring for themselves during pregnancy. They may:

- Eat poorly

- Not gain enough weight
- Have trouble sleeping
- Miss prenatal visits
- Not follow medical instructions
- Use harmful substances, like tobacco, alcohol, or illegal drugs

Depression during pregnancy can raise the risk of:

- Problems during pregnancy or delivery
- Having a low-birth-weight baby
- Premature birth

Untreated postpartum depression can affect your ability to parent. You may:

- Lack energy
- Have trouble focusing
- Feel moody
- Not be able to meet your child's needs

As a result, you may feel guilty and lose confidence in yourself as a mother. These feelings can make your depression worse.

Researchers believe postpartum depression in a mother can affect her baby. It can cause the baby to have:

- Delays in language development
- Problems with mother-child bonding
- Behavior problems
- Increased crying

It helps if your partner or another caregiver can help meet the baby's needs while you are depressed.

All children deserve the chance to have a healthy mom. And all moms deserve the chance to enjoy their life and their children. If you are feeling depressed during pregnancy or after having a baby, don't suffer alone. Please tell a loved one and call your doctor right away.

Chapter 36

Pregnancy Loss

Chapter Contents

Section 36.1

Ectopic Pregnancy

"Ectopic Pregnancy," © 2018 Omnigraphics.
Reviewed August 2017.

What Is an Ectopic Pregnancy?

Normally, a fertilized egg gets implanted and develops in the main uterine cavity. However, sometimes a fertilized egg implants itself in another place, often the fallopian tubes (the structures leading from the ovaries to the uterus). This is called an ectopic or tubular pregnancy. Ectopic pregnancies can also occur in the ovaries, cervix, or the abdominal cavity. Since these other anatomical structures lack the space and nourishing environment of the uterus, an ectopic pregnancy will not be viable. Also, ectopic pregnancies must be removed immediately, because, if not treated, the growing embryonic tissue will damage the mother's reproductive organs, resulting in serious and potentially life-threatening blood loss.

What Are the Risk Factors for an Ectopic Pregnancy?

All women have a slight risk of ectopic pregnancy. However, the risk increases with the following factors:

- Becoming pregnant over the age of 35
- History of:
  - ectopic pregnancy
  - endometriosis
  - pelvic surgery, abdominal surgery, or multiple abortions
  - sexually transmitted diseases (STDs)
- Structural abnormalities in the fallopian tubes that restrict the movement of eggs
- Conception that occurs in spite of tubal ligation or intrauterine device

- Conception assisted by fertility drugs or procedures
- Hormonal imbalances
- Smoking
- Abnormal development of a fertilized egg

What Are the Symptoms of an Ectopic Pregnancy?

The symptoms of an ectopic pregnancy are similar to those in the early stages of a normal pregnancy. As with a normal pregnancy, a woman will experience a missed period, nausea, and tenderness in the breasts. A pregnancy test will be positive. However, an ectopic pregnancy does not proceed normally. The first indication is slight vaginal bleeding or brown watery discharge accompanied by dull pelvic pain. However, the pain in the pelvis may spread to the abdomen and become sharp and stabbing. A woman may also experience shoulder pain or an urge to move her bowels if blood has leaked from the fallopian tube and pooled in the abdominal cavity where it irritates related nerves. If the fallopian tube is completely ruptured, resulting in heavy bleeding in the abdominal cavity, lightheadedness, fainting, and shock will occur.

When Should You Call for Emergency Help?

Given the potential life-threatening complications of an ectopic pregnancy, emergency help should be sought out immediately should you experience:

- Severe pain in the abdomen and pelvic areas accompanied by vaginal bleeding
- Fainting and lightheadedness
- Pain in the shoulders

How Is an Ectopic Pregnancy Diagnosed?

The doctor will perform an initial pregnancy test and pelvic examination. Since an ectopic pregnancy cannot be detected by a physical examination alone, the doctor will also order an ultrasound test. When the pregnancy is too early to see via imaging, the doctor will monitor the patient using blood tests until the condition can be confirmed using an ultrasound. One of the ultrasound tests frequently used is a transvaginal ultrasound, which uses a wand-like device placed in the vagina to produce images of the uterus and fallopian tubes to detect an ectopic pregnancy.

How Is an Ectopic Pregnancy Treated?

An ectopic pregnancy is treated by removing the implanted embryo via the following methods:

- Medication. If the ectopic pregnancy has been detected early, doctors will use an injection of the drug methotrexate to stop cell growth in the embryo and dissolve the tissue. They will then monitor levels of the pregnancy hormone chorionic gonadotropin (HCG) in the patient's blood. If the levels are high, indicating that the fetal tissue has not been completely removed, the doctor will administer a second injection of the same drug.

- Surgery. Doctors can also use laparoscopic surgery to remove an ectopic embryo. An incision is made in or near the naval and a tube is inserted with surgical tools and a camera with a light source. The embryo is then removed and any damage to the fallopian tube repaired. If heavy bleeding and heavy damage to the fallopian tube has occurred, the surgeon may remove the fallopian tube as well. After surgery, the patient is monitored for levels of the human chorionic gonadotropin (HCG) hormone to confirm that all ectopic tissue was removed. Otherwise, a methotrexate injection is administered.

How Can an Ectopic Pregnancy Be Prevented?

An ectopic pregnancy cannot be prevented but the risk factors can be controlled.

- Limit the number of sexual partners

- Do not engage in unprotected sex

- Quit smoking

What Is the Outlook after an Ectopic Pregnancy?

The outlook after an ectopic pregnancy depends on what effect it has had on the fallopian tubes or other reproductive organs. If the fallopian tubes are intact and damage has been minimal, the chances of having a normal pregnancy in the future are good. You will be advised to wait for two to three months before trying to get pregnant again. About 65 percent of women who have undergone treatment for ectopic pregnancy successfully become pregnant within 18 months of treatment. In some cases, in vitro fertilization (IVF) treatment may be necessary. The risk for a repeat ectopic pregnancy exists but is significantly less at 10 percent.

How Can You Cope after an Ectopic Pregnancy?

The loss of a pregnancy is devastating. It is important to recognize the loss and give yourself time to grieve. Seek the support of your partner, friend, or loved one. Contact a support group, grief counselor, or a mental health provider for support if needed.

Women who have been treated for ectopic pregnancies often go on to have healthy pregnancies later. If one fallopian tube was removed during treatment, the other fallopian tube can still function as part of a normal pregnancy. IVF treatment could be an option for women who have lost both fallopian tubes due to ectopic pregnancies.

Plan your pregnancy ahead of time and discuss it with your doctor. You can be reassured of a normal pregnancy with the help of blood tests and ultrasound imaging early in your pregnancy.

References

1. Johnson, Traci C., MD. "What to Know about Ectopic Pregnancy," WebMD, LLC, January 21, 2017.

2. "Ectopic Pregnancy," NHS Choices, March 2, 2016.

3. Selner, Marissa, Nall, Rachel. "Ectopic Pregnancy," Healthline, October 13, 2015.

4. "Ectopic Pregnancy," Mayo Foundation for Medical Education and Research (MFMER), January 20, 2015.

Section 36.2

Stillbirth

This section includes text excerpted from "Facts about
Stillbirth," Centers for Disease Control and
Prevention (CDC), February 22, 2017.

A stillbirth is the death or loss of a baby before or during delivery. Both miscarriage and stillbirth describe pregnancy loss, but they differ according to when the loss occurs. In the United States, a miscarriage is usually defined as loss of a baby before the 20th week of pregnancy, and a stillbirth is loss of a baby after 20 weeks of pregnancy.

Stillbirth is further classified as either early, late, or term.

- An **early** stillbirth is a fetal death occurring between 20 and 27 completed weeks of pregnancy.

- A **late** stillbirth occurs between 28 and 36 completed pregnancy weeks.

- A **term** stillbirth occurs between 37 or more completed pregnancy weeks.

How Many Babies Are Stillborn?

Stillbirth affects about 1 percent of all pregnancies, and each year about 24,000 babies are stillborn in the United States. That is about the same number of babies that die during the first year of life and it is more than 10 times as many deaths as the number that occur from sudden infant death syndrome (SIDS).

Because of advances in medical technology over the last 30 years, prenatal care (medical care during pregnancy) has improved, which has dramatically reduced the number of late and term stillbirth. However, the rate of early stillbirth has remained about the same over time.

What Increases the Risk of Stillbirth?

The causes of many stillbirths are unknown. Therefore, families are often left grieving without answers to their questions. Stillbirth is not a cause of death, but rather a term that means a baby's death during the pregnancy. Some women blame themselves, but rarely are these deaths caused by something a woman did or did not do. Known causes of stillbirth generally fall into one of three broad categories:

- Problems with the baby (birth defects or genetic problems)
- Problems with the placenta or umbilical cord (this is where the mother and baby exchange oxygen and nutrients)
- Certain conditions in the mother (for example, uncontrolled diabetes, high blood pressure, or obesity)

Stillbirth with an unknown cause is called "unexplained stillbirth." Having an unexplained stillbirth is more likely to occur the further along a woman is in her pregnancy.

Although stillbirth occurs in families of all races, ethnicities, and income levels, and to women of all ages, some women are at higher risk for having a stillbirth. Some of the factors that increase the risk for a stillbirth include the mother:

- being of black race
- being a teenager
- being 35 years of age or older
- being unmarried
- being obese
- smoking cigarettes during pregnancy
- having certain medical conditions, such as high blood pressure or diabetes
- having multiple pregnancies
- having had a previous pregnancy loss

These factors are also associated with other poor pregnancy outcomes, such as preterm birth.

What Can Be Done?

Centers for Disease Control and Prevention (CDC) works to learn more about who might have a stillbirth and why. CDC does this by tracking how often stillbirth occurs and researching what causes stillbirth and how to prevent it. Knowledge about the potential causes of stillbirth can be used to develop recommendations, policies, and services to help prevent stillbirth. While we continue to learn more about stillbirth, much work remains. Stillbirth is not often viewed as a public health issue, so increased awareness is key. Additionally, healthcare providers need increased training in using stillbirth evaluation guidelines, providing access to grief counseling, and discussing with families why a stillborn evaluation is important.

Section 36.3

Miscarriage

This section contains text excerpted from the following sources: Text beginning with the heading "What Is Miscarriage?" is excerpted from "Pregnancy Loss: Condition Information," *Eunice Kennedy Shriver* National Institute of Child Health and Human Development (NICHD), December 4, 2012. Reviewed August 2017; Text beginning with the heading "Coping with Loss" is excerpted from "Pregnancy Loss," Office on Women's Health (OWH), U.S. Department of Health and Human Services (HHS), February 1, 2017.

What Is Miscarriage?

A miscarriage, also called pregnancy loss or spontaneous abortion, is the unexpected loss of a fetus before the 20th week of pregnancy, or gestation. (Gestation is the period of pregnancy from conception to birth.) The loss of a pregnancy after the 20th week of gestation is called a stillbirth and can occur before or during delivery.

What Are the Symptoms of Miscarriage?

Symptoms of miscarriage may include vaginal spotting or bleeding; abdominal pain or abdominal cramps; low back pain; or fluid, tissue, or clot-like material passing from the vagina. Although vaginal bleeding is a common symptom when a woman has a miscarriage, many pregnant women have spotting early during their pregnancy because of other factors but do not miscarry. Regardless, pregnant women who have any of the symptoms of miscarriage should contact their healthcare providers immediately.

How Many People Are Affected by or at Risk for Miscarriage?

The estimated rate of miscarriage is 15 percent to 20 percent in women who know they are pregnant, but as many as half of all fertilized eggs may spontaneously abort, often before the women realize they are pregnant. Women who have had previous miscarriages are at a higher risk for miscarriage. The risk of miscarriage also increases with maternal age beginning at age 30 and becoming greater after age 35.

What Causes Miscarriage?

Miscarriage occurs due to many different causes, some of them known and others unknown. Frequently, miscarriages occur when a pregnancy is not developing normally. More than half of all miscarriages are caused by a chromosomal abnormality in the fetus (typically due to the wrong number of chromosomes, the structures in a cell that contain the genetic information), which is more common with increasing age of the parents, particularly among women who are older than age 35.

Other possible causes of pregnancy loss or miscarriage are maternal health issues or exposure to chemicals. Maternal health issues include chronic disease, such as diabetes, thyroid disease, or polycystic ovary syndrome (PCOS), or problems associated with the immune system, such as an autoimmune disorder. Other maternal health issues that can increase the risk of miscarriage include infection, hormone problems, obesity, or problems of the placenta, cervix, or uterus. Exposure to environmental toxins, drug use or alcohol use, smoking, or the consumption of 200 milligrams or more of caffeine per day (equal to about one 12-ounce cup of coffee) also can increase the risk of miscarriage.

How Do Healthcare Providers Diagnose Miscarriage?

If a pregnant woman experiences any of the symptoms of miscarriage, such as crampy abdominal or back pain, light spotting, or bleeding, she should contact her healthcare provider immediately. For diagnosis, the woman may need to undergo a blood test to check for the level of hCG, the pregnancy hormone, or an internal pelvic examination to determine if her cervix is dilated or thinned, which can be a sign of a miscarriage; or depending on the length of time since her last menstrual period, and the level of pregnancy hormone in the blood, she may need to have an ultrasound test so that her healthcare provider can observe the pregnancy and the maternal reproductive organs, such as the uterus and placenta. If a woman has had more than one miscarriage, she may choose to have blood tests performed to check for chromosome abnormalities or hormone problems, or to detect immune system disorders that may interfere with a healthy pregnancy.

What Are the Treatments for Miscarriage?

In most cases, no treatment is necessary for women who miscarry early in their pregnancy, because the bleeding associated with miscarriage usually empties the uterus of pregnancy-associated tissue. In some cases, however, a woman may need to undergo a surgical procedure called a dilation and curettage (D&C) to remove any pregnancy-associated tissue remaining in the uterus. A D&C is performed if the woman is bleeding heavily or if an ultrasound test detects any remaining tissue in the uterus.

An alternative to a D&C is the use of a medication called misoprostol that helps the tissue pass out of the uterus. The use of misoprostol has proven to be effective in 84 percent of the cases studied. Other treatments after a woman miscarries may include control of mild to moderate bleeding, prevention of infection, pain relief, and emotional support. If heavy bleeding occurs, the woman should contact her healthcare provider immediately.

Is There a Cure for Miscarriage?

In many cases, a woman can do little to prevent a miscarriage. However, having preconception and prenatal care (before becoming pregnant and during pregnancy) is the best prevention available for all complications associated with pregnancy. Miscarriages caused by systemic disease often can be prevented by detection and treatment of the disease before pregnancy occurs. A woman also can decrease her risk of miscarriage by avoiding environmental hazards, such as infectious diseases, X-rays, drugs and alcohol, and high levels of caffeine.

Coping with Loss

After the loss, you might be stunned or shocked. You might be asking, "Why me?" You might feel guilty that you did or didn't do something to cause your pregnancy to end. You might feel cheated and angry. Or you might feel extremely sad as you come to terms with the baby that will never be. These emotions are all normal reactions to loss. With time, you will be able to accept the loss and move on. You will never forget your baby. But you will be able to put this chapter behind you and look forward to life ahead. To help get you through this difficult time, try some of these ideas:

- **Turn to loved ones and friends for support.** Share your feelings and ask for help when you need it.

- **Talk to your partner about your loss.** Keep in mind that women and men cope with loss in different ways.

- **Take care of yourself.** Eating healthy foods, keeping active, and getting enough sleep will help restore energy and well-being.

- **Join a support group.** A support group might help you to feel less alone.

- **Do something in remembrance of your baby.**

- **Seek help from a grief counselor,** especially if your grief doesn't ease with time.

Trying Again

Give yourself plenty of time to heal emotionally. It could take a few months or even a year. Once you and your partner are emotionally ready to try again, confirm with your doctor that you are in good physical health and that your body is ready for pregnancy. Following a miscarriage, most healthy women do not need to wait before trying to conceive again. You might worry that pregnancy loss could happen again. But take heart in knowing that most women who have gone through pregnancy loss go on to have healthy babies.

Part Five

Gynecological and High-Prevalence Cancers in Women

Chapter 37

Breast Cancer

The breast is made up of lobes and ducts. Each breast has 15 to 20 sections called lobes. Each lobe has many smaller sections called lobules. Lobules end in dozens of tiny bulbs that can make milk. The lobes, lobules, and bulbs are linked by thin tubes called ducts.

Each breast also has blood vessels and lymph vessels. The lymph vessels carry an almost colorless fluid called lymph. Lymph vessels carry lymph between lymph nodes. Lymph nodes are small bean-shaped structures that are found throughout the body. They filter substances in lymph and help fight infection and disease. Clusters of lymph nodes are found near the breast in the axilla (under the arm), above the collarbone, and in the chest.

What Is Breast Cancer?

Breast cancer is a disease in which malignant (cancer) cells form in the tissues of the breast. The most common type of breast cancer is ductal carcinoma, which begins in the cells of the ducts. Breast cancer can also begin in the cells of the lobules and in other tissues in the breast. Ductal carcinoma in situ is a condition in which abnormal cells are found in the lining of the ducts but they haven't spread outside the duct. Breast cancer that has spread from where it began in the ducts or lobules to surrounding tissue is called invasive breast cancer. In

This chapter includes text excerpted from "Breast Cancer Treatment (PDQ®)– Patient Version," National Cancer Institute (NCI), May 5, 2017.

inflammatory breast cancer, the breast looks red and swollen and feels warm because the cancer cells block the lymph vessels in the skin.

In the United States, breast cancer is the second most common cancer in women after skin cancer. It can occur in both women and men, but it is rare in men. Each year there are about 100 times more new cases of breast cancer in women than in men.

What Are the Risk Factors for Breast Cancer?

A family history of breast cancer and other factors increase the risk of breast cancer.

Anything that increases your chance of getting a disease is called a risk factor. Having a risk factor does not mean that you will get cancer; not having risk factors doesn't mean that you will not get cancer. Talk to your doctor if you think you may be at risk for breast cancer.

Risk factors for breast cancer include the following:

- A personal history of invasive breast cancer, ductal carcinoma in situ (DCIS), or lobular carcinoma in situ (LCIS).

- A personal history of benign (noncancer) breast disease.

- A family history of breast cancer in a first-degree relative (mother, daughter, or sister).

- Inherited changes in the *BRCA1* or *BRCA2* genes or in other genes that increase the risk of breast cancer.

- Breast tissue that is dense on a mammogram.

- Exposure of breast tissue to estrogen made by the body. This may be caused by:

  - Menstruating at an early age.

  - Older age at first birth or never having given birth.

  - Starting menopause at a later age.

- Taking hormones such as estrogen combined with progestin for symptoms of menopause.

- Treatment with radiation therapy to the breast/chest.

- Drinking alcohol.

- Obesity.

Older age is the main risk factor for most cancers. The chance of getting cancer increases as you get older.

What Is the Role of Genes in Breast Cancer?

Breast cancer is sometimes caused by inherited gene mutations (changes). The genes in cells carry the hereditary information that is received from a person's parents. Hereditary breast cancer makes up about 5 to 10 percent of all breast cancer. Some mutated genes related to breast cancer are more common in certain ethnic groups.

Women who have certain gene mutations, such as a *BRCA1* or *BRCA2* mutation, have an increased risk of breast cancer. These women also have an increased risk of ovarian cancer, and may have an increased risk of other cancers.

There are tests that can detect (find) mutated genes. These genetic tests are sometimes done for members of families with a high risk of cancer.

What Are the Protective Factors for Breast Cancer

The use of certain medicines and other factors decrease the risk of breast cancer.

Anything that decreases your chance of getting a disease is called a protective factor.

Protective factors for breast cancer include the following:

- Taking any of the following:

  - Estrogen-only hormone therapy after a hysterectomy.

  - Selective estrogen receptor modulators (SERMs).

  - Aromatase inhibitors.

- Less exposure of breast tissue to estrogen made by the body. This can be a result of:

  - Early pregnancy.

  - Breastfeeding.

- Getting enough exercise.

- Having any of the following procedures:

  - Mastectomy to reduce the risk of cancer.

  - Oophorectomy to reduce the risk of cancer.

  - Ovarian ablation.

What Are the Signs and Symptoms of Breast Cancer?

Signs of breast cancer include a lump or change in the breast. These and other signs may be caused by breast cancer or by other conditions. Check with your doctor if you have any of the following:

- A lump or thickening in or near the breast or in the underarm area.

- A change in the size or shape of the breast.

- A dimple or puckering in the skin of the breast.

- A nipple turned inward into the breast.

- Fluid, other than breast milk, from the nipple, especially if it's bloody.

- Scaly, red, or swollen skin on the breast, nipple, or areola (the dark area of skin around the nipple).

- Dimples in the breast that look like the skin of an orange, called peau d'orange.

What Are the Tests Used to Diagnose Cancer?

Tests that examine the breasts are used to detect (find) and diagnose breast cancer.

Check with your doctor if you notice any changes in your breasts. The following tests and procedures may be used:

- **Physical exam and history.** An exam of the body to check general signs of health, including checking for signs of disease, such as lumps or anything else that seems unusual. A history of the patient's health habits and past illnesses and treatments will also be taken.

- **Clinical breast exam (CBE).** An exam of the breast by a doctor or other health professional. The doctor will carefully feel the breasts and under the arms for lumps or anything else that seems unusual.

- **Mammogram:** An X-ray of the breast.

- **Ultrasound exam.** A procedure in which high-energy sound waves (ultrasound) are bounced off internal tissues or organs and make echoes. The echoes form a picture of body tissues called a sonogram. The picture can be printed to be looked at later.

- **MRI (magnetic resonance imaging).** A procedure that uses a magnet, radio waves, and a computer to make a series of detailed pictures of both breasts. This procedure is also called nuclear magnetic resonance imaging (NMRI).

- **Blood chemistry studies.** A procedure in which a blood sample is checked to measure the amounts of certain substances released into the blood by organs and tissues in the body. An unusual (higher or lower than normal) amount of a substance can be a sign of disease.

- **Biopsy.** The removal of cells or tissues so they can be viewed under a microscope by a pathologist to check for signs of cancer. If a lump in the breast is found, a biopsy may be done.

There are four types of biopsy used to check for breast cancer:

- **Excisional biopsy:** The removal of an entire lump of tissue.

- **Incisional biopsy:** The removal of part of a lump or a sample of tissue.

- **Core biopsy:** The removal of tissue using a wide needle.

- **Fine-needle aspiration (FNA) biopsy:** The removal of tissue or fluid, using a thin needle.

What Are the Tests Conducted after Cancer is Detected?

If cancer is found, tests are done to study the cancer cells. Decisions about the best treatment are based on the results of these tests. The tests give information about:

- how quickly the cancer may grow.

- how likely it is that the cancer will spread through the body.

- how well certain treatments might work.

- how likely the cancer is to recur (come back).

Tests include the following:

- **Estrogen and progesterone receptor test:** A test to measure the amount of estrogen and progesterone (hormones) receptors in cancer tissue. If there are more estrogen and progesterone receptors than normal, the cancer is called estrogen and/or progesterone receptor positive. This type of breast cancer may grow more quickly. The test results show whether treatment to block estrogen and progesterone may stop the cancer from growing.

- **Human epidermal growth factor type 2 receptor (HER2/ neu) test:** A laboratory test to measure how many *HER2/neu* genes there are and how much HER2/neu protein is made in a sample of tissue. If there are more *HER2/neu* genes or higher levels of HER2/neu protein than normal, the cancer is called HER2/neu positive. This type of breast cancer may grow more quickly and is more likely to spread to other parts of the body. The cancer may be treated with drugs that target the *HER2/ neu* protein, such as trastuzumab and pertuzumab.

- **Multigene tests:** Tests in which samples of tissue are studied to look at the activity of many genes at the same time. These tests may help predict whether cancer will spread to other parts of the body or recur (come back).

- There are many types of multigene tests. The following multigene tests have been studied in clinical trials:

    - **Oncotype DX.** This test helps predict whether stage I or stage II breast cancer that is estrogen receptor positive and node negative will spread to other parts of the body. If the risk that the cancer will spread is high, chemotherapy may be given to lower the risk.

    - **MammaPrint.** This test helps predict whether stage I or stage II breast cancer that is node negative will spread to other parts of the body. If the risk that the cancer will spread is high, chemotherapy may be given to lower the risk.

Based on these tests, breast cancer is described as one of the following types:

- Hormone receptor positive (estrogen and/or progesterone receptor positive) or hormone receptor negative (estrogen and/or progesterone receptor negative).

- HER2/neu positive or HER2/neu negative.

- Triple negative (estrogen receptor, progesterone receptor, and HER2/neu negative).

This information helps the doctor decide which treatments will work best for your cancer.

What Are the Factors Affecting Prognosis and Treatment?

Certain factors affect prognosis (chance of recovery) and treatment options.

The prognosis (chance of recovery) and treatment options depend on the following:

- The stage of the cancer (the size of the tumor and whether it is in the breast only or has spread to lymph nodes or other places in the body).

- The type of breast cancer.

- Estrogen receptor and progesterone receptor levels in the tumor tissue.

- Human epidermal growth factor type 2 receptor (HER2/neu) levels in the tumor tissue.

- Whether the tumor tissue is triple negative (cells that do not have estrogen receptors, progesterone receptors, or high levels of HER2/neu).

- How fast the tumor is growing.

- How likely the tumor is to recur (come back).

- A woman's age, general health, and menopausal status (whether a woman is still having menstrual periods).

- Whether the cancer has just been diagnosed or has recurred (come back).

What Is the Treatment for Breast Cancer?

There are different types of treatment for patients with breast cancer. Different types of treatment are available for patients with breast cancer. Some treatments are standard (the currently used treatment), and some are being tested in clinical trials. A treatment clinical trial is a research study meant to help improve current treatments or obtain information on new treatments for patients with cancer. When clinical trials show that a new treatment is better than the standard treatment, the new treatment may become the standard treatment. Patients may want to think about taking part in a clinical trial. Some clinical trials are open only to patients who have not started treatment.

The following are the five types of standard treatment:

1. Surgery: Breast-conserving surgery, total mastectomy, and modified radical mastectomy

2. Radiation Therapy: External radiation therapy and internal radiation therapy

3. Chemotherapy

4. Hormone Therapy

5. Targeted Therapy

What Are the New Types of Treatment Being Tested in Clinical Trials?

High-Dose Chemotherapy with Stem Cell Transplant

High-dose chemotherapy with stem cell transplant is a way of giving high doses of chemotherapy and replacing blood -forming cells destroyed by the cancer treatment. Stem cells (immature blood cells) are removed from the blood or bone marrow of the patient or a donor and are frozen and stored. After the chemotherapy is completed, the stored stem cells are thawed and given back to the patient through an infusion. These reinfused stem cells grow into (and restore) the body's blood cells.

Studies have shown that high-dose chemotherapy followed by stem cell transplant does not work better than standard chemotherapy in the treatment of breast cancer. Doctors have decided that, for now, high-dose chemotherapy should be tested only in clinical trials. Before taking part in such a trial, women should talk with their doctors about the serious side effects, including death, that may be caused by high-dose chemotherapy.

What Are the Side Effects of Treatment for Breast Cancer?

Some treatments for breast cancer may cause side effects that continue or appear months or years after treatment has ended. These are called late effects.

Late effects of radiation therapy are not common, but may include:

- Inflammation of the lung after radiation therapy to the breast, especially when chemotherapy is given at the same time.

- Arm lymphedema, especially when radiation therapy is given after lymph node dissection.

- In women younger than 45 years who receive radiation therapy to the chest wall after mastectomy, there may be a higher risk of developing breast cancer in the other breast.

Late effects of chemotherapy depend on the drugs used, but may include:

- Heart failure.

- Blood clots.

- Premature menopause.

- Second cancer, such as leukemia.

Late effects of targeted therapy with trastuzumab, lapatinib, or pertuzumab may include:

- Heart problems such as heart failure.

How Does a Patient Take Part in a Clinical Trial for Breast Cancer Treatment?

For some patients, taking part in a clinical trial may be the best treatment choice. Clinical trials are part of the cancer research process. Clinical trials are done to find out if new cancer treatments are safe and effective or better than the standard treatment.

Many of today's standard treatments for cancer are based on earlier clinical trials. Patients who take part in a clinical trial may receive the standard treatment or be among the first to receive a new treatment.

Patients who take part in clinical trials also help improve the way cancer will be treated in the future. Even when clinical trials do not lead to effective new treatments, they often answer important questions and help move research forward.

Patients can enter clinical trials before, during, or after starting their cancer treatment. Some clinical trials only include patients who have not yet received treatment. Other trials test treatments for patients whose cancer has not gotten better. There are also clinical trials that test new ways to stop cancer from recurring (coming back) or reduce the side effects of cancer treatment.

Clinical trials are taking place in many parts of the country.

Follow-Up Tests May Be Needed

Some of the tests that were done to diagnose the cancer or to find out the stage of the cancer may be repeated. Some tests will be repeated in order to see how well the treatment is working. Decisions about whether to continue, change, or stop treatment may be based on the results of these tests.

Some of the tests will continue to be done from time to time after treatment has ended. The results of these tests can show if your condition has changed or if the cancer has recurred (come back). These tests are sometimes called follow-up tests or check-ups.

Chapter 38

Gynecological Cancers

Chapter Contents

Section 38.1

Cervical Cancer

This section includes text excerpted from "Cervical
Cancer Treatment (PDQ®)—Patient Version," National
Cancer Institute (NCI), July 14, 2016.

General Information about Cervical Cancer

Cervical cancer is a disease in which malignant (cancer) cells form
in the tissues of the cervix.

The cervix is the lower, narrow end of the uterus (the hollow, pear-
shaped organ where a fetus grows). The cervix leads from the uterus
to the vagina (birth canal).

Cervical cancer usually develops slowly over time. Before cancer
appears in the cervix, the cells of the cervix go through changes known
as dysplasia, in which abnormal cells begin to appear in the cervical tissue. Over time, the abnormal cells may become cancer cells and start to
grow and spread more deeply into the cervix and to surrounding areas.

Cervical cancer in children is rare.

Human Papillomavirus (HPV) Infection Is the Major Risk Factor for Cervical Cancer

Anything that increases your chance of getting a disease is called a
risk factor. Having a risk factor does not mean that you will get cancer; not having risk factors doesn't mean that you will not get cancer.
Talk to your doctor if you think you may be at risk for cervical cancer.

Risk factors for cervical cancer include the following:

- Being infected with human papillomavirus (HPV). This is the
  most important risk factor for cervical cancer.

- Being exposed to the drug DES (diethylstilbestrol) while in the
  mother's womb.

In women who are infected with HPV, the following risk factors
add to the increased risk of cervical cancer:

- Giving birth to many children.

- Smoking cigarettes.

- Using oral contraceptives ("the Pill") for a long time.

There are also risk factors that increase the risk of HPV infection:

- Having a weakened immune system caused by immunosuppression. Immunosuppression weakens the body's ability to fight infections and other diseases. The body's ability to fight HPV infection may be lowered by long-term immunosuppression from:

  - being infected with human immunodeficiency virus (HIV).

  - taking medicine to help prevent organ rejection after a transplant.

- Being sexually active at a young age.

- Having many sexual partners.

Older age is a main risk factor for most cancers. The chance of getting cancer increases as you get older.

There Are Usually No Signs or Symptoms of Early Cervical Cancer but It Can Be Detected Early with Regular Check-Ups

Early cervical cancer may not cause signs or symptoms. Women should have regular check-ups, including tests to check for human papillomavirus (HPV) or abnormal cells in the cervix. The prognosis (chance of recovery) is better when the cancer is found early.

Signs and Symptoms of Cervical Cancer Include Vaginal Bleeding and Pelvic Pain

These and other signs and symptoms may be caused by cervical cancer or by other conditions. Check with your doctor if you have any of the following:

- Vaginal bleeding (including bleeding after sexual intercourse)

- Unusual vaginal discharge

- Pelvic pain

- Pain during sexual intercourse

Tests That Examine the Cervix Are Used to Detect (Find) and Diagnose Cervical Cancer

The following procedures may be used:

- Physical exam and history
- Pelvic exam
- Pap test
- Human papillomavirus (HPV) test
- Endocervical curettage
- Colposcopy
- Biopsy

Certain Factors Affect Prognosis (Chance of Recovery) and Treatment Options

The prognosis (chance of recovery) depends on the following:

- The stage of the cancer (the size of the tumor and whether it affects part of the cervix or the whole cervix, or has spread to the lymph nodes or other places in the body).
- The type of cervical cancer.
- The patient's age and general health.
- Whether the patient has a certain type of human papillomavirus (HPV).
- Whether the patient has human immunodeficiency virus (HIV).
- Whether the cancer has just been diagnosed or has recurred (come back).

Treatment options depend on the following:

- The stage of the cancer.
- The type of cervical cancer.
- The patient's desire to have children.
- The patient's age.

Treatment of cervical cancer during pregnancy depends on the stage of the cancer and the stage of the pregnancy. For cervical cancer found early or for cancer found during the last trimester of pregnancy, treatment may be delayed until after the baby is born.

Stages of Cervical Cancer

After cervical cancer has been diagnosed, tests are done to find out if cancer cells have spread within the cervix or to other parts of the body.

The process used to find out if cancer has spread within the cervix or to other parts of the body is called staging. The information gathered from the staging process determines the stage of the disease. It is important to know the stage in order to plan treatment.

The following tests and procedures may be used in the staging process:

- Computerized tomography scan (CT scan; CAT scan)

- PET scan (positron emission tomography scan)

- MRI (magnetic resonance imaging)

- Ultrasound exam

- Chest X-ray

- Cystoscopy

- Laparoscopy

- Pretreatment surgical staging

The results of these tests are viewed together with the results of the original tumor biopsy to determine the cervical cancer stage.

There Are Three Ways That Cancer Spreads in the Body

Cancer can spread through:

1. Tissue

2. Lymph system

3. Blood

Cancer May Spread from Where It Began to Other Parts of the Body

When cancer spreads to another part of the body, it is called metastasis. Cancer cells break away from where they began (the primary tumor) and travel through the lymph system or blood.

The metastatic tumor is the same type of cancer as the primary tumor. For example, if cervical cancer spreads to the lung, the cancer cells in the lung are actually cervical cancer cells. The disease is metastatic cervical cancer, not lung cancer.

The Following Stages Are Used for Cervical Cancer

Carcinoma in Situ (Stage 0)

In carcinoma in situ (stage 0), abnormal cells are found in the innermost lining of the cervix. These abnormal cells may become cancer and spread into nearby normal tissue.

Stage I

In stage I, cancer is found in the cervix only.

Stage I is divided into stages IA and IB, based on the amount of cancer that is found.

- Stage IA:

  A very small amount of cancer that can only be seen with a microscope is found in the tissues of the cervix.

  Stage IA is divided into stages IA1 and IA2, based on the size of the tumor.

  - In stage IA1, the cancer is not more than 3 millimeters deep and not more than 7 millimeters wide.

  - In stage IA2, the cancer is more than 3 but not more than 5 millimeters deep, and not more than 7 millimeters wide.

- Stage IB:

  Stage IB is divided into stages IB1 and IB2, based on the size of the tumor.

- In stage IB1:

  - the cancer can only be seen with a microscope and is more than 5 millimeters deep and more than 7 millimeters wide; **or**

  - the cancer can be seen without a microscope and is not more than 4 centimeters.

- In stage IB2, the cancer can be seen without a microscope and is more than 4 centimeters.

Stage II

In stage II, cancer has spread beyond the uterus but not onto the pelvic wall (the tissues that line the part of the body between the hips) or to the lower third of the vagina.

Stage II is divided into stages IIA and IIB, based on how far the cancer has spread.

- Stage IIA: Cancer has spread beyond the cervix to the upper two thirds of the vagina but not to tissues around the uterus. Stage IIA is divided into stages IIA1 and IIA2, based on the size of the tumor.

    - In stage IIA1, the tumor can be seen without a microscope and is not more than 4 centimeters.

    - In stage IIA2, the tumor can be seen without a microscope and is more than 4 centimeters.

- Stage IIB: Cancer has spread beyond the cervix to the tissues around the uterus but not onto the pelvic wall.

Stage III

In stage III, cancer has spread to the lower third of the vagina, and/or onto the pelvic wall, and/or has caused kidney problems.

Stage III is divided into stages IIIA and IIIB, based on how far the cancer has spread.

- Stage IIIA: Cancer has spread to the lower third of the vagina but not onto the pelvic wall.

- Stage IIIB:

    - Cancer has spread onto the pelvic wall; **or**

    - the tumor has become large enough to block one or both ureters (tubes that connect the kidneys to the bladder) and has caused one or both kidneys to get bigger or stop working.

Stage IV

In stage IV, cancer has spread beyond the pelvis, or can be seen in the lining of the bladder and/or rectum, or has spread to other parts of the body.

Stage IV is divided into stages IVA and IVB, based on where the cancer has spread.

- Stage IVA: Cancer has spread to nearby organs, such as the bladder or rectum.

- Stage IVB: Cancer has spread to other parts of the body, such as the liver, lungs, bones, or distant lymph nodes.

Recurrent Cervical Cancer

Recurrent cervical cancer is cancer that has recurred (come back) after it has been treated. The cancer may come back in the cervix or in other parts of the body.

Treatment Option Overview

There are different types of treatment for patients with cervical cancer.

Different types of treatment are available for patients with cervical cancer. Some treatments are standard (the currently used treatment), and some are being tested in clinical trials. A treatment clinical trial is a research study meant to help improve current treatments or obtain information on new treatments for patients with cancer. When clinical trials show that a new treatment is better than the standard treatment, the new treatment may become the standard treatment. Patients may want to think about taking part in a clinical trial. Some clinical trials are open only to patients who have not started treatment.

Four Types of Standard Treatment Are Used

1. Surgery

    Surgery (removing the cancer in an operation) is sometimes used to treat cervical cancer. The following surgical procedures may be used:

    - Conization: A procedure to remove a cone-shaped piece of tissue from the cervix and cervical canal.

        - Cold-knife conization: A surgical procedure that uses a scalpel (sharp knife) to remove abnormal tissue or cancer.

        - Loop electrosurgical excision procedure (LEEP): A surgical procedure that uses electrical current passed through a thin wire loop as a knife to remove abnormal tissue or cancer.

- Laser surgery: A surgical procedure that uses electrical current passed through a thin wire loop as a knife to remove abnormal tissue or cancer.

- Total hysterectomy: Surgery to remove the uterus, including the cervix.

- Radical hysterectomy: Surgery to remove the uterus, cervix, part of the vagina, and a wide area of ligaments and tissues around these organs. The ovaries, fallopian tubes, or nearby lymph nodes may also be removed.

- Modified radical hysterectomy: Surgery to remove the uterus, cervix, upper part of the vagina, and ligaments and tissues that closely surround these organs. Nearby lymph nodes may also be removed.

- Radical trachelectomy: Surgery to remove the cervix, nearby tissue and lymph nodes, and the upper part of the vagina. The uterus and ovaries are not removed.

- Bilateral salpingo-oophorectomy: Surgery to remove both ovaries and both fallopian tubes.

- Pelvic exenteration: Surgery to remove the lower colon, rectum, and bladder. The cervix, vagina, ovaries, and nearby lymph nodes are also removed.

2. Radiation therapy

Radiation therapy is a cancer treatment that uses high-energy X-rays or other types of radiation to kill cancer cells or keep them from growing.

- External radiation therapy uses a machine outside the body to send radiation toward the cancer. This type of radiation therapy includes the following:

  - Intensity-modulated radiation therapy (IMRT): IMRT is a type of 3-dimensional (3-D) radiation therapy that uses a computer to make pictures of the size and shape of the tumor. Thin beams of radiation of different intensities (strengths) are aimed at the tumor from many angles. This type of external radiation therapy causes less damage to nearby healthy tissue.

- Internal radiation therapy uses a radioactive substance sealed in needles, seeds, wires, or catheters that are placed directly into or near the cancer.

3. Chemotherapy

Chemotherapy is a cancer treatment that uses drugs to stop the growth of cancer cells, either by killing the cells or by stopping them from dividing.

4. Targeted therapy

Targeted therapy is a type of treatment that uses drugs or other substances to identify and attack specific cancer cells without harming normal cells.

- Monoclonal antibody therapy: Monoclonal antibody therapy uses antibodies made in the laboratory from a single type of immune system cell. These antibodies can identify substances on cancer cells or normal substances that may help cancer cells grow. The antibodies attach to the substances and kill the cancer cells, block their growth, or keep them from spreading.

Follow-Up Tests May Be Needed

Some of the tests that were done to diagnose the cancer or to find out the stage of the cancer may be repeated. Some tests will be repeated in order to see how well the treatment is working. Decisions about whether to continue, change, or stop treatment may be based on the results of these tests.

Some of the tests will continue to be done from time to time after treatment has ended. The results of these tests can show if your condition has changed or if the cancer has recurred (come back). These tests are sometimes called follow-up tests or check-ups.

Your doctor will ask if you have any of the following signs or symptoms, which may mean the cancer has come back:

- Pain in the abdomen, back, or leg.

- Swelling in the leg.

- Trouble urinating.

- Cough.

- Feeling tired.

For cervical cancer, follow-up tests are usually done every 3 to 4 months for the first 2 years, followed by check-ups every 6 months. The check-up includes a current health history and exam of the body to check for signs and symptoms of recurrent cervical cancer and for late effects of treatment.

Treatment Options by Stage

Carcinoma in Situ (Stage 0)

Treatment of carcinoma in situ (stage 0) may include the following:

- Conization, such as cold-knife conization, loop electrosurgical excision procedure (LEEP), or laser surgery.
- Hysterectomy for women who cannot or no longer want to have children. This is done only if the tumor cannot be completely removed by conization.
- Internal radiation therapy for women who cannot have surgery.

Stage IA Cervical Cancer

Stage IA cervical cancer is separated into stage IA1 and IA2. Treatment for stage IA1 may include the following:

- Conization.
- Total hysterectomy with or without bilateral salpingo-oophorectomy.

Treatment for stage IA2 may include the following:

- Modified radical hysterectomy and removal of lymph nodes.
- Radical trachelectomy.
- Internal radiation therapy for women who cannot have surgery.

Stages IB and IIA Cervical Cancer

Treatment of stage IB and stage IIA cervical cancer may include the following:

- Radiation therapy with chemotherapy given at the same time.
- Radical hysterectomy and removal of pelvic lymph nodes with or without radiation therapy to the pelvis, plus chemotherapy.
- Radical trachelectomy.
- Chemotherapy followed by surgery.
- Radiation therapy alone.

Stages IIB, III, and IVA Cervical Cancer

Treatment of stage IIB, stage III, and stage IVA cervical cancer may include the following:

- Radiation therapy with chemotherapy given at the same time.

- Surgery to remove pelvic lymph nodes followed by radiation therapy with or without chemotherapy.

- Internal radiation therapy.

- A clinical trial of chemotherapy to shrink the tumor followed by surgery.

- A clinical trial of chemotherapy and radiation therapy given at the same time, followed by chemotherapy.

Stage IVB Cervical Cancer

Treatment of stage IVB cervical cancer may include the following:

- Radiation therapy as palliative therapy to relieve symptoms caused by the cancer and improve quality of life.

- Chemotherapy and targeted therapy.

- Chemotherapy as palliative therapy to relieve symptoms caused by the cancer and improve quality of life.

- Clinical trials of new anticancer drugs or drug combinations.

Treatment Options for Recurrent Cervical Cancer

Treatment of recurrent cervical cancer may include the following:

- Radiation therapy and chemotherapy.

- Chemotherapy and targeted therapy.

- Chemotherapy as palliative therapy to relieve symptoms caused by the cancer and improve quality of life.

- Pelvic exenteration.

- Clinical trials of new anticancer drugs or drug combinations.

Cervical Cancer during Pregnancy

Treatment of cervical cancer during pregnancy depends on the stage of the cancer and how long the patient has been pregnant. A biopsy and imaging tests may be done to determine the stage of the disease. To avoid exposing the fetus to radiation, MRI (magnetic resonance imaging) is used.

Treatment Options for Cervical Cancer during Pregnancy

Carcinoma in Situ (Stage 0) during Pregnancy

Usually, no treatment is needed for carcinoma in situ (stage 0) during pregnancy. A colposcopy may be done to check for invasive cancer.

Stage I Cervical Cancer during Pregnancy

Pregnant women with slow-growing stage I cervical cancer may be able to delay treatment until the second trimester of pregnancy or after delivery.

Pregnant women with fast-growing stage I cervical cancer may need immediate treatment. Treatment may include:

- Conization.

- Radical trachelectomy.

Women should be tested to find out if the cancer has spread to the lymph nodes. If cancer has spread to the lymph nodes, immediate treatment may be needed.

Stage II, III, and IV Cervical Cancer during Pregnancy

Treatment for stage II, stage III, and stage IV cervical cancer during pregnancy may include the following:

- Chemotherapy to shrink the tumor in the second or third trimester of pregnancy. Surgery or radiation therapy may be done after delivery.

- Radiation therapy plus chemotherapy. Talk with your doctor about the effects of radiation on the fetus. It may be necessary to end the pregnancy before treatment begins.

Section 38.2

Ovarian Cancer

This section includes text excerpted from "Ovarian Cancer,"
Office on Women's Health (OWH), U.S. Department of
Health and Human Services (HHS), March 18, 2014.

Ovarian cancer forms in tissues of the ovary. (An ovary is one of a pair of female reproductive glands in which the ova, or eggs, are formed.)

Tumors in the ovaries can be benign, which means they are not cancer, or they can be malignant, which means they are cancer.

Cancers that start in the ovaries can spread to other parts of the body. This is called metastasis. Cancer that starts in the ovaries and spreads to other parts of the body is still called ovarian cancer.

Who Gets Ovarian Cancer?

Around one in every 60 women in the United States will develop ovarian cancer. Most ovarian cancers are diagnosed in women over 60, but this disease can also affect younger women. Among women in the United States, ovarian cancer is rare. Most ovarian cancers are diagnosed among women ages 55 to 64, but ovarian cancer can also affect younger women.

Are Some Women More at Risk for Ovarian Cancer?

Women with a high risk of ovarian cancer are those with a harmful mutation on the *BRCA1* or *BRCA2* genes. These mutations can be found with a blood test. Women with a family or personal history of breast or ovarian cancer also have a higher risk of ovarian cancer.

If you have family members in multiple generations with breast cancer or ovarian cancer, see your doctor to learn more about your risk of ovarian cancer. Research shows that certain steps, such as surgery to remove the ovaries and the fallopian tubes, may help prevent ovarian cancer in women who are at high risk. The sooner ovarian cancer is found and treated, the better your chance for recovery. But ovarian cancer is hard to detect early, because its symptoms are also the symptoms of many other illnesses.

What Are the Symptoms of Ovarian Cancer?

The following may be symptoms of ovarian cancer if they continue or get worse over time:

- Pain in the pelvis or abdomen (belly)
- Bloating in the abdomen
- Urinary urgency (needing to pee right away)
- Urinary frequency (having to pee often)
- Constipation or diarrhea
- Feeling full quickly while eating
- Having difficulty eating
- Vaginal bleeding or other discharge that is different than normal
- Back pain

If you have any of these symptoms, talk to your doctor. He or she can determine if the cause is cancer or something else. Your doctor also may ask you to visit a gynecologic oncologist. This is a doctor who focuses on cancers of the female pelvis.

Should I Be Screened for Ovarian Cancer?

The U.S. Preventive Services Task Force (USPSTF) recommends against screening women who are not at high risk for ovarian cancer. The USPSTF found that testing for ovarian cancer may do more harm than good. Current testing methods, like pelvic exams, ultrasound, and blood tests, can lead to "false positives" (results that say a woman has ovarian cancer when she really does not have ovarian cancer). These incorrect results can lead to surgeries that are not needed and that can be risky.

Some women, like those who are at high risk, can talk to their doctor about their risk and what they can do to help prevent ovarian cancer.

Section 38.3

Endometrial Cancer

This section includes text excerpted from "Endometrial Cancer Treatment (PDQ®)–Patient Version," National Cancer Institute (NCI), April 6, 2017.

General Information about Endometrial Cancer

Endometrial cancer is a disease in which malignant (cancer) cells form in the tissues of the endometrium.

The endometrium is the lining of the uterus, a hollow, muscular organ in a woman's pelvis. The uterus is where a fetus grows. In most nonpregnant women, the uterus is about 3 inches long. The lower, narrow end of the uterus is the cervix, which leads to the vagina.

Cancer of the endometrium is different from cancer of the muscle of the uterus, which is called sarcoma of the uterus.

Obesity and Having Metabolic Syndrome May Increase the Risk of Endometrial Cancer

Anything that increases your risk of getting a disease is called a risk factor. Having a risk factor does not mean that you will get cancer; not having risk factors doesn't mean that you will not get cancer. Talk with your doctor if you think you may be at risk. Risk factors for endometrial cancer include the following:

- Having endometrial hyperplasia.

- Being obese.

- Having metabolic syndrome, a set of conditions that occur together, including extra fat around the abdomen, high blood sugar, high blood pressure, high levels of triglycerides and low levels of high-density lipoproteins in the blood.

- Never giving birth.

- Beginning menstruation at an early age.

- Reaching menopause at an older age.

- Having polycystic ovarian syndrome (PCOS).

- Having a mother, sister, or daughter with uterine cancer.

- Having a certain gene change that is linked to Lynch syndrome (hereditary nonpolyposis colon cancer).

- Having hyperinsulinemia (high levels of insulin in the blood).

Taking Tamoxifen for Breast Cancer or Taking Estrogen Alone (without Progesterone) Can Increase the Risk of Endometrial Cancer

Endometrial cancer may develop in breast cancer patients who have been treated with tamoxifen. A patient who takes this drug and has abnormal vaginal bleeding should have a follow-up exam and a biopsy of the endometrial lining if needed. Women taking estrogen (a hormone that can affect the growth of some cancers) alone also have an increased risk of endometrial cancer. Taking estrogen combined with progesterone (another hormone) does not increase a woman's risk of endometrial cancer.

Signs and Symptoms of Endometrial Cancer Include Unusual Vaginal Bleeding or Pain in the Pelvis

These and other signs and symptoms may be caused by endometrial cancer or by other conditions. Check with your doctor if you have any of the following:

- Vaginal bleeding or discharge not related to menstruation (periods).

- Vaginal bleeding after menopause.

- Difficult or painful urination.

- Pain during sexual intercourse.

- Pain in the pelvic area.

Tests That Examine the Endometrium Are Used to Detect (Find) and Diagnose Endometrial Cancer

Because endometrial cancer begins inside the uterus, it does not usually show up in the results of a Pap test. For this reason, a sample of endometrial tissue must be removed and checked under a microscope to look for cancer cells. One of the following procedures may be used:

- Endometrial biopsy

- Dilatation and curettage

- Hysteroscopy

Other tests and procedures used to diagnose endometrial cancer include the following:

- Physical exam and history

- Transvaginal ultrasound exam

Certain Factors Affect Prognosis (Chance of Recovery) and Treatment Options

The prognosis (chance of recovery) and treatment options depend on the following:

- The stage of the cancer (whether it is in the endometrium only, involves the uterus wall, or has spread to other places in the body).

- How the cancer cells look under a microscope.

- Whether the cancer cells are affected by progesterone.

Endometrial cancer can usually be cured because it is usually diagnosed early.

Stages of Endometrial Cancer

After endometrial cancer has been diagnosed, tests are done to find out if cancer cells have spread within the uterus or to other parts of the body.

The process used to find out whether the cancer has spread within the uterus or to other parts of the body is called staging. The information gathered from the staging process determines the stage of the disease. It is important to know the stage in order to plan treatment. Certain tests and procedures are used in the staging process. A hysterectomy (an operation in which the uterus is removed) will usually be done to treat endometrial cancer. Tissue samples are taken from the area around the uterus and checked under a microscope for signs of cancer to help find out whether the cancer has spread.

The following procedures may be used in the staging process:

- Pelvic exam
- Chest X-ray
- computed tomography scan (CT scan; CAT scan)
- MRI (magnetic resonance imaging)
- PET scan (positron emission tomography scan)
- Lymph node dissection

There Are Three Ways That Cancer Spreads in the Body

Cancer can spread through:

1. Tissue
2. Lymph system
3. Blood

Cancer May Spread from Where It Began to Other Parts of the Body

When cancer spreads to another part of the body, it is called metastasis. Cancer cells break away from where they began (the primary tumor) and travel through the lymph system or blood.

The metastatic tumor is the same type of cancer as the primary tumor. For example, if endometrial cancer spreads to the lung, the cancer cells in the lung are actually endometrial cancer cells. The disease is metastatic endometrial cancer, not lung cancer.

The Following Stages Are Used for Endometrial Cancer

Stage I

In stage I, cancer is found in the uterus only. Stage I is divided into stages IA and IB, based on how far the cancer has spread.

- Stage IA: Cancer is in the endometrium only or less than halfway through the myometrium (muscle layer of the uterus).
- Stage IB: Cancer has spread halfway or more into the myometrium.

Stage II

In stage II, cancer has spread into connective tissue of the cervix, but has not spread outside the uterus.

Stage III

In stage III, cancer has spread beyond the uterus and cervix, but has not spread beyond the pelvis. Stage III is divided into stages IIIA, IIIB, and IIIC, based on how far the cancer has spread within the pelvis.

- Stage IIIA: Cancer has spread to the outer layer of the uterus and/or to the fallopian tubes, ovaries, and ligaments of the uterus.

- Stage IIIB: Cancer has spread to the vagina and/or to the parametrium (connective tissue and fat around the uterus).

- Stage IIIC: Cancer has spread to lymph nodes in the pelvis and/or around the aorta (largest artery in the body, which carries blood away from the heart).

Stage IV

In stage IV, cancer has spread beyond the pelvis. Stage IV is divided into stages IVA and IVB, based on how far the cancer has spread.

- Stage IVA: Cancer has spread to the bladder and/or bowel wall.

- Stage IVB: Cancer has spread to other parts of the body beyond the pelvis, including the abdomen and/or lymph nodes in the groin.

Endometrial Cancer May Be Grouped for Treatment as Follows

Low-Risk Endometrial Cancer

Grades 1 and 2 tumors are usually considered low-risk. They usually do not spread to other parts of the body.

High-Risk Endometrial Cancer

Grade 3 tumors are considered high-risk. They often spread to other parts of the body. Uterine papillary serous, clear cell, and carcinosarcoma are three subtypes of endometrial cancer that are considered grade 3.

Recurrent Endometrial Cancer

Recurrent endometrial cancer is cancer that has recurred (come back) after it has been treated. The cancer may come back in the uterus, the pelvis, in lymph nodes in the abdomen, or in other parts of the body.

Treatment Option Overview

Different types of treatment are available for patients with endometrial cancer. Some treatments are standard (the currently used treatment), and some are being tested in clinical trials. A treatment clinical trial is a research study meant to help improve current treatments or obtain information on new treatments for patients with cancer. When clinical trials show that a new treatment is better than the standard treatment, the new treatment may become the standard treatment. Patients may want to think about taking part in a clinical trial. Some clinical trials are open only to patients who have not started treatment.

Five Types of Standard Treatment Are Used

1. Surgery

    Surgery (removing the cancer in an operation) is the most common treatment for endometrial cancer. The following surgical procedures may be used:

    - Total hysterectomy: Surgery to remove the uterus, including the cervix.

    - Bilateral salpingo-oophorectomy: Surgery to remove both ovaries and both fallopian tubes.

    - Radical hysterectomy: Surgery to remove the uterus, cervix, and part of the vagina. The ovaries, fallopian tubes, or nearby lymph nodes may also be removed.

    - Lymph node dissection: A surgical procedure in which the lymph nodes are removed from the pelvic area and a sample of tissue is checked under a microscope for signs of cancer.

2. Radiation therapy

    Radiation therapy is a cancer treatment that uses high-energy X-rays or other types of radiation to kill cancer cells or keep them from growing.

- External radiation therapy uses a machine outside the body to send radiation toward the cancer.

- Internal radiation therapy uses a radioactive substance sealed in needles, seeds, wires, or catheters that are placed directly into or near the cancer.

3. Chemotherapy

    Chemotherapy is a cancer treatment that uses drugs to stop the growth of cancer cells, either by killing the cells or by stopping the cells from dividing.

4. Hormone therapy

    Hormone therapy is a cancer treatment that removes hormones or blocks their action and stops cancer cells from growing.

5. Targeted therapy

    Targeted therapy is a type of treatment that uses drugs or other substances to identify and attack specific cancer cells without harming normal cells.

    - Monoclonal antibody therapy uses antibodies made in the laboratory from a single type of immune system cell. These antibodies can identify substances on cancer cells or normal substances that may help cancer cells grow. The antibodies attach to the substances and kill the cancer cells, block their growth, or keep them from spreading.

    - mTOR inhibitors block a protein called mTOR, which helps control cell division. mTOR inhibitors may keep cancer cells from growing and prevent the growth of new blood vessels that tumors need to grow.

    - Signal transduction inhibitors block signals that are passed from one molecule to another inside a cell. Blocking these signals may kill cancer cells.

Follow-Up Tests May Be Needed

Some of the tests that were done to diagnose the cancer or to find out the stage of the cancer may be repeated. Some tests will be repeated in order to see how well the treatment is working. Decisions about whether to continue, change, or stop treatment may be based on the results of these tests.

Some of the tests will continue to be done from time to time after treatment has ended. The results of these tests can show if your condition has changed or if the cancer has recurred (come back). These tests are sometimes called follow-up tests or check-ups.

Treatment Options by Stage

Stage I and Stage II Endometrial Cancer

Low-Risk Endometrial Cancer (Grade 1 or Grade 2)

Treatment of low-risk stage I endometrial cancer and stage II endometrial cancer may include the following:

- Surgery (total hysterectomy and bilateral salpingo-oophorectomy). Lymph nodes in the pelvis and abdomen may also be removed and viewed under a microscope to check for cancer cells.

- Surgery (total hysterectomy and bilateral salpingo-oophorectomy, with or without removal of lymph nodes in the pelvis and abdomen) followed by internal radiation therapy. In certain cases, external radiation therapy to the pelvis may be used in place of internal radiation therapy.

- Radiation therapy alone for patients who cannot have surgery.

- A clinical trial of a new chemotherapy regimen.

If cancer has spread to the cervix, a radical hysterectomy with bilateral salpingo-oophorectomy may be done.

High-Risk Endometrial Cancer (Grade 3)

Treatment of high-risk stage I endometrial cancer and stage II endometrial cancer may include the following:

- Surgery (radical hysterectomy and bilateral salpingo-oophorectomy). Lymph nodes in the pelvis and abdomen may also be removed and viewed under a microscope to check for cancer cells.

- Surgery (radical hysterectomy and bilateral salpingo-oophorectomy) followed by chemotherapy and sometimes radiation therapy.

- A clinical trial of a new chemotherapy regimen.

Stage III, Stage IV, and Recurrent Endometrial Cancer

Treatment of stage III endometrial cancer, stage IV endometrial cancer, and recurrent endometrial cancer may include the following:

- Surgery (radical hysterectomy and removal of lymph nodes in the pelvis so they can be viewed under a microscope to check for cancer cells) followed by adjuvant chemotherapy and/or radiation therapy.

- Chemotherapy and internal and external radiation therapy for patients who cannot have surgery.

- Hormone therapy for patients who cannot have surgery or radiation therapy.

- Targeted therapy with mTOR inhibitors (everolimus or ridaforolimus) or a monoclonal antibody (bevacizumab).

- A clinical trial of a new treatment regimen that may include combination chemotherapy, targeted therapy, such as an mTOR inhibitor (everolimus) or signal transduction inhibitor (metformin), and/or hormone therapy, for patients with advanced or recurrent endometrial cancer.

Section 38.4

Vaginal Cancer

This section includes text excerpted from "Vaginal Cancer Treatment (PDQ®)–Patient Version," National Cancer Institute (NCI), July 14, 2016.

General Information about Vaginal Cancer

Vaginal cancer is a disease in which malignant (cancer) cells form in the vagina.

The vagina is the canal leading from the cervix (the opening of uterus) to the outside of the body. At birth, a baby passes out of the body through the vagina (also called the birth canal).

Vaginal cancer is not common. There are two main types of vaginal cancer:

1. Squamous cell carcinoma: Cancer that forms in squamous cells, the thin, flat cells lining the vagina. Squamous cell vaginal cancer spreads slowly and usually stays near the vagina, but may spread to the lungs, liver, or bone. This is the most common type of vaginal cancer.

2. Adenocarcinoma: Cancer that begins in glandular (secretory) cells. Glandular cells in the lining of the vagina make and release fluids such as mucus. Adenocarcinoma is more likely than squamous cell cancer to spread to the lungs and lymph nodes. A rare type of adenocarcinoma is linked to being exposed to diethylstilbestrol (DES) before birth. Adenocarcinomas that are not linked with being exposed to DES are most common in women after menopause.

Age and Being Exposed to the Drug DES (Diethylstilbestrol) before Birth Affect a Woman's Risk of Vaginal Cancer

Anything that increases your risk of getting a disease is called a risk factor. Having a risk factor does not mean that you will get cancer; not having risk factors doesn't mean that you will not get cancer. Talk with your doctor if you think you may be at risk. Risk factors for vaginal cancer include the following:

* Being aged 60 or older.

* Being exposed to DES while in the mother's womb. In the 1950s, the drug DES was given to some pregnant women to prevent miscarriage (premature birth of a fetus that cannot survive). Women who were exposed to DES before birth have an increased risk of vaginal cancer. Some of these women develop a rare form of vaginal cancer called clear cell adenocarcinoma.

* Having human papillomavirus (HPV) infection.

* Having a history of abnormal cells in the cervix or cervical cancer.

* Having a history of abnormal cells in the uterus or cancer of the uterus.

* Having had a hysterectomy for health problems that affect the uterus.

Signs and Symptoms of Vaginal Cancer Include Pain or Abnormal Vaginal Bleeding

Vaginal cancer often does not cause early signs or symptoms. It may be found during a routine pelvic exam and Pap test. Signs and symptoms may be caused by vaginal cancer or by other conditions. Check with your doctor if you have any of the following:

- Bleeding or discharge not related to menstrual periods.

- Pain during sexual intercourse.

- Pain in the pelvic area.

- A lump in the vagina.

- Pain when urinating.

- Constipation.

Tests That Examine the Vagina and Other Organs in the Pelvis Are Used to Detect (Find) and Diagnose Vaginal Cancer

The following tests and procedures may be used:

- Physical exam and history

- Pelvic exam

- Pap test

- Colposcopy

- Biopsy

Certain Factors Affect Prognosis (Chance of Recovery) and Treatment Options

The prognosis (chance of recovery) depends on the following:

- The stage of the cancer (whether it is in the vagina only or has spread to other areas).

- The size of the tumor.

- The grade of tumor cells (how different they look from normal cells under a microscope).

- Where the cancer is within the vagina.

- Whether there are signs or symptoms at diagnosis.

- The patient's age and general health.
- Whether the cancer has just been diagnosed or has recurred (come back).

    When found in early stages, vaginal cancer can often be cured. Treatment options depend on the following:

- The stage and size of the cancer.
- Whether the cancer is close to other organs that may be damaged by treatment.
- Whether the tumor is made up of squamous cells or is an adenocarcinoma.
- Whether the patient has a uterus or has had a hysterectomy.
- Whether the patient has had past radiation treatment to the pelvis.

Stages of Vaginal Cancer

After vaginal cancer has been diagnosed, tests are done to find out if cancer cells have spread within the vagina or to other parts of the body.

The process used to find out if cancer has spread within the vagina or to other parts of the body is called staging. The information gathered from the staging process determines the stage of the disease. It is important to know the stage in order to plan treatment. The following procedures may be used in the staging process:

- Chest X-ray
- Computerized tomography scan (CT scan; CAT scan)
- MRI (magnetic resonance imaging)
- PET scan (positron emission tomography scan)
- Cystoscopy
- Ureteroscopy
- Proctoscopy
- Biopsy

There Are Three Ways That Cancer Spreads in the Body

Cancer can spread through:

1. Tissue

503

2. Lymph system

3. Blood

Cancer May Spread from Where It Began to Other Parts of the Body

When cancer spreads to another part of the body, it is called metastasis. Cancer cells break away from where they began (the primary tumor) and travel through the lymph system or blood.

The metastatic tumor is the same type of cancer as the primary tumor. For example, if vaginal cancer spreads to the lung, the cancer cells in the lung are actually vaginal cancer cells. The disease is metastatic vaginal cancer, not lung cancer.

In Vaginal Intraepithelial Neoplasia (VAIN), Abnormal Cells Are Found in Tissue Lining the inside of the Vagina

These abnormal cells are not cancer. Vaginal intraepithelial neoplasia (VAIN) is grouped based on how deep the abnormal cells are in the tissue lining the vagina:

- VAIN 1: Abnormal cells are found in the outermost one third of the tissue lining the vagina.

- VAIN 2: Abnormal cells are found in the outermost two-thirds of the tissue lining the vagina.

- VAIN 3: Abnormal cells are found in more than two-thirds of the tissue lining the vagina. When abnormal cells are found throughout the tissue lining, it is called carcinoma in situ.

VAIN may become cancer and spread into the vaginal wall. VAIN is sometimes called stage 0.

The Following Stages Are Used for Vaginal Cancer

Stage I

In stage I, cancer is found in the vaginal wall only.

Stage II

In stage II, cancer has spread through the wall of the vagina to the tissue around the vagina. Cancer has not spread to the wall of the pelvis.

Stage III

In stage III, cancer has spread to the wall of the pelvis.

Stage IV

Stage IV is divided into stage IVA and stage IVB:

- Stage IVA: Cancer may have spread to one or more of the following areas:
  - The lining of the bladder.
  - The lining of the rectum.
  - Beyond the area of the pelvis that has the bladder, uterus, ovaries, and cervix.
- Stage IVB: Cancer has spread to parts of the body that are not near the vagina, such as the lung or bone.

Recurrent Vaginal Cancer

Recurrent vaginal cancer is cancer that has recurred (come back) after it has been treated. The cancer may come back in the vagina or in other parts of the body.

Treatment Option Overview

Different types of treatments are available for patients with vaginal cancer. Some treatments are standard (the currently used treatment), and some are being tested in clinical trials. A treatment clinical trial is a research study meant to help improve current treatments or obtain information on new treatments for patients with cancer. When clinical trials show that a new treatment is better than the standard treatment, the new treatment may become the standard treatment. Patients may want to think about taking part in a clinical trial. Some clinical trials are open only to patients who have not started treatment.

Three Types of Standard Treatment Are Used

1. Surgery

   Surgery is the most common treatment of vaginal cancer. The following surgical procedures may be used:

   - Laser surgery: A surgical procedure that uses a laser beam (a narrow beam of intense light) as a knife to make bloodless cuts in tissue or to remove a surface lesion such as a tumor.

- Wide local excision: A surgical procedure that takes out the cancer and some of the healthy tissue around it.

- Vaginectomy: Surgery to remove all or part of the vagina.

- Total hysterectomy: Surgery to remove the uterus, including the cervix.

- Lymph node dissection: A surgical procedure in which lymph nodes are removed and a sample of tissue is checked under a microscope for signs of cancer.

- Pelvic exenteration: Surgery to remove the lower colon, rectum, bladder, cervix, vagina, and ovaries. Nearby lymph nodes are also removed.

2. Radiation therapy

   Radiation therapy is a cancer treatment that uses high-energy X-rays or other types of radiation to kill cancer cells or keep them from growing.

   - External radiation therapy uses a machine outside the body to send radiation toward the cancer.

   - Internal radiation therapy uses a radioactive substance sealed in needles, seeds, wires, or catheters that are placed directly into or near the cancer.

3. Chemotherapy

   Chemotherapy is a cancer treatment that uses drugs to stop the growth of cancer cells, either by killing the cells or by stopping them from dividing.

New Types of Treatment Are Being Tested in Clinical Trials

Radiosensitizers

Radiosensitizers are drugs that make tumor cells more sensitive to radiation therapy. Combining radiation therapy with radiosensitizers may kill more tumor cells.

Follow-Up Tests May Be Needed

Some of the tests that were done to diagnose the cancer or to find out the stage of the cancer may be repeated. Some tests will be repeated in order to see how well the treatment is working. Decisions about whether to continue, change, or stop treatment may be based on the results of these tests.

Treatment Options by Stage

Vaginal Intraepithelial Neoplasia (VAIN)

Treatment of vaginal intraepithelial neoplasia (VAIN) 1 is usually watchful waiting.

Treatment of VAIN 2 and 3 may include the following:

- Watchful waiting.

- Laser surgery.

- Wide local excision, with or without a skin graft.

- Partial or total vaginectomy, with or without a skin graft.

- Topical chemotherapy.

- Internal radiation therapy.

- A clinical trial of a new topical chemotherapy drug.

Stage I Vaginal Cancer

Treatment of stage I squamous cell vaginal cancer may include the following:

- Internal radiation therapy.

- External radiation therapy, especially for large tumors or the lymph nodes near tumors in the lower part of the vagina.

- Wide local excision or vaginectomy with vaginal reconstruction. Radiation therapy may be given after the surgery.

- Vaginectomy and lymph node dissection, with or without vaginal reconstruction. Radiation therapy may be given after the surgery.

Treatment of stage I vaginal adenocarcinoma may include the following:

- Vaginectomy, hysterectomy, and lymph node dissection. This may be followed by vaginal reconstruction and/or radiation therapy.

- Internal radiation therapy. External radiation therapy may also be given to the lymph nodes near tumors in the lower part of the vagina.

- A combination of therapies that may include wide local excision with or without lymph node dissection and internal radiation therapy.

Stage II Vaginal Cancer

Treatment of stage II vaginal cancer is the same for squamous cell cancer and adenocarcinoma. Treatment may include the following:

- Both internal and external radiation therapy to the vagina. External radiation therapy may also be given to the lymph nodes near tumors in the lower part of the vagina.

- Vaginectomy or pelvic exenteration. Internal and/or external radiation therapy may also be given.

Stage III Vaginal Cancer

Treatment of stage III vaginal cancer is the same for squamous cell cancer and adenocarcinoma. Treatment may include the following:

- External radiation therapy. Internal radiation therapy may also be given.

- Surgery (rare) followed by external radiation therapy. Internal radiation therapy may also be given.

Stage IVA Vaginal Cancer

Treatment of stage IVA vaginal cancer is the same for squamous cell cancer and adenocarcinoma. Treatment may include the following:

- External radiation therapy and/or internal radiation therapy.

- Surgery (rare) followed by external radiation therapy and/or internal radiation therapy.

Stage IVB Vaginal Cancer

Treatment of stage IVB vaginal cancer is the same for squamous cell cancer and adenocarcinoma. Treatment may include the following:

- Radiation therapy as palliative therapy, to relieve symptoms and improve the quality of life. Chemotherapy may also be given.

- A clinical trial of anticancer drugs and/or radiosensitizers.

Treatment Options for Recurrent Vaginal Cancer

Treatment of recurrent vaginal cancer may include the following:

- Pelvic exenteration.

- Radiation therapy.

- A clinical trial of anticancer drugs and/or radiosensitizers.

Although no anticancer drugs have been shown to help patients with recurrent vaginal cancer live longer, they are often treated with regimens used for cervical cancer.

Section 38.5

Vulvar Cancers

This section includes text excerpted from "Vulvar Cancer Treatment (PDQ®)–Patient Version," National Cancer Institute (NCI), July 14, 2016.

General Information about Vulvar Cancer

Vulvar cancer is a rare disease in which malignant (cancer) cells form in the tissues of the vulva.

Vulvar cancer forms in a woman's external genitalia. The vulva includes:

- Inner and outer lips of the vagina.

- Clitoris (sensitive tissue between the lips).

- Opening of the vagina and its glands.

- Mons pubis (the rounded area in front of the pubic bones that becomes covered with hair at puberty).

- Perineum (the area between the vulva and the anus).

Vulvar cancer most often affects the outer vaginal lips. Less often, cancer affects the inner vaginal lips, clitoris, or vaginal glands.

Vulvar cancer usually forms slowly over a number of years. Abnormal cells can grow on the surface of the vulvar skin for a long time. This condition is called vulvar intraepithelial neoplasia (VIN). Because it is possible for VIN to become vulvar cancer, it is very important to get treatment.

Having Vulvar Intraepithelial Neoplasia or HPV Infection Can Affect the Risk of Vulvar Cancer

Anything that increases your risk of getting a disease is called a risk factor. Having a risk factor does not mean that you will get cancer; not having risk factors doesn't mean that you will not get cancer. Talk with your doctor if you think you may be at risk. Risk factors for vulvar cancer include the following:

- Having vulvar intraepithelial neoplasia (VIN).

- Having human papillomavirus (HPV) infection.

- Having a history of genital warts.

Other possible risk factors include the following:

- Having many sexual partners.

- Having first sexual intercourse at a young age.

- Having a history of abnormal Pap tests (Pap smears).

Signs of Vulvar Cancer Include Bleeding or Itching

Vulvar cancer often does not cause early signs or symptoms. Signs and symptoms may be caused by vulvar cancer or by other conditions. Check with your doctor if you have any of the following:

- A lump or growth on the vulva.

- Changes in the vulvar skin, such as color changes or growths that look like a wart or ulcer.

- Itching in the vulvar area, that does not go away.

- Bleeding not related to menstruation (periods).

- Tenderness in the vulvar area.

Tests That Examine the Vulva Are Used to Detect (Find) and Diagnose Vulvar Cancer

The following tests and procedures may be used:

- Physical exam and history
- Biopsy

Certain Factors Affect Prognosis (Chance of Recovery) and Treatment Options

The prognosis (chance of recovery) and treatment options depend on the following:

- The stage of the cancer.
- The patient's age and general health.
- Whether the cancer has just been diagnosed or has recurred (come back).

Stages of Vulvar Cancer

After vulvar cancer has been diagnosed, tests are done to find out if cancer cells have spread within the vulva or to other parts of the body.

The process used to find out if cancer has spread within the vulva or to other parts of the body is called staging. The information gathered from the staging process determines the stage of the disease. It is important to know the stage in order to plan treatment. The following tests and procedures may be used in the staging process:

- Pelvic exam
- Colposcopy
- Cystoscopy
- Proctoscopy
- X-rays
- Intravenous pyelogram (IVP)
- Computerized tomography scan (CT scan; CAT scan)
- MRI (magnetic resonance imaging)
- PET scan (positron emission tomography scan)
- Sentinel lymph node biopsy

There Are Three Ways That Cancer Spreads in the Body

Cancer can spread through:

1. Tissue

2. Lymph system

3. Blood

Cancer May Spread from Where It Began to Other Parts of the Body

When cancer spreads to another part of the body, it is called metastasis. Cancer cells break away from where they began (the primary tumor) and travel through the lymph system or blood.

The metastatic tumor is the same type of cancer as the primary tumor. For example, if vulvar cancer spreads to the lung, the cancer cells in the lung are actually vulvar cancer cells. The disease is metastatic vulvar cancer, not lung cancer.

In vulvar intraepithelial neoplasia (VIN), abnormal cells are found on the surface of the vulvar skin.

These abnormal cells are not cancer. Vulvar intraepithelial neoplasia (VIN) may become cancer and spread into nearby tissue. VIN is sometimes called stage 0 or carcinoma in situ.

The Following Stages Are Used for Vulvar Cancer

Stage I

In stage I, cancer has formed. The tumor is found only in the vulva or perineum (area between the rectum and the vagina). Stage I is divided into stages IA and IB.

- In stage IA, the tumor is 2 centimeters or smaller and has spread 1 millimeter or less into the tissue of the vulva. Cancer has not spread to the lymph nodes.

- In stage IB, the tumor is larger than 2 centimeters or has spread more than 1 millimeter into the tissue of the vulva. Cancer has not spread to the lymph nodes.

Stage II

In stage II, the tumor is any size and has spread into the lower part of the urethra, the lower part of the vagina, or the anus. Cancer has not spread to the lymph nodes.

Stage III

In stage III, the tumor is any size and may have spread into the lower part of the urethra, the lower part of the vagina, or the anus. Cancer has spread to one or more nearby lymph nodes. Stage III is divided into stages IIIA, IIIB, and IIIC.

- In stage IIIA, cancer is found in 1 or 2 lymph nodes that are smaller than 5 millimeters or in one lymph node that is 5 millimeters or larger.

- In stage IIIB, cancer is found in 2 or more lymph nodes that are 5 millimeters or larger, or in 3 or more lymph nodes that are smaller than 5 millimeters.

- In stage IIIC, cancer is found in lymph nodes and has spread to the outside surface of the lymph nodes.

Stage IV

In stage IV, the tumor has spread into the upper part of the urethra, the upper part of the vagina, or to other parts of the body. Stage IV is divided into stages IVA and IVB.

- In stage IVA:
  - cancer has spread into the lining of the upper urethra, the upper vagina, the bladder, or the rectum, or has attached to the pelvic bone; or
  - cancer has spread to nearby lymph nodes and the lymph nodes are not moveable or have formed an ulcer.

- In stage IVB, cancer has spread to lymph nodes in the pelvis or to other parts of the body.

Recurrent Vulvar Cancer

Recurrent vulvar cancer is cancer that has recurred (come back) after it has been treated. The cancer may come back in the vulva or in other parts of the body.

Treatment Option Overview

Different types of treatments are available for patients with vulvar cancer. Some treatments are standard (the currently used treatment), and some are being tested in clinical trials. A treatment clinical trial is a research study meant to help improve current treatments or obtain information on new treatments for patients with cancer. When clinical trials show that a new treatment is better than the standard treatment, the new treatment may become the standard treatment. Patients may want to think about taking part in a clinical trial. Some clinical trials are open only to patients who have not started treatment.

Four Types of Standard Treatment Are Used

1. Surgery

    Surgery is the most common treatment for vulvar cancer. The goal of surgery is to remove all the cancer without any loss of the woman's sexual function. One of the following types of surgery may be done:

    - Laser surgery: A surgical procedure that uses a laser beam (a narrow beam of intense light) as a knife to make bloodless cuts in tissue or to remove a surface lesion such as a tumor.

    - Wide local excision: A surgical procedure to remove the cancer and some of the normal tissue around the cancer.

    - Radical local excision: A surgical procedure to remove the cancer and a large amount of normal tissue around it. Nearby lymph nodes in the groin may also be removed.

    - Ultrasound surgical aspiration (USA): A surgical procedure to break the tumor up into small pieces using very fine vibrations. The small pieces of tumor are washed away and removed by suction.

    - Vulvectomy: A surgical procedure to remove part or all of the vulva:

      - Skinning vulvectomy: The top layer of vulvar skin where the cancer is found is removed.

      - Modified radical vulvectomy: Surgery to remove part of the vulva. Nearby lymph nodes may also be removed.

      - Radical vulvectomy: Surgery to remove the entire vulva. Nearby lymph nodes are also removed.

    - Pelvic exenteration: A surgical procedure to remove the lower colon, rectum, and bladder. The cervix, vagina, ovaries, and nearby lymph nodes are also removed.

2. Radiation therapy

   Radiation therapy is a cancer treatment that uses high-energy X-rays or other types of radiation to kill cancer cells or keep them from growing.

   - External radiation therapy uses a machine outside the body to send radiation toward the cancer.

   - Internal radiation therapy uses a radioactive substance sealed in needles, seeds, wires, or catheters that are placed directly into or near the cancer.

3. Chemotherapy

   Chemotherapy is a cancer treatment that uses drugs to stop the growth of cancer cells, either by killing the cells or by stopping the cells from dividing.

4. Biologic therapy

   Biologic therapy is a treatment that uses the patient's immune system to fight cancer. Substances made by the body or made in a laboratory are used to boost, direct, or restore the body's natural defenses against cancer.

   - Imiquimod is a biologic therapy that may be used to treat vulvar lesions and is applied to the skin in a cream.

Follow-Up Tests May Be Needed

Some of the tests that were done to diagnose the cancer or to find out the stage of the cancer may be repeated. Some tests will be repeated in order to see how well the treatment is working. Decisions about whether to continue, change, or stop treatment may be based on the results of these tests.

Some of the tests will continue to be done from time to time after treatment has ended. The results of these tests can show if your condition has changed or if the cancer has recurred (come back). These tests are sometimes called follow-up tests or check-ups.

It is important to have regular follow-up exams to check for recurrent vulvar cancer.

Treatment Options by Stage

Vulvar Intraepithelial Neoplasia (VIN)

Treatment of vulvar intraepithelial neoplasia (VIN) may include the following:

- Removal of single lesions or wide local excision.
- Laser surgery.
- Ultrasound surgical aspiration.
- Skinning vulvectomy with or without a skin graft.
- Biologic therapy with topical imiquimod.

Stage I Vulvar Cancer

Treatment of stage I vulvar cancer may include the following:

- Wide local excision for lesions that are less than 1 millimeter deep.
- Radical local excision and removal of nearby lymph nodes.
- Radical local excision and sentinel lymph node biopsy. If cancer is found in the sentinel lymph node, nearby lymph nodes are also removed.
- Radiation therapy for patients who cannot have surgery.

Stage II Vulvar Cancer

Treatment of stage II vulvar cancer may include the following:

- Radical local excision and removal of nearby lymph nodes.
- Modified radical vulvectomy or radical vulvectomy for large tumors. Nearby lymph nodes may be removed. Radiation therapy may be given after surgery.
- Radical local excision and sentinel lymph node biopsy. If cancer is found in the sentinel lymph node, nearby lymph nodes are also removed.
- Radiation therapy for patients who cannot have surgery.

Stage III Vulvar Cancer

Treatment of stage III vulvar cancer may include the following:

- Modified radical vulvectomy or radical vulvectomy. Nearby lymph nodes may be removed. Radiation therapy may be given after surgery.
- Radiation therapy or chemotherapy and radiation therapy followed by surgery.

- Radiation therapy with or without chemotherapy for patients who cannot have surgery.

Stage IV Vulvar Cancer

Treatment of stage IVA vulvar cancer may include the following:

- Radical vulvectomy and pelvic exenteration.
- Radical vulvectomy followed by radiation therapy.
- Radiation therapy or chemotherapy and radiation therapy followed by surgery.
- Radiation therapy with or without chemotherapy for patients who cannot have surgery.

There is no standard treatment for stage IVB vulvar cancer. Treatment may include a clinical trial of a new treatment.

Treatment Options for Recurrent Vulvar Cancer

Treatment of recurrent vulvar cancer may include the following:

- Wide local excision with or without radiation therapy to treat cancer that has come back in the same area.
- Radical vulvectomy and pelvic exenteration to treat cancer that has come back in the same area.
- Chemotherapy and radiation therapy with or without surgery.
- Radiation therapy followed by surgery or chemotherapy.
- Radiation therapy as palliative treatment to relieve symptoms and improve quality of life.
- A clinical trial of a new treatment.

Chapter 39

Colon and Rectal Cancers

Colorectal cancer is cancer that starts in the colon or rectum. The colon and the rectum are parts of the large intestine, which is the lower part of the body's digestive system. During digestion, food moves through the stomach and small intestine into the colon. The colon absorbs water and nutrients from the food and stores waste matter (stool). Stool moves from the colon into the rectum before it leaves the body.

Most colorectal cancers are adenocarcinomas (cancers that begin in cells that make and release mucus and other fluids). Colorectal cancer often begins as a growth called a polyp, which may form on the inner wall of the colon or rectum. Some polyps become cancer over time. Finding and removing polyps can prevent colorectal cancer.

Colorectal cancer is the fourth most common type of cancer diagnosed in the United States. Deaths from colorectal cancer have decreased with the use of colonoscopies and fecal occult blood tests, which check for blood in the stool.

General Information about Colon Cancer

Colon cancer is a disease in which malignant (cancer) cells form in the tissues of the colon.

The colon is part of the body's digestive system. The digestive system removes and processes nutrients (vitamins, minerals,

This chapter includes text excerpted from "Colorectal Cancer—Patient Version," National Cancer Institute (NCI), February 27, 2017.

carbohydrates, fats, proteins, and water) from foods and helps pass waste material out of the body. The digestive system is made up of the esophagus, stomach, and the small and large intestines. The colon (large bowel) is the first part of the large intestine and is about 5 feet long. Together, the rectum and anal canal make up the last part of the large intestine and are about 6–8 inches long. The anal canal ends at the anus (the opening of the large intestine to the outside of the body). Gastrointestinal stromal tumors can occur in the colon.

Health History Affects the Risk of Developing Colon Cancer

Anything that increases your chance of getting a disease is called a risk factor. Having a risk factor does not mean that you will get cancer; not having risk factors doesn't mean that you will not get cancer. Talk to your doctor if you think you may be at risk for colorectal cancer.

Risk factors for colorectal cancer include the following:

- Having a family history of colon or rectal cancer in a first-degree relative (parent, sibling, or child).

- Having a personal history of cancer of the colon, rectum, or ovary.

- Having a personal history of high-risk adenomas (colorectal polyps that are 1 centimeter or larger in size or that have cells that look abnormal under a microscope).

- Having inherited changes in certain genes that increase the risk of familial adenomatous polyposis (FAP) or Lynch syndrome (hereditary nonpolyposis colorectal cancer).

- Having a personal history of chronic ulcerative colitis or Crohn's disease for 8 years or more.

- Having three or more alcoholic drinks per day.

- Smoking cigarettes.

- Being black.

- Being obese.

Older age is a main risk factor for most cancers. The chance of getting cancer increases as you get older.

Signs of Colon Cancer Include Blood in the Stool or a Change in Bowel Habits

These and other signs and symptoms may be caused by colon cancer or by other conditions. Check with your doctor if you have any of the following:

- A change in bowel habits.
- Blood (either bright red or very dark) in the stool.
- Diarrhea, constipation, or feeling that the bowel does not empty all the way.
- Stools that are narrower than usual.
- Frequent gas pains, bloating, fullness, or cramps.
- Weight loss for no known reason.
- Feeling very tired.
- Vomiting.

Tests That Examine the Colon and Rectum Are Used to Detect (Find) and Diagnose Colon Cancer

The following tests and procedures may be used:

- Physical exam and history
- Digital rectal exam
- Fecal occult blood test (FOBT)
  - Guaiac FOBT
  - Immunochemical FOBT
- Barium enema
- Sigmoidoscopy
- Colonoscopy
- Virtual colonoscopy
- Biopsy

Certain Factors Affect Prognosis (Chance of Recovery) and Treatment Options

The prognosis (chance of recovery) and treatment options depend on the following:

- The stage of the cancer (whether the cancer is in the inner lining of the colon only or has spread through the colon wall, or has spread to lymph nodes or other places in the body).

- Whether the cancer has blocked or made a hole in the colon.

- Whether there are any cancer cells left after surgery.

- Whether the cancer has recurred.

- The patient's general health.

The prognosis also depends on the blood levels of carcinoembryonic antigen (CEA) before treatment begins. CEA is a substance in the blood that may be increased when cancer is present.

Stages of Colon Cancer

After colon cancer has been diagnosed, tests are done to find out if cancer cells have spread within the colon or to other parts of the body.

The process used to find out if cancer has spread within the colon or to other parts of the body is called staging. The information gathered from the staging process determines the stage of the disease. It is important to know the stage in order to plan treatment.

The following tests and procedures may be used in the staging process:

- CT scan (CAT scan)
- MRI (magnetic resonance imaging)
- PET scan (positron emission tomography scan)
- Chest X-ray
- Surgery
- Lymph node biopsy
- Complete blood count (CBC)
- Carcinoembryonic antigen (CEA) assay

There Are Three Ways That Cancer Spreads in the Body

Cancer can spread through:

1. Tissue

2. Lymph system

3. Blood

Cancer May Spread from Where It Began to Other Parts of the Body

When cancer spreads to another part of the body, it is called metastasis. Cancer cells break away from where they began (the primary tumor) and travel through the lymph system or blood.

The metastatic tumor is the same type of cancer as the primary tumor. For example, if colon cancer spreads to the lung, the cancer cells in the lung are actually colon cancer cells. The disease is metastatic colon cancer, not lung cancer.

The Following Stages Are Used for Colon Cancer

Stage 0 (Carcinoma in Situ)

In stage 0, abnormal cells are found in the mucosa (innermost layer) of the colon wall. These abnormal cells may become cancer and spread. Stage 0 is also called carcinoma in situ.

Stage I

In stage I, cancer has formed in the mucosa (innermost layer) of the colon wall and has spread to the submucosa (layer of tissue under the mucosa). Cancer may have spread to the muscle layer of the colon wall.

Stage II

Stage II colon cancer is divided into stage IIA, stage IIB, and stage IIC.

- Stage IIA: Cancer has spread through the muscle layer of the colon wall to the serosa (outermost layer) of the colon wall.

- Stage IIB: Cancer has spread through the serosa (outermost layer) of the colon wall but has not spread to nearby organs.

- Stage IIC: Cancer has spread through the serosa (outermost layer) of the colon wall to nearby organs.

Stage III

Stage III colon cancer is divided into stage IIIA, stage IIIB, and stage IIIC.

In stage IIIA:

- Cancer has spread through the mucosa (innermost layer) of the colon wall to the submucosa (layer of tissue under the mucosa) and may have spread to the muscle layer of the colon wall. Cancer has spread to at least one but not more than 3 nearby lymph nodes or cancer cells have formed in tissues near the lymph nodes; or

- Cancer has spread through the mucosa (innermost layer) of the colon wall to the submucosa (layer of tissue under the mucosa). Cancer has spread to at least 4 but not more than 6 nearby lymph nodes.

In stage IIIB:

- Cancer has spread through the muscle layer of the colon wall to the serosa (outermost layer) of the colon wall or has spread through the serosa but not to nearby organs. Cancer has spread to at least one but not more than 3 nearby lymph nodes or cancer cells have formed in tissues near the lymph nodes; or

- Cancer has spread to the muscle layer of the colon wall or to the serosa (outermost layer) of the colon wall. Cancer has spread to at least 4 but not more than 6 nearby lymph nodes; or

- Cancer has spread through the mucosa (innermost layer) of the colon wall to the submucosa (layer of tissue under the mucosa) and may have spread to the muscle layer of the colon wall. Cancer has spread to 7 or more nearby lymph nodes.

In stage IIIC:

- Cancer has spread through the serosa (outermost layer) of the colon wall but has not spread to nearby organs. Cancer has spread to at least 4 but not more than 6 nearby lymph nodes; or

- Cancer has spread through the muscle layer of the colon wall to the serosa (outermost layer) of the colon wall or has spread through the serosa but has not spread to nearby organs. Cancer has spread to 7 or more nearby lymph nodes; or

- Cancer has spread through the serosa (outermost layer) of the colon wall and has spread to nearby organs. Cancer has spread to one or more nearby lymph nodes or cancer cells have formed in tissues near the lymph nodes.

Stage IV

Stage IV colon cancer is divided into stage IVA and stage IVB.

- Stage IVA: Cancer may have spread through the colon wall and may have spread to nearby organs or lymph nodes. Cancer has spread to one organ that is not near the colon, such as the liver, lung, or ovary, or to a distant lymph node.

- Stage IVB: Cancer may have spread through the colon wall and may have spread to nearby organs or lymph nodes. Cancer has spread to more than one organ that is not near the colon or into the lining of the abdominal wall.

Recurrent Colon Cancer

Recurrent colon cancer is cancer that has recurred (come back) after it has been treated. The cancer may come back in the colon or in other parts of the body, such as the liver, lungs, or both.

Treatment Option Overview

Different types of treatment are available for patients with colon cancer. Some treatments are standard (the currently used treatment), and some are being tested in clinical trials. A treatment clinical trial is a research study meant to help improve current treatments or obtain information on new treatments for patients with cancer. When clinical trials show that a new treatment is better than the standard treatment, the new treatment may become the standard treatment. Patients may want to think about taking part in a clinical trial. Some clinical trials are open only to patients who have not started treatment.

Six Types of Standard Treatment Are Used

1. Surgery

   Surgery (removing the cancer in an operation) is the most common treatment for all stages of colon cancer. A doctor may remove the cancer using one of the following types of surgery:

   - Local excision: If the cancer is found at a very early stage, the doctor may remove it without cutting through the abdominal wall. Instead, the doctor may put a tube with a cutting tool through the rectum into the colon and cut the cancer out. This is called a local excision.

   - Resection of the colon with anastomosis: If the cancer is larger, the doctor will perform a partial colectomy (removing

the cancer and a small amount of healthy tissue around it).
The doctor may then perform an anastomosis (sewing the
healthy parts of the colon together).

- Resection of the colon with colostomy: If the doctor is not
able to sew the 2 ends of the colon back together, a stoma (an
opening) is made on the outside of the body for waste to pass
through. This procedure is called a colostomy.

2. Radiofrequency ablation

Radiofrequency ablation is the use of a special probe with tiny
electrodes that kill cancer cells.

3. Cryosurgery

Cryosurgery is a treatment that uses an instrument to freeze
and destroy abnormal tissue.

4. Chemotherapy

Chemotherapy is a cancer treatment that uses drugs to stop
the growth of cancer cells, either by killing the cells or by stopping them from dividing.

5. Radiation therapy

Radiation therapy is a cancer treatment that uses high-energy
X-rays or other types of radiation to kill cancer cells or keep
them from growing.

- External radiation therapy uses a machine outside the body
to send radiation toward the cancer.

- Internal radiation therapy uses a radioactive substance
sealed in needles, seeds, wires, or catheters that are placed
directly into or near the cancer.

6. Targeted therapy

Targeted therapy is a type of treatment that uses drugs or
other substances to identify and attack specific cancer cells
without harming normal cells.

- Monoclonal antibodies: Monoclonal antibodies are made in
the laboratory from a single type of immune system cell.
These antibodies can identify substances on cancer cells or
normal substances that may help cancer cells grow. The
antibodies attach to the substances and kill the cancer cells,
block their growth, or keep them from spreading.

- Bevacizumab and ramucirumab are types of monoclonal antibodies that bind to a protein called vascular endothelial growth factor (VEGF). This may prevent the growth of new blood vessels that tumors need to grow.

- Cetuximab and panitumumab are types of monoclonal antibodies that bind to a protein called epidermal growth factor receptor (EGFR) on the surface of some types of cancer cells. This may stop cancer cells from growing and dividing.

- Angiogenesis inhibitors: Angiogenesis inhibitors stop the growth of new blood vessels that tumors need to grow.

  - Ziv-aflibercept is a vascular endothelial growth factor trap that blocks an enzyme needed for the growth of new blood vessels in tumors.

  - Regorafenib is used to treat colorectal cancer that has spread to other parts of the body and has not gotten better with other treatment. It blocks the action of certain proteins, including vascular endothelial growth factor. This may help keep cancer cells from growing and may kill them.

Follow-Up Tests May Be Needed

Some of the tests that were done to diagnose the cancer or to find out the stage of the cancer may be repeated. Some tests will be repeated in order to see how well the treatment is working. Decisions about whether to continue, change, or stop treatment may be based on the results of these tests.

Some of the tests will continue to be done from time to time after treatment has ended. The results of these tests can show if your condition has changed or if the cancer has recurred (come back). These tests are sometimes called follow-up tests or check-ups.

Treatment Options for Colon Cancer

Stage 0 (Carcinoma in Situ)

Treatment of stage 0 (carcinoma in situ) may include the following types of surgery:

- Local excision or simple polypectomy

- Resection and anastomosis

Stage I Colon Cancer

Treatment of stage I colon cancer usually includes the following:

- Resection and anastomosis

Stage II Colon Cancer

Treatment of stage II colon cancer may include the following:

- Resection and anastomosis

Stage III Colon Cancer

Treatment of stage III colon cancer may include the following:

- Resection and anastomosis which may be followed by chemotherapy.

- Clinical trials of new chemotherapy regimens after surgery

Stage IV and Recurrent Colon Cancer

Treatment of stage IV and recurrent colon cancer may include the following:

- Local excision for tumors that have recurred.

- Resection with or without anastomosis.

- Surgery to remove parts of other organs, such as the liver, lungs, and ovaries, where the cancer may have recurred or spread. Treatment of cancer that has spread to the liver may also include the following:

  - Chemotherapy given before surgery to shrink the tumor, after surgery, or both before and after.

  - Radiofrequency ablation or cryosurgery, for patients who cannot have surgery.

  - Chemoembolization of the hepatic artery.

- Radiation therapy or chemotherapy may be offered to some patients as palliative therapy to relieve symptoms and improve quality of life.

- Chemotherapy and/or targeted therapy with a monoclonal antibody or an angiogenesis inhibitor.

- Clinical trials of chemotherapy and/or targeted therapy.

General Information about Rectal Cancer

Rectal cancer is a disease in which malignant (cancer) cells form in the tissues of the rectum.

Health History Affects the Risk of Developing Rectal Cancer

Anything that increases your chance of getting a disease is called a risk factor. Having a risk factor does not mean that you will get cancer; not having risk factors doesn't mean that you will not get cancer. Talk to your doctor if you think you may be at risk for colorectal cancer.

Risk factors for colorectal cancer include the following:

- Having a family history of colon or rectal cancer in a first-degree relative (parent, sibling, or child).

- Having a personal history of cancer of the colon, rectum, or ovary.

- Having a personal history of high-risk adenomas (colorectal polyps that are 1 centimeter or larger in size or that have cells that look abnormal under a microscope).

- Having inherited changes in certain genes that increase the risk of familial adenomatous polyposis (FAP) or Lynch syndrome (hereditary nonpolyposis colorectal cancer).

- Having a personal history of chronic ulcerative colitis or Crohn's disease for 8 years or more.

- Having three or more alcoholic drinks per day.

- Smoking cigarettes.

- Being black.

- Being obese.

Older age is a main risk factor for most cancers. The chance of getting cancer increases as you get older.

Signs of Rectal Cancer Include a Change in Bowel Habits or Blood in the Stool

These and other signs and symptoms may be caused by rectal cancer or by other conditions. Check with your doctor if you have any of the following:

- Blood (either bright red or very dark) in the stool.

- A change in bowel habits.
  - Diarrhea.
  - Constipation.
  - Feeling that the bowel does not empty completely.
  - Stools that are narrower or have a different shape than usual.
- General abdominal discomfort (frequent gas pains, bloating, fullness, or cramps).
- Change in appetite.
- Weight loss for no known reason.
- Feeling very tired.

Tests That Examine the Rectum and Colon Are Used to Detect (Find) and Diagnose Rectal Cancer

Tests used to diagnose rectal cancer include the following:

- Physical exam and history
- Digital rectal exam (DRE)
- Colonoscopy
- Biopsy
  - Reverse transcription–polymerase chain reaction (RT–PCR) test
  - Immunohistochemistry
- Carcinoembryonic antigen (CEA) assay

Certain Factors Affect Prognosis (Chance of Recovery) and Treatment Options

The prognosis (chance of recovery) and treatment options depend on the following:

- The stage of the cancer (whether it affects the inner lining of the rectum only, involves the whole rectum, or has spread to lymph nodes, nearby organs, or other places in the body).
- Whether the tumor has spread into or through the bowel wall.

- Where the cancer is found in the rectum.

- Whether the bowel is blocked or has a hole in it.

- Whether all of the tumor can be removed by surgery.

- The patient's general health.

- Whether the cancer has just been diagnosed or has recurred (come back).

Stages of Rectal Cancer

After rectal cancer has been diagnosed, tests are done to find out if cancer cells have spread within the rectum or to other parts of the body.

The process used to find out whether cancer has spread within the rectum or to other parts of the body is called staging. The information gathered from the staging process determines the stage of the disease. It is important to know the stage in order to plan treatment.

The following tests and procedures may be used in the staging process:

- Chest X-ray

- Colonoscopy

- Computed tomography scan (CT scan, CAT scan)

- MRI (magnetic resonance imaging)

- PET scan (positron emission tomography scan)

- Endorectal ultrasound

There Are Three Ways That Cancer Spreads in the Body

Cancer can spread through:

1. Tissue

2. Lymph system

3. Blood

Cancer May Spread from Where It Began to Other Parts of the Body

When cancer spreads to another part of the body, it is called metastasis. Cancer cells break away from where they began (the primary tumor) and travel through the lymph system or blood.

When cancer spreads to another part of the body, it is called metastasis. Cancer cells break away from where they began (the primary tumor) and travel through the lymph system or blood.

The Following Stages Are Used for Rectal Cancer

Stage 0 (Carcinoma in Situ)

In stage 0, abnormal cells are found in the mucosa (innermost layer) of the rectum wall. These abnormal cells may become cancer and spread. Stage 0 is also called carcinoma in situ.

Stage I

In stage I, cancer has formed in the mucosa (innermost layer) of the rectum wall and has spread to the submucosa (layer of tissue under the mucosa). Cancer may have spread to the muscle layer of the rectum wall.

Stage II

Stage II rectal cancer is divided into stage IIA, stage IIB, and stage IIC.

- **Stage IIA**: Cancer has spread through the muscle layer of the rectum wall to the serosa (outermost layer) of the rectum wall.

- **Stage IIB:** Cancer has spread through the serosa (outermost layer) of the rectum wall but has not spread to nearby organs.

- **Stage IIC:** Cancer has spread through the serosa (outermost layer) of the rectum wall to nearby organs.

Stage III

Stage III rectal cancer is divided into stage IIIA, stage IIIB, and stage IIIC.
Stage IIIA:

- Cancer has spread through the mucosa (innermost layer) of the rectum wall to the submucosa (layer of tissue under the mucosa) and may have spread to the muscle layer of the rectum wall. Cancer has spread to at least one but not more than 3 nearby lymph nodes or cancer cells have formed in tissues near the lymph nodes; or

- Cancer has spread through the mucosa (innermost layer) of the rectum wall to the submucosa (layer of tissue under the mucosa). Cancer has spread to at least 4 but not more than 6 nearby lymph nodes.

Stage IIIB:

Cancer has spread through the muscle layer of the rectum wall to the serosa (outermost layer) of the rectum wall or has spread through the serosa but not to nearby organs. Cancer has spread to at least one but not more than 3 nearby lymph nodes or cancer cells have formed in tissues near the lymph nodes; or

Cancer has spread to the muscle layer of the rectum wall or to the serosa (outermost layer) of the rectum wall. Cancer has spread to at least 4 but not more than 6 nearby lymph nodes; or

Cancer has spread through the mucosa (innermost layer) of the rectum wall to the submucosa (layer of tissue under the mucosa) and may have spread to the muscle layer of the rectum wall. Cancer has spread to 7 or more nearby lymph nodes.

Stage IIIC:

Cancer has spread through the serosa (outermost layer) of the rectum wall but has not spread to nearby organs. Cancer has spread to at least 4 but not more than 6 nearby lymph nodes; or

Cancer has spread through the muscle layer of the rectum wall to the serosa (outermost layer) of the rectum wall or has spread through the serosa but has not spread to nearby organs. Cancer has spread to 7 or more nearby lymph nodes; or

Cancer has spread through the serosa (outermost layer) of the rectum wall and has spread to nearby organs. Cancer has spread to one or more nearby lymph nodes or cancer cells have formed in tissues near the lymph nodes.

Stage IV

Stage IV rectal cancer is divided into stage IVA and stage IVB.

- **Stage IVA:** Cancer may have spread through the rectum wall and may have spread to nearby organs or lymph nodes. Cancer has spread to one organ that is not near the rectum, such as the liver, lung, or ovary, or to a distant lymph node.

- **Stage IVB:** Cancer may have spread through the rectum wall and may have spread to nearby organs or lymph nodes. Cancer has spread to more than one organ that is not near the rectum or into the lining of the abdominal wall.

Recurrent Rectal Cancer

Recurrent rectal cancer is cancer that has recurred (come back) after it has been treated. The cancer may come back in the rectum or in other parts of the body, such as the colon, pelvis, liver, or lungs.

Treatment Option Overview

There are different types of treatment for patients with rectal cancer.

Different types of treatment are available for patients with rectal cancer. Some treatments are standard (the currently used treatment), and some are being tested in clinical trials. A treatment clinical trial is a research study meant to help improve current treatments or obtain information on new treatments for patients with cancer. When clinical trials show that a new treatment is better than the standard treatment, the new treatment may become the standard treatment. Patients may want to think about taking part in a clinical trial. Some clinical trials are open only to patients who have not started treatment.

Five Types of Standard Treatment Are Used

1. Surgery

    Surgery is the most common treatment for all stages of rectal cancer. The cancer is removed using one of the following types of surgery:

    -   Polypectomy: If the cancer is found in a polyp (a small piece of bulging tissue), the polyp is often removed during a colonoscopy.

    -   Local excision: If the cancer is found on the inside surface of the rectum and has not spread into the wall of the rectum, the cancer and a small amount of surrounding healthy tissue is removed.

    -   Resection: If the cancer has spread into the wall of the rectum, the section of the rectum with cancer and nearby healthy tissue is removed. Sometimes the tissue between the rectum and the abdominal wall is also removed.

- Radiofrequency ablation: The use of a special probe with tiny electrodes that kill cancer cells.

- Cryosurgery: The use of a special probe with tiny electrodes that kill cancer cells.

- Pelvic exenteration: If the cancer has spread to other organs near the rectum, the lower colon, rectum, and bladder are removed. In women, the cervix, vagina, ovaries, and nearby lymph nodes may be removed.

After the cancer is removed, the surgeon will either:

- do an anastomosis (sew the healthy parts of the rectum together, sew the remaining rectum to the colon, or sew the colon to the anus); or

- make a stoma (an opening) from the rectum to the outside of the body for waste to pass through. This procedure is done if the cancer is too close to the anus and is called a colostomy. A bag is placed around the stoma to collect the waste. Sometimes the colostomy is needed only until the rectum has healed, and then it can be reversed. If the entire rectum is removed, however, the colostomy may be permanent.

Radiation therapy and/or chemotherapy may be given before surgery to shrink the tumor, make it easier to remove the cancer, and help with bowel control after surgery. Treatment given before surgery is called neoadjuvant therapy. Even if all the cancer that can be seen at the time of the operation is removed, some patients may be given radiation therapy and/or chemotherapy after surgery to kill any cancer cells that are left. Treatment given after the surgery, to lower the risk that the cancer will come back, is called adjuvant therapy.

2. Radiation therapy

Radiation therapy is a cancer treatment that uses high-energy X-rays or other types of radiation to kill cancer cells or keep them from growing.

- External radiation therapy uses a machine outside the body to send radiation toward the cancer.

- Internal radiation therapy uses a radioactive substance sealed in needles, seeds, wires, or catheters that are placed directly into or near the cancer.

535

3. Chemotherapy

    Chemotherapy is a cancer treatment that uses drugs to stop the growth of cancer cells, either by killing the cells or by stopping the cells from dividing.

4. Active surveillance

    Active surveillance is closely following a patient's condition without giving any treatment unless there are changes in test results. It is used to find early signs that the condition is getting worse. In active surveillance, patients are given certain exams and tests to check if the cancer is growing. When the cancer begins to grow, treatment is given to cure the cancer. Tests include the following:

    - Digital rectal exam

    - MRI

    - Endoscopy

    - Sigmoidoscopy

    - CT scan

    - Carcinoembryonic antigen (CEA) assay

5. Targeted therapy

    Targeted therapy is a type of treatment that uses drugs or other substances to identify and attack specific cancer cells without harming normal cells.

    - Monoclonal antibodies: Monoclonal antibody therapy uses antibodies made in the laboratory from a single type of immune system cell. These antibodies can identify substances on cancer cells or normal substances that may help cancer cells grow. The antibodies attach to the substances and kill the cancer cells, block their growth, or keep them from spreading.

        - Bevacizumab and ramucirumab are types of monoclonal antibodies that bind to a protein called vascular endothelial growth factor (VEGF). This may prevent the growth of new blood vessels that tumors need to grow.

        - Cetuximab and panitumumab are types of monoclonal antibodies that bind to a protein called epidermal growth factor receptor (EGFR) on the surface of some types of cancer cells. This may stop cancer cells from growing and dividing.

- Angiogenesis inhibitors: Angiogenesis inhibitors stop the growth of new blood vessels that tumors need to grow.

  - Ziv-aflibercept is a vascular endothelial growth factor trap that blocks an enzyme needed for the growth of new blood vessels in tumors.

  - Regorafenib is used to treat colorectal cancer that has spread to other parts of the body and has not gotten better with other treatment. It blocks the action of certain proteins, including vascular endothelial growth factor. This may help keep cancer cells from growing and may kill them.

Follow-Up Tests May Be Needed

Some of the tests that were done to diagnose the cancer or to find out the stage of the cancer may be repeated. Some tests will be repeated in order to see how well the treatment is working. Decisions about whether to continue, change, or stop treatment may be based on the results of these tests.

Some of the tests will continue to be done from time to time after treatment has ended. The results of these tests can show if your condition has changed or if the cancer has recurred (come back). These tests are sometimes called follow-up tests or check-ups.

After treatment for rectal cancer, a blood test to measure amounts of carcinoembryonic antigen (a substance in the blood that may be increased when cancer is present) may be done to see if the cancer has come back.

Treatment Options by Stage

Stage 0 (Carcinoma in Situ)

Treatment of stage 0 may include the following:

- Simple polypectomy.
- Local excision.
- Resection (when the tumor is too large to remove by local excision).

Stage I Rectal Cancer

Treatment of stage I rectal cancer may include the following:

- Local excision.
- Resection.
- Resection with radiation therapy and chemotherapy after surgery.

Stages II and III Rectal Cancer

Treatment of stage II and stage III rectal cancer may include the following:

- Surgery.
- Chemotherapy combined with radiation therapy, followed by surgery.
- Short-course radiation therapy followed by surgery and chemotherapy.
- Resection followed by chemotherapy combined with radiation therapy.
- Chemotherapy combined with radiation therapy, followed by active surveillance. Surgery may be done if the cancer recurs (comes back).
- A clinical trial of a new treatment.

Stage IV and Recurrent Rectal Cancer

Treatment of stage IV and recurrent rectal cancer may include the following:

- Surgery with or without chemotherapy or radiation therapy.
- Systemic chemotherapy with or without targeted therapy (a monoclonal antibody or angiogenesis inhibitor).
- Chemotherapy to control the growth of the tumor.
- Radiation therapy, chemotherapy, or a combination of both, as palliative therapy to relieve symptoms and improve the quality of life.
- Placement of a stent to help keep the rectum open if it is partly blocked by the tumor, as palliative therapy to relieve symptoms and improve the quality of life.
- A clinical trial of a new anticancer drug.

Chapter 40

Lung Cancer

Non-Small Cell Lung Cancer

The lungs are a pair of cone-shaped breathing organs inside the chest. The lungs bring oxygen into the body when breathing in and send carbon dioxide out of the body when breathing out.

The two main types of lung cancer are non-small cell lung cancer and small cell lung cancer. The types are based on the way the cells look under a microscope. Non-small cell lung cancer is much more common than small cell lung cancer.

Most cases of lung cancer are caused by smoking. Lung cancer is the leading cause of death from cancer in the United States.

For most patients with lung cancer, current treatments do not cure the cancer.

Types of Non-Small Cell Lung Cancer

There are several types of non-small cell lung cancer. Each type of non-small cell lung cancer has different kinds of cancer cells. The cancer cells of each type grow and spread in different ways. The types of non-small cell lung cancer are named for the kinds of cells found in the cancer and how the cells look under a microscope:

- **Squamous cell carcinoma.** Cancer that begins in squamous cells, which are thin, flat cells that look like fish scales. This is also called epidermoid carcinoma.

This chapter includes text excerpted from "Lung Cancer—Patient Version," National Cancer Institute (NCI), April 13, 2017.

- **Large cell carcinoma.** Cancer that may begin in several types of large cells.

- **Adenocarcinoma.** Cancer that begins in the cells that line the alveoli and make substances such as mucus.

Other less common types of non-small cell lung cancer are: pleomorphic, carcinoid tumor, salivary gland carcinoma, and unclassified carcinoma.

Smoking Is the Major Risk Factor for Non-Small Cell Lung Cancer

Anything that increases your chance of getting a disease is called a risk factor. Having a risk factor does not mean that you will get cancer; not having risk factors doesn't mean that you will not get cancer. Talk to your doctor if you think you may be at risk for lung cancer.

Risk factors for lung cancer include the following:

- Smoking cigarettes, pipes, or cigars, now or in the past. This is the most important risk factor for lung cancer. The earlier in life a person starts smoking, the more often a person smokes, and the more years a person smokes, the greater the risk of lung cancer.

- Being exposed to secondhand smoke.

- Being exposed to radiation from any of the following:

  - Radiation therapy to the breast or chest.

  - Radon in the home or workplace.

  - Imaging tests such as computerized tomography (CT) scan.

  - Atomic bomb radiation.

- Being exposed to asbestos, chromium, nickel, beryllium, arsenic, soot, or tar in the workplace.

- Living where there is air pollution.

- Having a family history of lung cancer.

- Being infected with the human immunodeficiency virus (HIV).

- Taking beta carotene supplements and being a heavy smoker.

Older age is the main risk factor for most cancers. The chance of getting cancer increases as you get older.

When smoking is combined with other risk factors, the risk of lung cancer is increased.

Signs of Non-Small Cell Lung Cancer

Signs of non-small cell lung cancer include a cough that doesn't go away and shortness of breath. Sometimes lung cancer does not cause any signs or symptoms. It may be found during a chest X-ray done for another condition. Signs and symptoms may be caused by lung cancer or by other conditions. Check with your doctor if you have any of the following:

- Chest discomfort or pain.
- A cough that doesn't go away or gets worse over time.
- Trouble breathing.
- Wheezing.
- Blood in sputum (mucus coughed up from the lungs).
- Hoarseness.
- Loss of appetite.
- Weight loss for no known reason.
- Feeling very tired.
- Trouble swallowing.
- Swelling in the face and/or veins in the neck.

Tests to Detect, Diagnose, and Stage Non-Small Cell Lung Cancer

Tests and procedures to detect, diagnose, and stage non-small cell lung cancer are often done at the same time. Some of the following tests and procedures may be used:

- Physical exam and history
- Laboratory tests
- Chest X-ray
- CT scan (CAT scan)
- Sputum cytology
- Fine-needle aspiration (FNA) biopsy of the lung
- Bronchoscopy

541

- Thoracoscopy

- Thoracentesis

- Light and electron microscopy

- Immunohistochemistry

Certain Factors Affect Prognosis and Treatment Options

The prognosis (chance of recovery) and treatment options depend on the following:

- The stage of the cancer (the size of the tumor and whether it is in the lung only or has spread to other places in the body).

- The type of lung cancer.

- Whether the cancer has mutations (changes) in certain genes, such as the epidermal growth factor receptor (EGFR) gene or the anaplastic lymphoma kinase (ALK) gene.

- Whether there are signs and symptoms such as coughing or trouble breathing.

- The patient's general health.

Stages of Non-Small Cell Lung Cancer

After lung cancer has been diagnosed, tests are done to find out if cancer cells have spread within the lungs or to other parts of the body.

The process used to find out if cancer has spread within the lungs or to other parts of the body is called staging. The information gathered from the staging process determines the stage of the disease. It is important to know the stage in order to plan treatment. Some of the tests used to diagnose non-small cell lung cancer are also used to stage the disease.

Other tests and procedures that may be used in the staging process include the following:

- MRI (magnetic resonance imaging)

- CT scan (CAT scan)

- PET scan (positron emission tomography scan)

- Radionuclide bone scan

- Pulmonary function test (PFT)

- Endoscopic ultrasound (EUS)
- Mediastinoscopy
- Anterior mediastinotomy
- Lymph node biopsy
- Bone marrow aspiration and biopsy

How Cancer Spreads

There are three ways that cancer spreads in the body. Cancer can spread through:

1. **Tissue.** The cancer spreads from where it began by growing into nearby areas.

2. **Lymph system.** The cancer spreads from where it began by getting into the lymph system. The cancer travels through the lymph vessels to other parts of the body.

3. **Blood.** The cancer spreads from where it began by getting into the blood. The cancer travels through the blood vessels to other parts of the body.

Cancer May Spread from Where It Began to Other Parts of the Body

When cancer spreads to another part of the body, it is called metastasis. Cancer cells break away from where they began (the primary tumor) and travel through the lymph system or blood.

The metastatic tumor is the same type of cancer as the primary tumor. For example, if non-small cell lung cancer spreads to the brain, the cancer cells in the brain are actually lung cancer cells. The disease is metastatic lung cancer, not brain cancer.

The following stages are used for non-small cell lung cancer:

Occult (Hidden) stage. In the occult (hidden) stage, cancer cannot be seen by imaging or bronchoscopy. Cancer cells are found in sputum (mucus coughed up from the lungs) or bronchial washing (a sample of cells taken from inside the airways that lead to the lung). Cancer may have spread to other parts of the body.

Stage 0 (Carcinoma in Situ). In stage 0, abnormal cells are found in the lining of the airways. These abnormal cells may become cancer and spread into nearby normal tissue. Stage 0 is also called carcinoma in situ.

Stage I. In stage I, cancer has formed. Stage I is divided into stages IA and IB:

- Stage IA: The tumor is in the lung only and is 3 centimeters or smaller.

- Stage IB: Cancer has not spread to the lymph nodes and one or more of the following is true:

  - The tumor is larger than 3 centimeters but not larger than 5 centimeters.

  - Cancer has spread to the main bronchus and is at least 2 centimeters below where the trachea joins the bronchus.

  - Cancer has spread to the innermost layer of the membrane that covers the lung.

  - Part of the lung has collapsed or developed pneumonitis (inflammation of the lung) in the area where the trachea joins the bronchus.

Stage II. Stage II is divided into stages IIA and IIB. Stage IIA and IIB are each divided into two sections depending on the size of the tumor, where the tumor is found, and whether there is cancer in the lymph nodes.

Stage IIA.

1. Cancer has spread to lymph nodes on the same side of the chest as the tumor. The lymph nodes with cancer are within the lung or near the bronchus. Also, one or more of the following is true:

    - The tumor is not larger than 5 centimeters.

    - Cancer has spread to the main bronchus and is at least 2 centimeters below where the trachea joins the bronchus.

    - Cancer has spread to the innermost layer of the membrane that covers the lung.

    - Part of the lung has collapsed or developed pneumonitis (inflammation of the lung) in the area where the trachea joins the bronchus.

    or

2. Cancer has not spread to lymph nodes and one or more of the following is true:

- The tumor is larger than 5 centimeters but not larger than 7 centimeters.

- Cancer has spread to the main bronchus and is at least 2 centimeters below where the trachea joins the bronchus.

- Cancer has spread to the innermost layer of the membrane that covers the lung.

- Part of the lung has collapsed or developed pneumonitis (inflammation of the lung) in the area where the trachea joins the bronchus.

Stage IIB

1. Cancer has spread to nearby lymph nodes on the same side of the chest as the tumor. The lymph nodes with cancer are within the lung or near the bronchus. Also, one or more of the following is true:

   - The tumor is larger than 5 centimeters but not larger than 7 centimeters.

   - Cancer has spread to the main bronchus and is at least 2 centimeters below where the trachea joins the bronchus.

   - Cancer has spread to the innermost layer of the membrane that covers the lung.

   - Part of the lung has collapsed or developed pneumonitis (inflammation of the lung) in the area where the trachea joins the bronchus.

   or

2. Cancer has not spread to lymph nodes and one or more of the following is true:

   - The tumor is larger than 7 centimeters.

   - Cancer has spread to the main bronchus (and is less than 2 centimeters below where the trachea joins the bronchus), the chest wall, the diaphragm, or the nerve that controls the diaphragm.

   - Cancer has spread to the membrane around the heart or lining the chest wall.

   - The whole lung has collapsed or developed pneumonitis (inflammation of the lung).

- There are one or more separate tumors in the same lobe of the lung.

Stage III

Stage IIIA. Stage IIIA is divided into three sections depending on the size of the tumor, where the tumor is found, and which lymph nodes have cancer (if any).

1. Cancer has spread to lymph nodes on the same side of the chest as the tumor. The lymph nodes with cancer are near the sternum (chest bone) or where the bronchus enters the lung. Also:

    - The tumor may be any size.

    - Part of the lung (where the trachea joins the bronchus) or the whole lung may have collapsed or developed pneumonitis (inflammation of the lung).

    - There may be one or more separate tumors in the same lobe of the lung.

    - Cancer may have spread to any of the following:

        - Main bronchus, but not the area where the trachea joins the bronchus.

        - Chest wall.

        - Diaphragm and the nerve that controls it.

        - Membrane around the lung or lining the chest wall.

        - Membrane around the heart.

    or

2. Cancer has spread to lymph nodes on the same side of the chest as the tumor. The lymph nodes with cancer are within the lung or near the bronchus. Also:

    - The tumor may be any size.

    - The whole lung may have collapsed or developed pneumonitis (inflammation of the lung).

    - There may be one or more separate tumors in any of the lobes of the lung with cancer.

    - Cancer may have spread to any of the following:

        - Main bronchus, but not the area where the trachea joins the bronchus.

- Chest wall.
- Diaphragm and the nerve that controls it.
- Membrane around the lung or lining the chest wall.
- Heart or the membrane around it.
- Major blood vessels that lead to or from the heart.
- Trachea.
- Esophagus.
- Nerve that controls the larynx (voice box).
- Sternum (chest bone) or backbone.
- Carina (where the trachea joins the bronchi).

or

3. Cancer has not spread to the lymph nodes and the tumor may be any size. Cancer has spread to any of the following:

- Heart.
- Major blood vessels that lead to or from the heart.
- Trachea.
- Esophagus.
- Nerve that controls the larynx (voice box).
- Sternum (chest bone) or backbone.
- Carina (where the trachea joins the bronchi).

Stage IIIB

Stage IIIB is divided into two sections depending on the size of the tumor, where the tumor is found, and which lymph nodes have cancer.

1. Cancer has spread to lymph nodes above the collarbone or to lymph nodes on the opposite side of the chest as the tumor. Also:

- The tumor may be any size.
- Part of the lung (where the trachea joins the bronchus) or the whole lung may have collapsed or developed pneumonitis (inflammation of the lung).
- There may be one or more separate tumors in any of the lobes of the lung with cancer.

- Cancer may have spread to any of the following:
  - Main bronchus.
  - Chest wall.
  - Diaphragm and the nerve that controls it.
  - Membrane around the lung or lining the chest wall.
  - Heart or the membrane around it.
  - Major blood vessels that lead to or from the heart.
  - Trachea.
  - Esophagus.
  - Nerve that controls the larynx (voice box).
  - Sternum (chest bone) or backbone.
  - Carina (where the trachea joins the bronchi).

or

2. Cancer has spread to lymph nodes on the same side of the chest as the tumor. The lymph nodes with cancer are near the sternum (chest bone) or where the bronchus enters the lung. Also:

- The tumor may be any size.
- There may be separate tumors in different lobes of the same lung.
- Cancer has spread to any of the following:
  - Heart.
  - Major blood vessels that lead to or from the heart.
  - Trachea.
  - Esophagus.
  - Nerve that controls the larynx (voice box).
  - Sternum (chest bone) or backbone.
  - Carina (where the trachea joins the bronchi).

Stage IV. In stage IV, the tumor may be any size and cancer may have spread to lymph nodes. One or more of the following is true:

- There are one or more tumors in both lungs.

- Cancer is found in fluid around the lungs or the heart.

- Cancer has spread to other parts of the body, such as the brain, liver, adrenal glands, kidneys, or bone.

Treatment Option Overview

Different types of treatments are available for patients with non-small cell lung cancer. Some treatments are standard (the currently used treatment), and some are being tested in clinical trials. A treatment clinical trial is a research study meant to help improve current treatments or obtain information on new treatments for patients with cancer. When clinical trials show that a new treatment is better than the standard treatment, the new treatment may become the standard treatment. Patients may want to think about taking part in a clinical trial. Some clinical trials are open only to patients who have not started treatment.

Nine types of standard treatment are used:

1. Surgery

    - Wedge resection: Surgery to remove a tumor and some of the normal tissue around it.

    - Lobectomy: Surgery to remove a whole lobe (section) of the lung.

    - Pneumonectomy: Surgery to remove one whole lung.

    - Sleeve resection: Surgery to remove part of the bronchus.

2. Radiation therapy

    Radiation therapy is a cancer treatment that uses high-energy X-rays or other types of radiation to kill cancer cells or keep them from growing.

    - External radiation therapy uses a machine outside the body to send radiation toward the cancer.

        - Stereotactic body radiation therapy is a type of external radiation therapy. Special equipment is used to place the patient in the same position for each radiation treatment. Once a day for several days, a radiation machine aims a larger than usual dose of radiation directly at the tumor. By having the patient in the same position for each treatment, there is less damage to nearby healthy tissue.

- Stereotactic radiosurgery is a type of external radiation therapy used to treat lung cancer that has spread to the brain. A rigid head frame is attached to the skull to keep the head still during the radiation treatment. A machine aims a single large dose of radiation directly at the tumor in the brain. This procedure does not involve surgery.

- Internal radiation therapy uses a radioactive substance sealed in needles, seeds, wires, or catheters that are placed directly into or near the cancer.

3. Chemotherapy

   Chemotherapy is a cancer treatment that uses drugs to stop the growth of cancer cells, either by killing the cells or by stopping them from dividing.

4. Targeted therapy

   Targeted therapy is a type of treatment that uses drugs or other substances to attack specific cancer cells.

   - Monoclonal antibodies: Monoclonal antibody therapy is a cancer treatment that uses antibodies made in the laboratory from a single type of immune system cell. These antibodies can identify substances on cancer cells or normal substances in the blood or tissues that may help cancer cells grow. The antibodies attach to the substances and kill the cancer cells, block their growth, or keep them from spreading.

   - Tyrosine kinase inhibitors: Tyrosine kinase inhibitors are small-molecule drugs that go through the cell membrane and work inside cancer cells to block signals that cancer cells need to grow and divide.

5. Laser therapy

   Laser therapy is a cancer treatment that uses a laser beam (a narrow beam of intense light) to kill cancer cells.

6. Photodynamic therapy (PDT)

   Photodynamic therapy (PDT) is a cancer treatment that uses a drug and a certain type of laser light to kill cancer cells.

7. Cryosurgery

   Cryosurgery is a treatment that uses an instrument to freeze and destroy abnormal tissue, such as carcinoma in situ.

8. Electrocautery

   Electrocautery is a treatment that uses a probe or needle heated by an electric current to destroy abnormal tissue.

9. Watchful waiting

   Watchful waiting is closely monitoring a patient's condition without giving any treatment until signs or symptoms appear or change.

Follow-Up Tests May Be Needed

Some of the tests that were done to diagnose the cancer or to find out the stage of the cancer may be repeated. Some tests will be repeated in order to see how well the treatment is working. Decisions about whether to continue, change, or stop treatment may be based on the results of these tests.

Some of the tests will continue to be done from time to time after treatment has ended. The results of these tests can show if your condition has changed or if the cancer has recurred (come back). These tests are sometimes called follow-up tests or check-ups.

Small Cell Lung Cancer

General Information about Small Cell Lung Cancer

There are two main types of small cell lung cancer. These two types include many different types of cells. The cancer cells of each type grow and spread in different ways. The types of small cell lung cancer are named for the kinds of cells found in the cancer and how the cells look when viewed under a microscope:

1. Small cell carcinoma (oat cell cancer).

2. Combined small cell carcinoma.

Smoking Is the Major Risk Factor for Small Cell Lung Cancer

Anything that increases your chance of getting a disease is called a risk factor. Having a risk factor does not mean that you will get cancer; not having risk factors doesn't mean that you will not get cancer. Talk to your doctor if you think you may be at risk for lung cancer.

Risk factors for lung cancer include the following:

• Smoking cigarettes, pipes, or cigars, now or in the past. This is the most important risk factor for lung cancer. The earlier in life a person starts smoking, the more often a person smokes, and the more years a person smokes, the greater the risk of lung cancer.

- Being exposed to secondhand smoke.

- Being exposed to radiation from any of the following:

  - Radiation therapy to the breast or chest.

  - Radon in the home or workplace.

  - Imaging tests such as CT scans.

  - Atomic bomb radiation.

- Being exposed to asbestos, chromium, nickel, beryllium, arsenic, soot, or tar in the workplace.

- Living where there is air pollution.

- Having a family history of lung cancer.

- Being infected with the human immunodeficiency virus (HIV).

- Taking beta carotene supplements and being a heavy smoker.

Older age is the main risk factor for most cancers. The chance of getting cancer increases as you get older.

When smoking is combined with other risk factors, the risk of lung cancer is increased.

Signs and Symptoms of Small Cell Lung Cancer

Signs and symptoms of small cell lung cancer include coughing, shortness of breath, and chest pain. These and other signs and symptoms may be caused by small cell lung cancer or by other conditions. Check with your doctor if you have any of the following:

- Chest discomfort or pain.

- A cough that doesn't go away or gets worse over time.

- Trouble breathing.

- Wheezing.

- Blood in sputum (mucus coughed up from the lungs).

- Hoarseness.

- Trouble swallowing.

- Loss of appetite.

- Weight loss for no known reason.

- Feeling very tired.
- Swelling in the face and/or veins in the neck.

Tests and Procedures to Detect, Diagnose, and Stage Small Cell Lung Cancer

The following tests and procedures may be used:
- Physical exam and history
- Laboratory tests
- Chest X-ray
- CT scan (CAT scan) of the brain, chest, and abdomen
- Sputum cytology
- Biopsy:
    - Fine-needle aspiration (FNA) biopsy of the lung
    - Bronchoscopy
    - Thoracoscopy
    - Thoracentesis
    - Mediastinoscopy
- Light and electron microscopy
- Immunohistochemistry

Factors Affecting Prognosis and Treatment Options

The prognosis (chance of recovery) and treatment options depend on the following:

- The stage of the cancer (whether it is in the chest cavity only or has spread to other places in the body).

- The patient's age, gender, and general health.

For certain patients, prognosis also depends on whether the patient is treated with both chemotherapy and radiation.

Stages of Small Cell Lung Cancer

After small cell lung cancer has been diagnosed, tests are done to find out if cancer cells have spread within the chest or to other parts of the body.

The process used to find out if cancer has spread within the chest or to other parts of the body is called staging. The information gathered from the staging process determines the stage of the disease. It is important to know the stage in order to plan treatment. Some of the tests used to diagnose small cell lung cancer are also used to stage the disease.

Other tests and procedures that may be used in the staging process include the following:

- MRI (magnetic resonance imaging) of the brain

- CT scan (CAT scan)

- PET scan (positron emission tomography scan)

- Bone scan

How Cancer Spreads

There are three ways that cancer spreads in the body. Cancer can spread through:

1. Tissue

2. Lymph system

3. Blood

Cancer May Spread from Where It Began to Other Parts of the Body

When cancer spreads to another part of the body, it is called metastasis. Cancer cells break away from where they began (the primary tumor) and travel through the lymph system or blood.

The metastatic tumor is the same type of cancer as the primary tumor. For example, if small cell lung cancer spreads to the brain, the cancer cells in the brain are actually lung cancer cells. The disease is metastatic small cell lung cancer, not brain cancer.

Stages Used for Small Cell Lung Cancer

The following stages are used for small cell lung cancer.

Limited-Stage Small Cell Lung Cancer. In limited-stage, cancer is in the lung where it started and may have spread to the area between the lungs or to the lymph nodes above the collarbone.

Limited-Stage Small Cell Lung Cancer. In limited-stage, cancer is in the lung where it started and may have spread to the area between the lungs or to the lymph nodes above the collarbone.

Treatment Option Overview

Different types of treatment are available for patients with small cell lung cancer. Some treatments are standard (the currently used treatment), and some are being tested in clinical trials. A treatment clinical trial is a research study meant to help improve current treatments or obtain information on new treatments for patients with cancer. When clinical trials show that a new treatment is better than the standard treatment, the new treatment may become the standard treatment. Patients may want to think about taking part in a clinical trial. Some clinical trials are open only to patients who have not started treatment.

Types of Standard Treatment

Five types of standard treatment are used.

1. Surgery

   Surgery may be used if the cancer is found in one lung and in nearby lymph nodes only. During surgery, the doctor will also remove lymph nodes to find out if they have cancer in them. Sometimes, surgery may be used to remove a sample of lung tissue to find out the exact type of lung cancer.

2. Chemotherapy

   Chemotherapy is a cancer treatment that uses drugs to stop the growth of cancer cells, either by killing the cells or by stopping them from dividing.

3. Radiation therapy

   Radiation therapy is a cancer treatment that uses high-energy X-rays or other types of radiation to kill cancer cells or keep them from growing.

   • External radiation therapy uses a machine outside the body to send radiation toward the cancer.

   • Internal radiation therapy uses a radioactive substance sealed in needles, seeds, wires, or catheters that are placed directly into or near the cancer.

4. Laser therapy

   Laser therapy is a cancer treatment that uses a laser beam (a narrow beam of intense light) to kill cancer cells.

5. Endoscopic stent placement

    An endoscope is a thin, tube-like instrument used to look at
    tissues inside the body. An endoscope has a light and a lens for
    viewing and may be used to place a stent in a body structure
    to keep the structure open. An endoscopic stent can be used to
    open an airway blocked by abnormal tissue.

Follow-Up Tests May Be Needed

Some of the tests that were done to diagnose the cancer or to find out
the stage of the cancer may be repeated. Some tests will be repeated
in order to see how well the treatment is working. Decisions about
whether to continue, change, or stop treatment may be based on the
results of these tests.

Some of the tests will continue to be done from time to time after
treatment has ended. The results of these tests can show if your condition has changed or if the cancer has recurred (come back). These
tests are sometimes called follow-up tests or check-ups.

Chapter 41

Skin Cancer

General Information about Skin Cancer

Skin cancer is a disease in which malignant (cancer) cells form in the tissues of the skin.

The skin is the body's largest organ. It protects against heat, sunlight, injury, and infection. Skin also helps control body temperature and stores water, fat, and vitamin D. The skin has several layers, but the two main layers are the epidermis (upper or outer layer) and the dermis (lower or inner layer). Skin cancer begins in the epidermis, which is made up of three kinds of cells:

1. **Squamous cells:** Thin, flat cells that form the top layer of the epidermis.

2. **Basal cells:** Round cells under the squamous cells.

3. **Melanocytes:** Cells that make melanin and are found in the lower part of the epidermis. Melanin is the pigment that gives skin its natural color. When skin is exposed to the sun, melanocytes make more pigment and cause the skin to darken.

Skin cancer can occur anywhere on the body, but it is most common in skin that is often exposed to sunlight, such as the face, neck, hands, and arms.

This chapter includes text excerpted from "Skin Cancer Treatment (PDQ®)—Patient Version," National Cancer Institute (NCI), June 21, 2017.

There Are Different Types of Cancer That Start in the Skin

The most common types are basal cell carcinoma and squamous cell carcinoma, which are nonmelanoma skin cancers. Nonmelanoma skin cancers rarely spread to other parts of the body. Melanoma is a much rarer type of skin cancer. It is more likely to invade nearby tissues and spread to other parts of the body. Actinic keratosis is a skin condition that sometimes becomes squamous cell carcinoma.

Skin Color and Being Exposed to Sunlight Can Increase the Risk of Nonmelanoma Skin Cancer and Actinic Keratosis

Anything that increases your chance of getting a disease is called a risk factor. Having a risk factor does not mean that you will get cancer; not having risk factors doesn't mean that you will not get cancer. Talk with your doctor if you think you may be at risk.

Risk factors for basal cell carcinoma and squamous cell carcinoma include the following:

- Being exposed to natural sunlight or artificial sunlight (such as from tanning beds) over long periods of time.

- Having a fair complexion, which includes the following:

  - Fair skin that freckles and burns easily, does not tan, or tans poorly.

  - Blue or green or other light-colored eyes.

  - Red or blond hair.

- Having actinic keratosis.

- Past treatment with radiation.

- Having a weakened immune system.

- Having certain changes in the genes that are linked to skin cancer.

- Being exposed to arsenic.

Risk factors for actinic keratosis include the following:

- Being exposed to natural sunlight or artificial sunlight (such as from tanning beds) over long periods of time.

  - Having a fair complexion, which includes the following:

  - Fair skin that freckles and burns easily, does not tan, or tans poorly.

- Blue or green or other light-colored eyes.
- Red or blond hair.

Although having a fair complexion is a risk factor for skin cancer and actinic keratosis, people of all skin colors can get skin cancer and actinic keratosis.

Nonmelanoma Skin Cancer and Actinic Keratosis Often Appear as a Change in the Skin

Not all changes in the skin are a sign of nonmelanoma skin cancer or actinic keratosis. Check with your doctor if you notice any changes in your skin.

Signs of nonmelanoma skin cancer include the following:

- A sore that does not heal.
- Areas of the skin that are:
  - Raised, smooth, shiny, and look pearly.
  - Firm and look like a scar, and may be white, yellow, or waxy.
  - Raised, and red or reddish-brown.
  - Scaly, bleeding or crusty.

Signs of actinic keratosis include the following:

- A rough, red, pink, or brown, raised, scaly patch on the skin that may be flat or raised.
- Cracking or peeling of the lower lip that is not helped by lip balm or petroleum jelly.

Tests or Procedures That Examine the Skin Are Used to Detect (Find) and Diagnose Nonmelanoma Skin Cancer and Actinic Keratosis

The following procedures may be used:

- Skin exam
- Skin biopsy:
  - Shave biopsy
  - Punch biopsy
  - Incisional biopsy
  - Excisional biopsy

Certain Factors Affect Prognosis (Chance of Recovery) and Treatment Options

The prognosis (chance of recovery) depends mostly on the stage of the cancer and the type of treatment used to remove the cancer.

Treatment options depend on the following:

- The stage of the cancer (whether it has spread deeper into the skin or to other places in the body).

- The type of cancer.

- The size of the tumor and what part of the body it affects.

- The patient's general health.

Stages of Skin Cancer

After nonmelanoma skin cancer has been diagnosed, tests are done to find out if cancer cells have spread within the skin or to other parts of the body.

The process used to find out if cancer has spread within the skin or to other parts of the body is called staging. The information gathered from the staging process determines the stage of the disease. It is important to know the stage in order to plan treatment.

The following tests and procedures may be used in the staging process:

- CT scan (CAT scan)

- MRI (magnetic resonance imaging)

- Lymph node biopsy

How Cancer Spreads

There are three ways that cancer spreads in the body. Cancer can spread through:

1. **Tissue.** The cancer spreads from where it began by growing into nearby areas.

2. **Lymph system.** The cancer spreads from where it began by getting into the lymph system. The cancer travels through the lymph vessels to other parts of the body.

3. **Blood**. The cancer spreads from where it began by getting into the blood. The cancer travels through the blood vessels to other parts of the body.

Cancer May Spread from Where It Began to Other Parts of the Body

When cancer spreads to another part of the body, it is called metastasis. Cancer cells break away from where they began (the primary tumor) and travel through the lymph system or blood.

The metastatic tumor is the same type of cancer as the primary tumor. For example, if skin cancer spreads to the lung, the cancer cells in the lung are actually skin cancer cells. The disease is metastatic skin cancer, not lung cancer.

Staging of Nonmelanoma Skin Cancer Depends on Whether the Tumor Has Certain "High-Risk" Features and If the Tumor Is on the Eyelid

Staging of nonmelanoma skin cancer depends on whether the tumor has certain "high-risk" features and if the tumor is on the eyelid. Staging for nonmelanoma skin cancer that is on the eyelid is different from staging for nonmelanoma skin cancer that affects other parts of the body.

The following are high-risk features for nonmelanoma skin cancer that is not on the eyelid:

- The tumor is thicker than 2 millimeters.

- The tumor is described as Clark level IV (has spread into the lower layer of the dermis) or Clark level V (has spread into the layer of fat below the skin).

- The tumor has grown and spread along nerve pathways.

- The tumor began on an ear or on a lip that has hair on it.

- The tumor has cells that look very different from normal cells under a microscope.

The following stages are used:

Stage 0 (Carcinoma in Situ). In stage 0, abnormal cells are found in the squamous cell or basal cell layer of the epidermis (topmost layer of the skin). These abnormal cells may become cancer and spread into nearby normal tissue. Stage 0 is also called carcinoma in situ.

Stage I. In stage I, cancer has formed. The tumor is not larger than 2 centimeters at its widest point and may have one high-risk feature.

Stage II. In stage II, the tumor is either:

- larger than 2 centimeters at its widest point; or

- any size and has two or more high-risk features.

Stage III. In stage III:

- The tumor has spread to the jaw, eye socket, or side of the skull. Cancer may have spread to one lymph node on the same side of the body as the tumor. The lymph node is not larger than 3 centimeters.

or

- Cancer has spread to one lymph node on the same side of the body as the tumor. The lymph node is not larger than 3 centimeters and one of the following is true:

  - the tumor is not larger than 2 centimeters at its widest point and may have one high-risk feature; or

  - the tumor is larger than 2 centimeters at its widest point; or

  - the tumor is any size and has two or more high-risk features.

Stage IV. In stage IV, one of the following is true:

- The tumor is any size and may have spread to the jaw, eye socket, or side of the skull. Cancer has spread to one lymph node on the same side of the body as the tumor and the affected node is larger than 3 centimeters but not larger than 6 centimeters, or cancer has spread to more than one lymph node on one or both sides of the body and the affected nodes are not larger than 6 centimeters; or

- The tumor is any size and may have spread to the jaw, eye socket, skull, spine, or ribs. Cancer has spread to one lymph node that is larger than 6 centimeters; or

- The tumor is any size and has spread to the base of the skull, spine, or ribs. Cancer may have spread to the lymph nodes; or

- Cancer has spread to other parts of the body, such as the lung.

Stages Used for Nonmelanoma Skin Cancer on the Eyelid

Stage 0 (Carcinoma in Situ). In stage 0, abnormal cells are found in the epidermis (topmost layer of the skin). These abnormal cells may become cancer and spread into nearby normal tissue. Stage 0 is also called carcinoma in situ.

Stage I. Stage I is divided into stages IA, IB, and IC.

- Stage IA: The tumor is 5 millimeters or smaller and has not spread to the connective tissue of the eyelid or to the edge of the eyelid where the lashes are.

- Stage IB: The tumor is larger than 5 millimeters but not larger than 10 millimeters or has spread to the connective tissue of the eyelid, or to the edge of the eyelid where the lashes are.

- Stage IC: The tumor is larger than 10 millimeters but not larger than 20 millimeters or has spread through the full thickness of the eyelid.

Stage II. In stage II, one of the following is true:

- The tumor is larger than 20 millimeters.

- The tumor has spread to nearby parts of the eye or eye socket.

- The tumor has spread to spaces around the nerves in the eyelid.

Stage III. Stage III is divided into stages IIIA, IIIB, and IIIC.

- Stage IIIA: To remove all of the tumor, the whole eye and part of the optic nerve must be removed. The bone, muscles, fat, and connective tissue around the eye may also be removed.

- Stage IIIB: The tumor may be anywhere in or near the eye and has spread to nearby lymph nodes.

- Stage IIIC: The tumor has spread to structures around the eye or in the face, or to the brain, and cannot be removed in surgery.

Stage IV. The tumor has spread to distant parts of the body.

Treatment Is Based on the Type of Nonmelanoma Skin Cancer or Other Skin Condition Diagnosed

Basal Cell Carcinoma

Basal cell carcinoma is the most common type of skin cancer. It usually occurs on areas of the skin that have been in the sun, most often the nose. Often this cancer appears as a raised bump that looks smooth and pearly. Another type looks like a scar and is flat and firm and may be white, yellow, or waxy. Basal cell carcinoma may spread to tissues around the cancer, but it usually does not spread to other parts of the body.

Squamous Cell Carcinoma

Squamous cell carcinoma occurs on areas of the skin that have been in the sun, such as the ears, lower lip, and the back of the hands. Squamous cell carcinoma may also appear on areas of the skin that have been burned or exposed to chemicals or radiation. Often this cancer appears as a firm red bump. The tumor may feel scaly, bleed, or form a crust. Squamous cell tumors may spread to nearby lymph nodes. Squamous cell carcinoma that has not spread can usually be cured.

Actinic keratosis

Actinic keratosis is a skin condition that is not cancer, but sometimes changes into squamous cell carcinoma. It usually occurs in areas that have been exposed to the sun, such as the face, the back of the hands, and the lower lip. It looks like rough, red, pink, or brown scaly patches on the skin that may be flat or raised, or the lower lip cracks and peels and is not helped by lip balm or petroleum jelly.

Treatment Option Overview

There are different types of treatment for patients with nonmelanoma skin cancer and actinic keratosis.

Different types of treatment are available for patients with nonmelanoma skin cancer and actinic keratosis. Some treatments are standard (the currently used treatment), and some are being tested in clinical trials. A treatment clinical trial is a research study meant to help improve current treatments or obtain information on new treatments for patients with cancer. When clinical trials show that a new treatment is better than the standard treatment, the new treatment may become the standard treatment. Patients may want to think about taking part in a clinical trial. Some clinical trials are open only to patients who have not started treatment.

Types of Standard Treatment

Six types of standard treatment are used:

1. Surgery

   - Mohs micrographic surgery: The tumor is cut from the skin in thin layers. During surgery, the edges of the tumor and each layer of tumor removed are viewed through a microscope to check for cancer cells. Layers continue to be removed until no more cancer cells are seen.

- Simple excision: The tumor is cut from the skin along with some of the normal skin around it.

- Shave excision: The abnormal area is shaved off the surface of the skin with a small blade.

- Electrodesiccation and curettage: The tumor is cut from the skin with a curette (a sharp, spoon-shaped tool). A needle-shaped electrode is then used to treat the area with an electric current that stops the bleeding and destroys cancer cells that remain around the edge of the wound.

- Cryosurgery: A treatment that uses an instrument to freeze and destroy abnormal tissue, such as carcinoma in situ.

- Laser surgery: A surgical procedure that uses a laser beam (a narrow beam of intense light) as a knife to make bloodless cuts in tissue or to remove a surface lesion such as a tumor.

- Dermabrasion: Removal of the top layer of skin using a rotating wheel or small particles to rub away skin cells.

2. Radiation therapy

Radiation therapy is a cancer treatment that uses high-energy X-rays or other types of radiation to kill cancer cells or keep them from growing.

- External radiation therapy uses a machine outside the body to send radiation toward the cancer.

- Internal radiation therapy uses a radioactive substance sealed in needles, seeds, wires, or catheters that are placed directly into or near the cancer.

3. Chemotherapy

Chemotherapy is a cancer treatment that uses drugs to stop the growth of cancer cells, either by killing the cells or by stopping them from dividing.

4. Photodynamic therapy

Photodynamic therapy (PDT) is a cancer treatment that uses a drug and a certain type of laser light to kill cancer cells.

5. Biologic therapy

Biologic therapy is a treatment that uses the patient's immune system to fight cancer. Substances made by the body or made in a laboratory are used to boost, direct, or restore the body's natural defenses against cancer.

6. Targeted therapy

Targeted therapy is a type of treatment that uses drugs or other substances to attack cancer cells.

Treatment Options for Nonmelanoma Skin Cancer

Basal Cell Carcinoma

Treatment of basal cell carcinoma may include the following:

- Simple excision
- Mohs micrographic surgery
- Radiation therapy
- Electrodesiccation and curettage
- Cryosurgery
- Photodynamic therapy
- Topical chemotherapy
- Topical biologic therapy with imiquimod
- Laser surgery

Treatment of recurrent basal cell carcinoma is usually Mohs micrographic surgery.

Treatment of basal cell carcinoma that is metastatic or cannot be treated with local therapy may include the following:

- Targeted therapy with a signal transduction inhibitor.
- Chemotherapy.
- A clinical trial of a new treatment.

Squamous Cell Carcinoma

Treatment of squamous cell carcinoma may include the following:

- Simple excision
- Mohs micrographic surgery
- Radiation therapy

- Electrodesiccation and curettage
- Cryosurgery

Treatment of recurrent squamous cell carcinoma may include the following:

- Simple excision
- Mohs micrographic surgery
- Radiation therapy

Treatment of squamous cell carcinoma that is metastatic or cannot be treated with local therapy may include the following:

- Chemotherapy
- Retinoid therapy and biologic therapy with interferon
- A clinical trial of a new treatment

Treatment Options for Actinic Keratosis

Actinic keratosis is not cancer but is treated because it may develop into cancer. Treatment of actinic keratosis may include the following:

- Topical chemotherapy
- Topical biologic therapy with imiquimod
- Cryosurgery
- Electrodesiccation and curettage
- Dermabrasion
- Shave excision
- Photodynamic therapy
- Laser surgery

Chapter 42

Thyroid Cancer

General Information about Thyroid Cancer

Thyroid cancer is a disease in which malignant (cancer) cells form in the tissues of the thyroid gland.

The thyroid is a gland at the base of the throat near the trachea (windpipe). It is shaped like a butterfly, with a right lobe and a left lobe. The isthmus, a thin piece of tissue, connects the two lobes. A healthy thyroid is a little larger than a quarter. It usually cannot be felt through the skin.

The thyroid uses iodine, a mineral found in some foods and in iodized salt, to help make several hormones. Thyroid hormones do the following:

- Control heart rate, body temperature, and how quickly food is changed into energy (metabolism).

- Control the amount of calcium in the blood.

Thyroid Nodules Are Common but Usually Are Not Cancer

Your doctor may find a lump (nodule) in your thyroid during a routine medical exam. A thyroid nodule is an abnormal growth of thyroid cells in the thyroid. Nodules may be solid or fluid-filled.

This chapter includes text excerpted from "Thyroid Cancer Treatment (PDQ®)—Patient Version," National Cancer Institute (NCI), April 27, 2017.

When a thyroid nodule is found, an ultrasound of the thyroid and a fine-needle aspiration biopsy are often done to check for signs of cancer. Blood tests to check thyroid hormone levels and for antithyroid antibodies in the blood may also be done to check for other types of thyroid disease.

Thyroid nodules usually don't cause symptoms or need treatment. Sometimes the thyroid nodules become large enough that it is hard to swallow or breathe and more tests and treatment are needed. Only a small number of thyroid nodules are diagnosed as cancer.

Types of Thyroid Cancer

There are four main types of thyroid cancer:

1. Papillary thyroid cancer: The most common type of thyroid cancer.

2. Follicular thyroid cancer.

3. Medullary thyroid cancer.

4. Anaplastic thyroid cancer.

Papillary and follicular thyroid cancer are sometimes called differentiated thyroid cancer. Medullary and anaplastic thyroid cancer are sometimes called poorly differentiated or undifferentiated thyroid cancer.

Age, Gender, and Being Exposed to Radiation Can Affect the Risk of Thyroid Cancer

Anything that increases your risk of getting a disease is called a risk factor. Having a risk factor does not mean that you will get cancer; not having risk factors doesn't mean that you will not get cancer. Talk with your doctor if you think you may be at risk.

Risk factors for thyroid cancer include the following:

- Being between 25 and 65 years old.

- Being female.

- Being exposed to radiation to the head and neck as an infant or child or being exposed to radiation from an atomic bomb. The cancer may occur as soon as 5 years after exposure.

- Having a history of goiter (enlarged thyroid).

- Having a family history of thyroid disease or thyroid cancer.

- Having certain genetic conditions such as familial medullary thyroid cancer (FMTC), multiple endocrine neoplasia type 2A syndrome (MEN2A), and multiple endocrine neoplasia type 2B syndrome (MEN2B).

- Being Asian.

Medullary Thyroid Cancer Is Sometimes Caused by a Change in a Gene That Is Passed from Parent to Child

The genes in cells carry hereditary information from parent to child. A certain change in the *RET* gene that is passed from parent to child (inherited) may cause medullary thyroid cancer.

There is a genetic test that is used to check for the changed gene. The patient is tested first to see if he or she has the changed gene. If the patient has it, other family members may also be tested to find out if they are at increased risk for medullary thyroid cancer. Family members, including young children, who have the changed gene may have a thyroidectomy (surgery to remove the thyroid). This can decrease the chance of developing medullary thyroid cancer.

Signs of Thyroid Cancer Include a Swelling or Lump in the Neck

Thyroid cancer may not cause early signs or symptoms. It is sometimes found during a routine physical exam. Signs or symptoms may occur as the tumor gets bigger. Other conditions may cause the same signs or symptoms. Check with your doctor if you have any of the following:

- A lump (nodule) in the neck.

- Trouble breathing.

- Trouble swallowing.

- Pain when swallowing.

- Hoarseness.

Tests That Examine the Thyroid, Neck, and Blood Are Used to Detect (Find) and Diagnose Thyroid Cancer

The following tests and procedures may be used:

- Physical exam and history

- Laryngoscopy

- Blood hormone studies

- Blood chemistry studies

- Ultrasound exam

- CT scan (CAT scan)

- Fine-needle aspiration biopsy of the thyroid

- Surgical biopsy

Certain Factors Affect Prognosis (Chance of Recovery) and Treatment Options

The prognosis (chance of recovery) and treatment options depend on the following:

- The age of the patient at the time of diagnosis.

- The type of thyroid cancer.

- The stage of the cancer.

- Whether the cancer was completely removed by surgery.

- Whether the patient has multiple endocrine neoplasia type 2B (MEN 2B).

- The patient's general health.

- Whether the cancer has just been diagnosed or has recurred (come back).

Stages of Thyroid Cancer

After thyroid cancer has been diagnosed, tests are done to find out if cancer cells have spread within the thyroid or to other parts of the body.

The process used to find out if cancer has spread within the thyroid or to other parts of the body is called staging. The information gathered from the staging process determines the stage of the disease. It is important to know the patient's age and the stage of the cancer in order to plan treatment.

The following tests and procedures may be used in the staging process:

- CT scan (CAT scan)

- Ultrasound exam

- Chest X-ray

- Bone scan

- Sentinel lymph node biopsy

There Are Three Ways That Cancer Spreads in the Body

Cancer can spread through:

1. Tissue. The cancer spreads from where it began by growing into nearby areas.

2. Lymph system. The cancer spreads from where it began by getting into the lymph system. The cancer travels through the lymph vessels to other parts of the body.

3. Blood. The cancer spreads from where it began by getting into the blood. The cancer travels through the blood vessels to other parts of the body.

Cancer May Spread from Where It Began to Other Parts of the Body

When cancer spreads to another part of the body, it is called metastasis. Cancer cells break away from where they began (the primary tumor) and travel through the lymph system or blood.

The metastatic tumor is the same type of cancer as the primary tumor. For example, if thyroid cancer spreads to the lung, the cancer cells in the lung are actually thyroid cancer cells. The disease is metastatic thyroid cancer, not lung cancer.

Stages Are Used to Describe Thyroid Cancer Based on the Type of Thyroid Cancer and the Age of the Patient

Papillary and Follicular Thyroid Cancer in Patients Younger Than 45 Years

- **Stage I.** In stage I papillary and follicular thyroid cancer, the tumor is any size and may have spread to nearby tissues and lymph nodes. Cancer has not spread to other parts of the body.

- **Stage II.** In stage II papillary and follicular thyroid cancer, the tumor is any size and cancer has spread from the thyroid to other parts of the body, such as the lungs or bone, and may have spread to lymph nodes.

Papillary and Follicular Thyroid Cancer in Patients 45 Years and Older

- **Stage I.** In stage I papillary and follicular thyroid cancer, cancer is found only in the thyroid and the tumor is 2 centimeters or smaller.

- **Stage II.** In stage II papillary and follicular thyroid cancer, cancer is only in the thyroid and the tumor is larger than 2 centimeters but not larger than 4 centimeters.

- **Stage III.** In stage III papillary and follicular thyroid cancer, either of the following is found:

  - the tumor is larger than 4 centimeters and only in the thyroid or the tumor is any size and cancer has spread to tissues just outside the thyroid, but not to lymph nodes; or

  - the tumor is any size and cancer may have spread to tissues just outside the thyroid and has spread to lymph nodes near the trachea or the larynx (voice box).

- **Stage IV.** Stage IV papillary and follicular thyroid cancer is divided into stages IVA, IVB, and IVC.

  - In stage IVA, either of the following is found:

  - the tumor is any size and cancer has spread outside the thyroid to tissues under the skin, the trachea, the esophagus, the larynx (voice box), and/or the recurrent laryngeal nerve (a nerve that goes to the larynx); cancer may have spread to lymph nodes near the trachea or the larynx; or

  - the tumor is any size and cancer may have spread to tissues just outside the thyroid. Cancer has spread to lymph nodes on one or both sides of the neck or between the lungs.

  - In stage IVB, cancer has spread to tissue in front of the spinal column or has surrounded the carotid artery or the blood vessels in the area between the lungs. Cancer may have spread to lymph nodes.

  - In stage IVC, the tumor is any size and cancer has spread to other parts of the body, such as the lungs and bones, and may have spread to lymph nodes.

Medullary Thyroid Cancer for All Ages

- **Stage 0.** Stage 0 medullary thyroid cancer is found only with a special screening test. No tumor can be found in the thyroid.

- **Stage I.** Stage I medullary thyroid cancer is found only in the thyroid and is 2 centimeters or smaller.

- **Stage II.** In stage II medullary thyroid cancer, either of the following is found:
  - the tumor is larger than 2 centimeters and only in the thyroid; or
  - the tumor is any size and has spread to tissues just outside the thyroid, but not to lymph nodes.

- **Stage III.** In stage III medullary thyroid cancer, the tumor is any size, has spread to lymph nodes near the trachea and the larynx (voice box), and may have spread to tissues just outside the thyroid.

- **Stage IV.** Stage IV medullary thyroid cancer is divided into stages IVA, IVB, and IVC.
  - In stage IVA, either of the following is found:
  - the tumor is any size and cancer has spread outside the thyroid to tissues under the skin, the trachea, the esophagus, the larynx (voice box), and/or the recurrent laryngeal nerve (a nerve that goes to the larynx); cancer may have spread to lymph nodes near the trachea or the larynx; or
  - the tumor is any size and cancer may have spread to tissues just outside the thyroid. Cancer has spread to lymph nodes on one or both sides of the neck or between the lungs.
  - In stage IVB, cancer has spread to tissue in front of the spinal column or has surrounded the carotid artery or the blood vessels in the area between the lungs. Cancer may have spread to lymph nodes.
- In stage IVC, the tumor is any size and cancer has spread to other parts of the body, such as the lungs and bones, and may have spread to lymph nodes.

Anaplastic Thyroid Cancer Is Considered Stage IV Thyroid Cancer

Anaplastic thyroid cancer grows quickly and has usually spread within the neck when it is found. Stage IV anaplastic thyroid cancer is divided into stages IVA, IVB, and IVC.

- In stage IVA, cancer is found in the thyroid and may have spread to lymph nodes.

- In stage IVB, cancer has spread to tissue just outside the thyroid and may have spread to lymph nodes.

- In stage IVC, cancer has spread to other parts of the body, such as the lungs and bones, and may have spread to lymph nodes.

Treatment Option Overview

Different types of treatment are available for patients with thyroid cancer. Some treatments are standard (the currently used treatment), and some are being tested in clinical trials. A treatment clinical trial is a research study meant to help improve current treatments or obtain information on new treatments for patients with cancer. When clinical trials show that a new treatment is better than the standard treatment, the new treatment may become the standard treatment. Patients may want to think about taking part in a clinical trial. Some clinical trials are open only to patients who have not started treatment.

Standard Treatment

Six types of standard treatment are used.

1. Surgery

    - Lobectomy: Removal of the lobe in which thyroid cancer is found. Lymph nodes near the cancer may also be removed and checked under a microscope for signs of cancer.

    - Near-total thyroidectomy: Removal of all but a very small part of the thyroid. Lymph nodes near the cancer may also be removed and checked under a microscope for signs of cancer.

    - Total thyroidectomy: Removal of the whole thyroid. Lymph nodes near the cancer may also be removed and checked under a microscope for signs of cancer.

    - Tracheostomy: Surgery to create an opening (stoma) into the windpipe to help you breathe.

2. Radiation therapy

    Radiation therapy is a cancer treatment that uses high-energy X-rays or other types of radiation to kill cancer cells or keep them from growing.

    - External radiation therapy uses a machine outside the body to send radiation toward the cancer. Sometimes the radiation is aimed directly at the tumor during surgery.

- Internal radiation therapy uses a radioactive substance sealed in needles, seeds, wires, or catheters that are placed directly into or near the cancer.

3. Chemotherapy

   Chemotherapy is a cancer treatment that uses drugs to stop the growth of cancer cells, either by killing the cells or by stopping them from dividing.

4. Thyroid hormone therapy

   Hormone therapy is a cancer treatment that removes hormones or blocks their action and stops cancer cells from growing.

5. Targeted therapy

   Targeted therapy is a type of treatment that uses drugs or other substances to identify and attack specific cancer cells without harming normal cells.

6. Watchful waiting

   Watchful waiting is closely monitoring a patient's condition without giving any treatment until signs or symptoms appear or change.

Part Six

Other Health Conditions with Issues of Significance to Women

Chapter 43

Alzheimer Disease

Alzheimer disease (AD) is an irreversible, progressive brain disorder that slowly destroys memory and thinking skills and, eventually, the ability to carry out the simplest tasks. In most people with Alzheimer, symptoms first appear in their mid-60s. Estimates vary, but experts suggest that more than 5 million Americans may have Alzheimer.

Alzheimer disease is currently ranked as the sixth leading cause of death in the United States, but recent estimates indicate that the disorder may rank third, just behind heart disease and cancer, as a cause of death for older people.

AD is the most common cause of dementia among older adults. Dementia is the loss of cognitive functioning—thinking, remembering, and reasoning—and behavioral abilities to such an extent that it interferes with a person's daily life and activities. Dementia ranges in severity from the mildest stage, when it is just beginning to affect a person's functioning, to the most severe stage, when the person must depend completely on others for basic activities of daily living.

The causes of dementia can vary, depending on the types of brain changes that may be taking place. Other dementias include Lewy body dementia, frontotemporal disorders, and vascular dementia. It is common for people to have mixed dementia—a combination of two or more disorders, at least one of which is dementia. For example, some people have both Alzheimer disease and vascular dementia.

Text in this chapter is excerpted from "Alzheimer's Disease: Fact Sheet," National Institute on Aging (NIA), August 2016.

Signs and Symptoms

Memory problems are typically one of the first signs of cognitive impairment related to Alzheimer disease. Some people with memory problems have a condition called mild cognitive impairment (MCI). In MCI, people have more memory problems than normal for their age, but their symptoms do not interfere with their everyday lives. Movement difficulties and problems with the sense of smell have also been linked to MCI. Older people with MCI are at greater risk for developing AD, but not all of them do. Some may even go back to normal cognition.

The first symptoms of AD vary from person to person. For many, decline in non-memory aspects of cognition, such as word-finding, vision/spatial issues, and impaired reasoning or judgment, may signal the very early stages of Alzheimer disease. Researchers are studying

biomarkers (biological signs of disease found in brain images, cerebrospinal fluid, and blood) to see if they can detect early changes in the brains of people with MCI and in cognitively normal people who may be at greater risk for AD. Studies indicate that such early detection may be possible, but more research is needed before these techniques can be relied upon to diagnose Alzheimer disease in everyday medical practice.

Mild Alzheimer Disease

As Alzheimer disease progresses, people experience greater memory loss and other cognitive difficulties. Problems can include wandering and getting lost, trouble handling money and paying bills, repeating questions, taking longer to complete normal daily tasks, and personality and behavior changes. People are often diagnosed at this stage.

Moderate Alzheimer Disease

In this stage, damage occurs in areas of the brain that control language, reasoning, sensory processing, and conscious thought. Memory loss and confusion grow worse, and people begin to have problems recognizing family and friends. They may be unable to learn new things, carry out multi step tasks such as getting dressed, or cope with new situations. In addition, people at this stage may have hallucinations, delusions, and paranoia and may behave impulsively.

Severe Alzheimer Disease

Ultimately, plaques and tangles spread throughout the brain, and brain tissue shrinks significantly. People with severe AD cannot communicate and are completely dependent on others for their care. Near the end, the person may be in bed most or all of the time as the body shuts down.

What Causes Alzheimer Disease (AD)?

Scientists don't yet fully understand what causes Alzheimer disease in most people. In people with early-onset Alzheimer, a genetic mutation is usually the cause. Late-onset Alzheimer arises from a complex series of brain changes that occur over decades. The causes probably include a combination of genetic, environmental, and lifestyle factors.

The importance of any one of these factors in increasing or decreasing the risk of developing AD may differ from person to person.

The Basics of AD

Scientists are conducting studies to learn more about plaques, tangles, and other biological features of Alzheimer disease. Advances in brain imaging techniques allow researchers to see the development and spread of abnormal amyloid and tau proteins in the living brain, as well as changes in brain structure and function. Scientists are also exploring the very earliest steps in the disease process by studying changes in the brain and body fluids that can be detected years before AD symptoms appear. Findings from these studies will help in understanding the causes of AD and make diagnosis easier.

One of the great mysteries of Alzheimer disease is why it largely strikes older adults. Research on normal brain aging is shedding light on this question. For example, scientists are learning how age-related changes in the brain may harm neurons and contribute to AD damage. These age-related changes include atrophy (shrinking) of certain parts of the brain, inflammation, production of unstable molecules called free radicals, and mitochondrial dysfunction (a breakdown of energy production within a cell).

Genetics

Most people with AD have the late-onset form of the disease, in which symptoms become apparent in their mid-60s. The apolipoprotein

E (APOE) gene is involved in late-onset Alzheimer. This gene has several forms. One of them, APOE ε4, increases a person's risk

of developing the disease and is also associated with an earlier age of disease onset. However, carrying the APOE4 form of the gene does not mean that a person will definitely develop Alzheimer disease, and some people with no APOE ε4 may also develop the disease.

Also, scientists have identified a number of regions of interest in the genome (an organism's complete set of DNA) that may increase a person's risk for late-onset Alzheimer to varying degrees.

Early-onset Alzheimer disease occurs in people age 30 to 60 and represents less than 5 percent of all people with AD. Most cases are caused by an inherited change in one of three genes, resulting in a type known as early-onset familial Alzheimer disease, or FAD. For others, the disease appears to develop without any specific, known cause, much as it does for people with late-onset disease.

Most people with Down syndrome develop AD. This may be because people with Down syndrome have an extra copy of chromosome 21, which contains the gene that generates harmful amyloid.

Health, Environmental, and Lifestyle Factors

Research suggests that a host of factors beyond genetics may play a role in the development and course of Alzheimer disease. There is a great deal of interest, for example, in the relationship between cognitive decline and vascular conditions such as heart disease, stroke, and high blood pressure, as well as metabolic conditions such as diabetes and obesity. Ongoing research will help us understand whether and how reducing risk factors for these conditions may also reduce the risk of AD.

A nutritious diet, physical activity, social engagement, and mentally stimulating pursuits have all been associated with helping people stay healthy as they age. These factors might also help reduce the risk of cognitive decline and Alzheimer disease. Clinical trials are testing some of these possibilities.

Diagnosis of AD

Doctors use several methods and tools to help determine whether a person who is having memory problems has "possible Alzheimer dementia" (dementia may be due to another cause) or "probable Alzheimer dementia" (no other cause for dementia can be found).

To diagnose AD, doctors may:

- Ask the person and a family member or friend questions about overall health, past medical problems, ability to carry out daily activities, and changes in behavior and personality
- Conduct tests of memory, problem solving, attention, counting, and language
- Carry out standard medical tests, such as blood and urine tests, to identify other possible causes of the problem
- Perform brain scans, such as computed tomography (CT), magnetic resonance imaging (MRI), or positron emission tomography (PET), to rule out other possible causes for symptoms.

These tests may be repeated to give doctors information about how the person's memory and other cognitive functions are changing over time.

Alzheimer disease can be definitively diagnosed only after death, by linking clinical measures with an examination of brain tissue in an autopsy.

People with memory and thinking concerns should talk to their doctor to find out whether their symptoms are due to AD or another cause, such as stroke, tumor, Parkinson disease, sleep disturbances, side effects of medication, an infection, or a non-Alzheimer dementia. Some of these conditions may be treatable and possibly reversible.

If the diagnosis is AD, beginning treatment early in the disease process may help preserve daily functioning for some time, even though the underlying disease process cannot be stopped or reversed. An early diagnosis also helps families plan for the future. They can take care of financial and legal matters, address potential safety issues, learn about living arrangements, and develop support networks.

In addition, an early diagnosis gives people greater opportunities to participate in clinical trials that are testing possible new treatments for Alzheimer disease or other research studies.

Treatment of AD

Alzheimer disease is complex, and it is unlikely that any one drug or other intervention will successfully treat it. Current approaches focus on helping people maintain mental function, manage behavioral symptoms, and slow or delay the symptoms of disease. Researchers hope to develop therapies targeting specific genetic, molecular, and cellular mechanisms so that the actual underlying cause of the disease can be stopped or prevented.

Maintaining Mental Function

Several medications are approved by the U.S. Food and Drug Administration (FDA) to treat symptoms of AD. Donepezil (Aricept®), rivastigmine (Exelon®), and galantamine (Razadyne®) are used to treat mild to moderate Alzheimer (donepezil can be used for severe Alzheimer as well). Memantine (Namenda®) is used to treat moderate to severe Alzheimer. These drugs work by regulating neurotransmitters, the brain chemicals that transmit messages between neurons. They may help maintain thinking, memory, and communication skills, and help with certain behavioral problems. However, these drugs don't change the underlying disease process. They are effective for some but not all people and may help only for a limited time.

Managing Behavior

Common behavioral symptoms of AD include sleeplessness, wandering, agitation, anxiety, and aggression. Scientists are learning why these symptoms occur and are studying new treatments—drug and nondrug—to manage them. Research has shown that treating behavioral symptoms can make people with AD more comfortable and makes things easier for caregivers.

Looking for New Treatments

Alzheimer disease research has developed to a point where scientists can look beyond treating symptoms to think about addressing underlying disease processes. In ongoing clinical trials, scientists are developing and testing several possible interventions, including immunization therapy, drug therapies, cognitive training, physical activity, and treatments used for cardiovascular disease and diabetes.

Support for Families and Caregivers

Caring for a person with Alzheimer disease can have high physical, emotional, and financial costs. The demands of day-to-day care, changes in family roles, and decisions about placement in a care facility can be difficult. There are several evidence-based approaches and programs that can help, and researchers are continuing to look for new and better ways to support caregivers.

Good coping skills, a strong support network, and respite care are other ways that help caregivers handle the stress of caring for a loved one with Alzheimer disease. For example, staying physically active provides physical and emotional benefits.

Chapter 44

Anemia and Bleeding Disorders

Chapter Contents

Section 44.1

Anemia

This section includes text excerpted from "Anemia,"
National Heart, Lung, and Blood Institute (NHLBI),
May 18, 2012. Reviewed August 2017.

What Is Anemia?

Anemia is a condition in which your blood has a lower than normal number of red blood cells.

Anemia also can occur if your red blood cells don't contain enough hemoglobin. Hemoglobin is an iron-rich protein that gives blood its red color. This protein helps red blood cells carry oxygen from the lungs to the rest of the body.

If you have anemia, your body doesn't get enough oxygen-rich blood. As a result, you may feel tired or weak. You also may have other symptoms, such as shortness of breath, dizziness, or headaches.

Severe or long-lasting anemia can damage your heart, brain, and other organs in your body. Very severe anemia may even cause death.

What Causes Anemia?

The three main causes of anemia are:

- Blood loss
- Lack of red blood cell production
    - Diet
    - Hormones
    - Diseases and disease treatments
    - Pregnancy
    - Aplastic anemia
- High rates of red blood cell destruction

For some people, the condition is caused by more than one of these factors.

Who Is at Risk for Anemia?

Anemia is a common condition. It occurs in all age, racial, and ethnic groups. Both women and men can have anemia. However, women of childbearing age are at higher risk for the condition because of blood loss from menstruation.

Anemia can develop during pregnancy due to low levels of iron and folic acid (folate) and changes in the blood. During the first 6 months of pregnancy, the fluid portion of a woman's blood (the plasma) increases faster than the number of red blood cells. This dilutes the blood and can lead to anemia.

Major Risk Factors

Factors that raise your risk for anemia include:

- A diet that is low in iron, vitamins, or minerals

- Blood loss from surgery or an injury

- Long-term or serious illnesses, such as kidney disease, cancer, diabetes, rheumatoid arthritis, HIV/AIDS, inflammatory bowel disease (including Crohn disease), liver disease, heart failure, and thyroid disease

- Long-term infections

- A family history of inherited anemia, such as sickle cell anemia or thalassemia

What Are the Signs and Symptoms of Anemia?

The most common symptom of anemia is fatigue (feeling tired or weak). If you have anemia, you may find it hard to find the energy to do normal activities.

Other signs and symptoms of anemia include:

- Shortness of breath

- Dizziness

- Headache

- Coldness in the hands and feet

- Pale skin

- Chest pain

These signs and symptoms can occur because your heart has to work harder to pump oxygen-rich blood through your body.

Mild to moderate anemia may cause very mild symptoms or none at all.

How Is Anemia Diagnosed?

Your doctor will diagnose anemia based on your medical and family histories, a physical exam, and results from tests and procedures.

Because anemia doesn't always cause symptoms, your doctor may find out you have it while checking for another condition.

- Medical and family histories
- Physical exam
- Diagnostic tests and procedures
  - Complete blood count
  - Other tests and procedures
  - Hemoglobin electrophoresis.
  - A reticulocyte count.
  - Tests for the level of iron in your blood and body.

How Is Anemia Treated?

Treatment for anemia depends on the type, cause, and severity of the condition. Treatments may include dietary changes or supplements, medicines, procedures, or surgery to treat blood loss.

Goals of Treatment

The goal of treatment is to increase the amount of oxygen that your blood can carry. This is done by raising the red blood cell count and/or hemoglobin level. (Hemoglobin is the iron-rich protein in red blood cells that carries oxygen to the body.)

Another goal is to treat the underlying cause of the anemia.

Dietary Changes and Supplements

Low levels of vitamins or iron in the body can cause some types of anemia. These low levels might be the result of a poor diet or certain diseases or conditions.

To raise your vitamin or iron level, your doctor may ask you to change your diet or take vitamin or iron supplements. Common vitamin supplements are vitamin B12 and folic acid (folate). Vitamin C sometimes is given to help the body absorb iron.

Medicines

Your doctor may prescribe medicines to help your body make more red blood cells or to treat an underlying cause of anemia. Some of these medicines include:

- Antibiotics to treat infections.

- Hormones to treat heavy menstrual bleeding in teenaged and adult women.

- A man-made version of erythropoietin to stimulate your body to make more red blood cells. This hormone has some risks. You and your doctor will decide whether the benefits of this treatment outweigh the risks.

- Medicines to prevent the body's immune system from destroying its own red blood cells.

- Chelation therapy for lead poisoning. Chelation therapy is used mainly in children. This is because children who have iron-deficiency anemia are at increased risk of lead poisoning.

Procedures

If your anemia is severe, your doctor may recommend a medical procedure. Procedures include blood transfusions and blood and marrow stem cell transplants.

Surgery

If you have serious or life-threatening bleeding that's causing anemia, you may need surgery. For example, you may need surgery to control ongoing bleeding due to a stomach ulcer or colon cancer.

If your body is destroying red blood cells at a high rate, you may need to have your spleen removed. The spleen is an organ that removes worn out red blood cells from the body. An enlarged or diseased spleen may remove more red blood cells than normal, causing anemia.

How Can Anemia Be Prevented?

You might be able to prevent repeat episodes of some types of anemia, especially those caused by lack of iron or vitamins. Dietary changes or supplements can prevent these types of anemia from occurring again.

Treating anemia's underlying cause may prevent the condition (or prevent repeat episodes). For example, if medicine is causing your anemia, your doctor may prescribe another type of medicine.

To prevent anemia from getting worse, tell your doctor about all of your signs and symptoms. Talk with your doctor about the tests you may need and follow your treatment plan.

You can't prevent some types of inherited anemia, such as sickle cell anemia. If you have an inherited anemia, talk with your doctor about treatment and ongoing care.

Section 44.2

Bleeding Disorders

This section includes text excerpted from "Bleeding Disorders," Office on Women's Health (OWH), U.S. Department of Health and Human Services (HHS), March 20, 2017.

What Is a Bleeding Disorder?

A bleeding disorder is a health problem that makes it difficult for a person to stop bleeding. Normally when a person is hurt, a blood clot forms to stop the bleeding quickly. For blood to clot, your body needs a type of blood cell called platelets and blood proteins called clotting factors.

If you have a bleeding disorder, your platelets or clotting factors do not work correctly or your body does not make enough platelets or clotting factors. This makes it easy for too much bleeding to happen during normal bodily functions such as a menstrual period. People with a bleeding disorder can also bleed too much or for too long after an injury, dental work, childbirth, or surgery.

Who Gets Bleeding Disorders?

Bleeding disorders affect both women and men. But bleeding disorders can cause more problems for women because of heavy bleeding during menstrual periods and the risk of dangerous bleeding after childbirth.

Does Heavy Bleeding during My Menstrual Period Mean That I Have a Bleeding Disorder?

It might. As many as one in 10 women with heavy periods may have some type of bleeding disorder.

But other causes of heavy periods include:

- **Certain health problems.** Heavy bleeding can be a sign of thyroid problems or uterine fibroids.

- **Reproductive problems.** In a normal menstrual cycle, your body discards your uterine lining with each period. If your hormones get out of balance or if you do not ovulate, the uterine lining can build up too much. This can cause heavy bleeding as the lining is discarded during the next menstrual period.

- **Certain medicines.** Some antiinflammatory medicines and blood thinners can lead to heavy or long periods.

Talk to your doctor or nurse if you have heavy periods.

How Can I Tell If I Have Heavy Bleeding during My Menstrual Period?

Your menstrual period is heavy if you:

- Soak through a pad or tampon every hour or two

- Have menstrual bleeding for more than 7 days in a row

- Have menstrual blood with clots larger than a quarter

Menstrual blood is a combination of tissues and blood, so it often comes out in large clumps or clots. These clots are different from the clotting factors that your body needs to help stop bleeding from a cut or other injury. Having many large menstrual blood clots (larger than a quarter) in your menstrual flow is a sign of abnormal or heavy bleeding.

Women with heavy menstrual bleeding often have to change their daily activities because of the bleeding. If you have to change your regular work or school schedule or activities because of too much bleeding during your period, then you probably have heavy menstrual bleeding that is not normal.

Talk to your doctor or nurse if you think you have heavy bleeding. Your doctor will want to do tests to find out what is causing the heavy bleeding. Treatments include medicines or surgery.

What Causes Bleeding Disorders?

Usually, bleeding disorders are inherited, passed down from parent to child when you are born. But it's possible to have a bleeding disorder even if your parents did not. Talk to your doctor or nurse about your risks if bleeding disorders run in your family.

Sometimes, bleeding disorders can be caused by other health problems or medicines you take:

- Liver disease. Your liver makes most of the blood clotting factors (proteins in the blood) you need.

- Kidney disease, especially in the advanced stages

- Side effects from certain medicines, such as blood thinners (anticoagulants), certain pain medicines, or long-term use of antibiotics

- Thyroid hormone imbalance

What Are Symptoms of Bleeding Disorders?

Some common symptoms of bleeding disorders include:

- Large bruises from a minor bump or injury

- Nosebleeds that are difficult to stop or happen often

- Heavy menstrual bleeding

- Heavy vaginal bleeding from other conditions, such as endometriosis

- Blood in stool or urine

- Bleeding too much or for a long time after an injury, surgery, or dental work

- Anemia, which causes you to become pale or feel tired or weak

- Bleeding into joints, muscles, and organs

If you have any of these symptoms, talk with your doctor or nurse. These can also be a symptom of another health problem.

What Types of Bleeding Disorders Affect Women?

Bleeding disorders in women and girls are often inherited, meaning the disorders run in families. Sometimes bleeding disorders happen when a girl or woman does not have any family history of a bleeding disorder. Women can also develop bleeding disorders as a side effect of certain medicines or from other health problems.

von Willebrand Disease (VWD)

von Willebrand disease (VWD) is the most common inherited bleeding disorder in women in the United States. Your blood contains a protein called von Willebrand factor. People with VWD either don't have enough von Willebrand factor or it doesn't work correctly. This can lead to heavy bleeding that can be difficult to stop. Women with VWD may have:

- Unusually heavy and long menstrual periods (this is the most common symptom)

- Nosebleeds that are difficult to stop or happen often

- Bleeding gums

- Blood in stool or urine

- Bleeding too much or for a long time after an injury, surgery, or dental work

- Easy bruising

- Heavy or prolonged bleeding during or after childbirth

Hemophilia

Hemophilia is another type of bleeding disorder that is well-known but rare. Hemophilia usually runs in families. Hemophilia affects both women and men, but most children born with hemophilia are male. Women can be carriers of hemophilia, meaning they have one active gene for hemophilia and one inactive gene for hemophilia. Women who are carriers of hemophilia can pass either the inactive or active hemophilia gene onto their children. Some women who are carriers have a mild or less serious form of hemophilia and are at risk for heavy bleeding and bleeding with pregnancy or after childbirth. If you have heavy bleeding, your doctor or nurse may test you for hemophilia.

How Do Bleeding Disorders Affect Pregnancy?

Women with bleeding disorders are at risk of complications during and after pregnancy:

- Iron-deficiency anemia

- Bleeding during pregnancy

- Dangerous bleeding after childbirth (called postpartum hemorrhage)

If you have a bleeding disorder (or think you have one) and are thinking of becoming pregnant, talk to your doctor first. You may also want to find a doctor who specializes in high-risk pregnancies. Because bleeding disorders run in families, your baby may also have a bleeding disorder.

How Are Bleeding Disorders Diagnosed?

To diagnose a bleeding disorder, your doctor will:

- Talk to you about your symptoms and any history of bleeding disorders in your family

- Do a physical exam

- Do blood tests. Your doctor may do tests on your blood to check for anemia caused by blood loss. Your doctor may also check the amount of platelets and white blood cells that you have and how well your liver and kidney are working. Other blood tests for blood clotting problems will tell your doctor whether you have a bleeding disorder and what type you have.

You may need to see a hematologist for special blood tests to detect a bleeding disorder. A hematologist is a doctor who specializes in problems with the blood.

How Are Bleeding Disorders Treated?

There is no cure for bleeding disorders, but for many people medicine can help control the symptoms. People with mild bleeding problems may only need treatment before or after surgery and dental work or after an injury. If your symptoms are more serious, you may need to take medicine more often.

Common treatments for bleeding disorders include:

- Birth control
- Iron supplements
- Hormones
- Antifibrinolytics
- Clotting factor concentrates

What Can Happen If Bleeding Disorders Are Not Treated?

Bleeding disorders can raise your risk for anemia and dangerous bleeding after surgery or childbirth. They can also affect your quality of life. Women with heavy menstrual bleeding may miss days of work or school due to side effects from blood loss, including fatigue, or the need to manage heavy bleeding.

Without treatment, bleeding disorders can also lead to:

- The need for blood transfusions
- Arthritis and breakdown of joints (because of bleeding in those areas)
- Bleeding into other areas of the body
- Hysterectomy or other surgery. Many women who do not know they have a bleeding disorder may get a hysterectomy or other procedure to help control heavy menstrual periods.

If you know you have a bleeding disorder, tell your doctor, nurse, midwife, and dentist to prevent dangerous complications.

Chapter 45

Arthritis (Osteoarthritis)

What Is Osteoarthritis?

Osteoarthritis is the most common type of arthritis and is seen especially among older people. Sometimes it is called degenerative joint disease. Osteoarthritis mostly affects cartilage, the hard but slippery tissue that covers the ends of bones where they meet to form a joint. Healthy cartilage allows bones to glide over one another. It also absorbs energy from the shock of physical movement. In osteoarthritis, the surface layer of cartilage breaks and wears away. This allows bones under the cartilage to rub together, causing pain, swelling, and loss of motion of the joint. Over time, the joint may lose its normal shape. Also, small deposits of bone—called osteophytes or bone spurs—may grow on the edges of the joint. Bits of bone or cartilage can break off and float inside the joint space. This causes more pain and damage.

People with osteoarthritis usually have joint pain and stiffness. Unlike some other forms of arthritis, such as rheumatoid arthritis, osteoarthritis affects only joint function. It does not affect skin tissue, the lungs, the eyes, or the blood vessels.

In rheumatoid arthritis, another common form of arthritis, the immune system attacks the tissues of the joints, leading to pain, inflammation, and eventually joint damage and malformation. It typically begins at a younger age than osteoarthritis, causes swelling and

---

This chapter includes text excerpted from *"Osteoarthritis,"* National Institute of Arthritis and Musculoskeletal and Skin Diseases (NIAMS), May 2016.

redness in joints, and may make people feel sick, tired, and feverish. Also, the joint involvement of rheumatoid arthritis is symmetrical; that is, if one joint is affected, the same joint on the opposite side of the body is usually similarly affected. Osteoarthritis, on the other hand, can occur in a single joint or can affect a joint on one side of the body much more severely.

Who Has Osteoarthritis?

Osteoarthritis is by far the most common type of arthritis, and the percentage of people who have it grows higher with age. An estimated 27 million Americans age 25 and older have osteoarthritis.

Although osteoarthritis becomes more common with age, younger people can develop it, usually as the result of a joint injury, a joint malformation, or a genetic defect in joint cartilage. Both women and men have the disease. Before age 45, more men than women have osteoarthritis; after age 45, it is more common in women. It is also more likely to occur in people who are overweight and in those with jobs that stress particular joints.

How Does Osteoarthritis Affect People?

People with osteoarthritis usually experience joint pain and stiffness. The most commonly affected joints are those at the ends of the fingers (closest to the nail), thumbs, neck, lower back, knees, and hips.

Osteoarthritis affects different people differently. It may progress quickly, but for most people, joint damage develops gradually over years. In some people, osteoarthritis is relatively mild and interferes little with day-to-day life; in others, it causes significant pain and disability.

How Do You Know If You Have Osteoarthritis?

Usually, osteoarthritis comes on slowly. Early in the disease, your joints may ache after physical work or exercise. Later on, joint pain may become more persistent. You may also experience joint stiffness, particularly when you first wake up in the morning or have been in one position for a long time.

Although osteoarthritis can occur in any joint, most often it affects the hands, knees, hips, and spine (either at the neck or lower back). Different characteristics of the disease can depend on the specific joint(s) affected. For information on the joints most often affected by osteoarthritis, see the following descriptions:

Hands: Osteoarthritis of the hands seems to have some hereditary characteristics; that is, it runs in families. If your mother or grandmother has or had osteoarthritis in their hands, you're at greater-than-average risk of having it too. Women are more likely than men to have osteoarthritis in the hands. For most women, it develops after menopause.

Knees: The knees are among the joints most commonly affected by osteoarthritis. Symptoms of knee osteoarthritis include stiffness, swelling, and pain, which make it hard to walk, climb, and get in and out of chairs and bathtubs. Osteoarthritis in the knees can lead to disability.

Hips: The hips are also common sites of osteoarthritis. As with knee osteoarthritis, symptoms of hip osteoarthritis include pain and stiffness of the joint itself. But sometimes pain is felt in the groin, inner thigh, buttocks, or even the knees. Osteoarthritis of the hip may limit moving and bending, making daily activities such as dressing and putting on shoes a challenge.

Spine: Osteoarthritis of the spine may show up as stiffness and pain in the neck or lower back. In some cases, arthritis-related changes in the spine can cause pressure on the nerves where they exit the spinal column, resulting in weakness, tingling, or numbness of the arms and legs. In severe cases, this can even affect bladder and bowel function.

How Do Doctors Diagnose Osteoarthritis?

No single test can diagnose osteoarthritis; however, sometimes doctors use tests to help confirm a diagnosis or rule out other conditions that could be causing your symptoms. Most doctors use a combination of the following methods:

- Clinical history
- Physical examination
- X-rays
- Magnetic resonance imaging (MRI)
- Other Tests:
  - Blood tests
  - Joint aspiration

How Is Osteoarthritis Treated?

Most successful treatment programs involve a combination of approaches tailored to the patient's needs, lifestyle, and health. Most programs include ways to manage pain and improve function. These approaches are described below

The Four Goals of Osteoarthritis Treatment

- to control pain
- to improve joint function
- to maintain normal body weight
- to achieve a healthy lifestyle.

Treatment Approaches to Osteoarthritis

- Exercises:
  - Strengthening exercises: These exercises strengthen muscles that support joints affected by arthritis. They can be performed with weights or with exercise bands, inexpensive devices that add resistance.
  - Aerobic activities: These are exercises, such as brisk walking or low-impact aerobics, that get your heart pumping and can keep your lungs and circulatory system in shape.
  - Range-of-motion activities: These keep your joints limber.
  - Balance and agility exercises: These help you maintain daily living skills.
- Weight control
- Nondrug pain relief techniques and alternative therapies
- Medications to control pain:
  - Over-the-counter pain relievers: Oral pain medications, such as acetaminophen, are often a first-line approach to relieve pain in people with osteoarthritis.
  - NSAIDs (nonsteroidal anti-inflammatory drugs): A large class of medications useful against both pain and inflammation, (NSAIDs) are a common arthritis treatment. Aspirin and ibuprofen are examples of NSAIDs.
  - Narcotic or central acting agents: Prescription pain relievers are sometimes prescribed when over-the-counter medications

don't provide sufficient relief or when people have certain medical problems that would make traditional NSAIDs or other first-line therapies unsafe. These medications can carry risks, including the potential for addiction.

- Corticosteroids: Corticosteroids are powerful anti-inflammatory hormones made naturally in the body or man-made for use as medicine. They may be injected into the affected joints to temporarily relieve pain.

- Hyaluronic acid substitutes: Sometimes called viscosupplements, hyaluronic acid substitutes are designed to replace a normal component of the joint involved in joint lubrication and nutrition. Depending on the particular product your doctor prescribes, it will be given in a series of three to five injections. These products are approved only for osteoarthritis of the knee.

- Surgery

Who Provides Care for People with Osteoarthritis?

Treating arthritis often requires a multidisciplinary or team approach. Many types of health professionals care for people with arthritis. You may choose a few or more of the following professionals to be part of your healthcare team:

- Primary care physicians

- Rheumatologists

- Orthopaedists

- Physical therapists

- Occupational therapists

- Dietitians

- Nurse educators

- Physiatrists (rehabilitation specialists)

- Licensed acupuncture therapists

- Psychologists

- Social workers

- Chiropractors

- Massage therapists

Chapter 46

Autoimmune and Related Diseases

Chapter Contents

Section 46.1

Autoimmune Diseases: An Overview

This section includes text excerpted from "Autoimmune Diseases,"
Office on Women's Health (OWH), U.S. Department of Health and
Human Services (HHS), April 28, 2017.

What Are Autoimmune Diseases?

Our bodies have an immune system, which is a complex network of special cells and organs that defends the body from germs and other foreign invaders. At the core of the immune system is the ability to tell the difference between self and nonself: what's you and what's foreign. A flaw can make the body unable to tell the difference between self and nonself. When this happens, the body makes autoantibodies that attack normal cells by mistake. At the same time, special cells called regulatory T cells fail to do their job of keeping the immune system in line. The result is a misguided attack on your own body. This causes the damage we know as autoimmune disease. The body parts that are affected depend on the type of autoimmune disease. There are more than 80 known types.

How Common Are Autoimmune Diseases?

Overall, autoimmune diseases are common, affecting more than 23.5 million Americans. They are a leading cause of death and disability. Some autoimmune diseases are rare, while others, such as Hashimoto disease, affect many people.

Who Gets Autoimmune Diseases?

Autoimmune diseases can affect anyone. Yet certain people are at greater risk, including:

- **Women of childbearing age**—More women than men have autoimmune diseases, which often start during their childbearing years.

- **People with a family history**—Some autoimmune diseases run in families, such as lupus and multiple sclerosis. It is also common for different types of autoimmune diseases to affect different members of a single family. Inheriting certain genes can make it more likely to get an autoimmune disease. But a combination of genes and other factors may trigger the disease to start.

- **People who are around certain things in the environment**—Certain events or environmental exposures may cause some autoimmune diseases, or make them worse. Sunlight, chemicals called solvents, and viral and bacterial infections are linked to many autoimmune diseases.

- **People of certain races or ethnic backgrounds**—Some autoimmune diseases are more common or affect certain groups of people more severely. For instance, type 1 diabetes is more common in white people. Lupus is most severe for African-American and Hispanic people.

How Do I Find out If I Have an Autoimmune Disease?

Getting a diagnosis can be a long and stressful process. Although each autoimmune disease is unique, many share some of the same symptoms. And many symptoms of autoimmune diseases are the same for other types of health problems too. This makes it hard for doctors to find out if you really have an autoimmune disease, and which one it might be. But if you are having symptoms that bother you, it's important to find the cause. Don't give up if you're not getting any answers. You can take these steps to help find out the cause of your symptoms:

- Write down a complete family health history that includes extended family and share it with your doctor.

- Record any symptoms you have, even if they seem unrelated, and share it with your doctor.

- See a specialist who has experience dealing with your most major symptom. For instance, if you have symptoms of inflammatory bowel disease, start with a gastroenterologist. Ask your regular doctor, friends, and others for suggestions.

- Get a second, third, or fourth opinion if need be. If your doctor doesn't take your symptoms seriously or tells you they are stress-related or in your head, see another doctor.

What Types of Doctors Treat Autoimmune Diseases?

Juggling your healthcare needs among many doctors and specialists can be hard. But specialists, along with your main doctor, may be helpful in managing some symptoms of your autoimmune disease. If you see a specialist, make sure you have a supportive main doctor to help you. Often, your family doctor may help you coordinate care if you need to see one or more specialists. Here are some specialists who treat autoimmune diseases:

- Nephrologist
- Rheumatologist
- Endocrinologist
- Neurologist
- Hematologist
- Gastroenterologist
- Dermatologist
- Physical therapist
- Occupational therapist
- Speech therapist
- Audiologist
- Vocational therapist
- Counselor for emotional support

Are There Medicines to Treat Autoimmune Diseases?

There are many types of medicines used to treat autoimmune diseases. The type of medicine you need depends on which disease you have, how severe it is, and your symptoms. Treatment can do the following:

- **Relieve symptoms**. Some people can use over-the-counter drugs for mild symptoms, like aspirin and ibuprofen for mild pain. Others with more severe symptoms may need prescription drugs to help relieve symptoms such as pain, swelling, depression, anxiety, sleep problems, fatigue, or rashes. For others, treatment may be as involved as having surgery.

- **Replace vital substances the body can no longer make on its own**. Some autoimmune diseases, like diabetes and thyroid disease, can affect the body's ability to make substances it needs to function. With diabetes, insulin injections are needed to regulate blood sugar. Thyroid hormone replacement restores thyroid hormone levels in people with underactive thyroid.

- **Suppress the immune system**. Some drugs can suppress immune system activity. These drugs can help control the disease process and preserve organ function. For instance, these drugs are used to control inflammation in affected kidneys in people with lupus to keep the kidneys working. Medicines used to suppress inflammation include chemotherapy given at lower doses than for cancer treatment and drugs used in patients who have had an organ transplant to protect against rejection. A class of drugs called anti-tumor necrosis factor (TNF) medications blocks inflammation in some forms of autoimmune arthritis and psoriasis.

New treatments for autoimmune diseases are being studied all the time.

Are There Alternative Treatments That Can Help?

Many people try some form of complementary and alternative medicine (CAM) at some point in their lives. Some examples of CAM are herbal products, chiropractic, acupuncture, and hypnosis. If you have an autoimmune disease, you might wonder if CAM therapies can help some of your symptoms. This is hard to know. Studies on CAM therapies are limited. Also, some CAM products can cause health problems or interfere with how the medicines you might need work. If you want to try a CAM treatment, be sure to discuss it with your doctor. Your doctor can tell you about the possible benefits and risks of trying CAM.

How Can I Deal with Flares?

Flares are the sudden and severe onset of symptoms. You might notice that certain triggers, such as stress or being out in the sun, cause your symptoms to flare. Knowing your triggers, following your treatment plan, and seeing your doctor regularly can help you to prevent flares or keep them from becoming severe. If you suspect a flare is coming, call your doctor. Don't try a "cure" you heard about from a friend or relative.

What Are Some Things I Can Do to Feel Better?

If you are living with an autoimmune disease, there are things you can do each day to feel better:

- Eat healthy, well-balanced meals
- Get regular physical activity. But be careful not to overdo it
- Get enough rest
- Reduce stress

You have some power to lessen your pain! Try using imagery for 15 minutes, two or three times each day.

- Put on your favorite calming music.

- Lie back on your favorite chair or sofa. Or if you are at work, sit back and relax in your chair.

- Close your eyes.

- Imagine your pain or discomfort.

- Imagine something that confronts this pain and watch it "destroy" the pain.

Section 46.2

Celiac Disease

This section includes text excerpted from "Definition and Facts for Celiac Disease," National Institute of Diabetes and Digestive and Kidney Diseases (NIDDK), June 2016.

Celiac disease is a digestive disorder that damages the small intestine. The disease is triggered by eating foods containing gluten. Gluten is a protein found naturally in wheat, barley, and rye, and is common in foods such as bread, pasta, cookies, and cakes. Many prepackaged foods, lip balms and lipsticks, hair and skin products, toothpastes, vitamin and nutrient supplements, and, rarely, medicines, contain gluten.

Celiac disease can be very serious. The disease can cause long-lasting digestive problems and keep your body from getting all the nutrients it needs. Celiac disease can also affect the body outside the intestine.

Celiac disease is different from gluten sensitivity or wheat intolerance. If you have gluten sensitivity, you may have symptoms similar to those of celiac disease, such as abdominal pain and tiredness. Unlike celiac disease, gluten sensitivity does not damage the small intestine.

Celiac disease is also different from a wheat allergy. In both cases, your body's immune system reacts to wheat. However, some symptoms in wheat allergies, such as having itchy eyes or a hard time breathing, are different from celiac disease. Wheat allergies also do not cause long-term damage to the small intestine.

How Common Is Celiac Disease?

As many as one in 141 Americans has celiac disease, although most don't know it.

Who Is More Likely to Develop Celiac Disease?

Although celiac disease affects children and adults in all parts of the world, the disease is more common in Caucasians and more often diagnosed in females. You are more likely to develop celiac disease if someone in your family has the disease. Celiac disease also is more common among people with certain other diseases, such as Down syndrome, Turner syndrome, and type 1 diabetes.

What Other Health Problems Do People with Celiac Disease Have?

If you have celiac disease, you also may be at risk for:

- Addison disease
- Hashimoto disease
- primary biliary cirrhosis
- type 1 diabetes

What Are the Symptoms of Celiac Disease?

Most people with celiac disease have one or more symptoms. However, some people with the disease may not have symptoms or feel sick. Sometimes health issues such as surgery, a pregnancy, childbirth, bacterial gastroenteritis, a viral infection, or severe mental stress can trigger celiac disease symptoms.

Adults are less likely to have digestive symptoms and, instead, may have one or more of the following:

- anemia
- a red, smooth, shiny tongue
- bone or joint pain
- depression or anxiety

- dermatitis herpetiformis
- headaches
- infertility or repeated miscarriage
- missed menstrual periods
- mouth problems such a canker sores or dry mouth
- seizures
- tingling numbness in the hands and feet
- tiredness
- weak and brittle bones

Adults who have digestive symptoms with celiac disease may have:

- abdominal pain and bloating
- intestinal blockages
- tiredness that lasts for long periods of time
- ulcers, or sores on the stomach or lining of the intestine

Celiac disease also can produce a reaction in which your immune system, or your body's natural defense system, attacks healthy cells in your body. This reaction can spread outside your digestive tract to other areas of your body, including your:

- bones
- joints
- nervous system
- skin
- spleen

Depending on how old you are when a doctor diagnoses your celiac disease, some symptoms, such as short height and tooth defects, will not improve.

What Causes Celiac Disease?

Research suggests that celiac disease only happens to individuals who have particular genes. These genes are common and are carried by about one-third of the population. Individuals also have to be eating food that contains gluten to get celiac disease. Researchers do not know exactly what triggers celiac disease in people at risk who eat gluten over a long period of time. Sometimes the disease runs in families. About 10 to 20 percent of close relatives of people with celiac disease also are affected.

Your chances of developing celiac disease increase when you have changes in your genes, or variants. Certain gene variants and other factors, such as things in your environment, can lead to celiac disease.

Diagnosis of Celiac Disease

How Do Doctors Diagnose Celiac Disease?

Celiac disease can be hard to diagnose because some of the symptoms are like symptoms of other diseases, such as irritable bowel syndrome (IBS) and lactose intolerance. Your doctor may diagnose celiac disease with a medical and family history, physical exam, and tests. Tests may include blood tests, genetic tests, and biopsy.

Do Doctors Screen for Celiac Disease?

Screening is testing for diseases when you have no symptoms. Doctors in the United States do not routinely screen people for celiac disease. However, blood relatives of people with celiac disease and those with type 1 diabetes should talk with their doctor about their chances of getting the disease.

Many researchers recommend routine screening of all family members, such as parents and siblings, for celiac disease. However, routine genetic screening for celiac disease is not usually helpful when diagnosing the disease.

Treatment for Celiac Disease

How Do Doctors Treat Celiac Disease?

A Gluten-Free Diet

Doctors treat celiac disease with a gluten-free diet. Gluten is a protein found naturally in wheat, barley, and rye that triggers a reaction if you have celiac disease. Symptoms greatly improve for most people with celiac disease who stick to a gluten-free diet. In recent years, grocery stores and restaurants have added many more gluten-free foods and products, making it easier to stay gluten free.

Your doctor may refer you to a dietitian who specializes in treating people with celiac disease. The dietitian will teach you how to avoid gluten while following a healthy diet. He or she will help you:

- check food and product labels for gluten

- design everyday meal plans

- make healthy choices about the types of foods to eat

For most people, following a gluten-free diet will heal damage in the small intestine and prevent more damage. You may see symptoms improve within days to weeks of starting the diet. The small intestine usually heals in 3 to 6 months in children. Complete healing can take several years in adults. Once the intestine heals, the villi, which were damaged by the disease, regrow and will absorb nutrients from food into the bloodstream normally.

Gluten-Free Diet and Dermatitis Herpetiformis

If you have dermatitis herpetiformis—an itchy, blistering skin rash—skin symptoms generally respond to a gluten-free diet. However, skin symptoms may return if you add gluten back into your diet. Medicines such as dapsone, taken by mouth, can control the skin symptoms. People who take dapsone need to have regular blood tests to check for side effects from the medicine.

Dapsone does not treat intestinal symptoms or damage, which is why you should stay on a gluten-free diet if you have the rash. Even when you follow a gluten-free diet, the rash may take months or even years to fully heal—and often comes back over the years.

Avoiding Medicines and Nonfood Products That May Contain Gluten

In addition to prescribing a gluten-free diet, your doctor will want you to avoid all hidden sources of gluten. If you have celiac disease, ask a pharmacist about ingredients in:

- Herbal and nutritional supplements

- Prescription and over-the-counter medicines

- Vitamin and mineral supplements

You also could take in or transfer from your hands to your mouth other products that contain gluten without knowing it. Products that may contain gluten include:

- Children's modeling dough, such as Play-Doh

- Cosmetics

- Lipstick, lip gloss, and lip balm

- Skin and hair products

- Toothpaste and mouthwash

- Communion wafers

Medications are rare sources of gluten. Even if gluten is present in a medicine, it is likely to be in such small quantities that it would not cause any symptoms.

Reading product labels can sometimes help you avoid gluten. Some product makers label their products as being gluten-free. If a product label doesn't list the product's ingredients, ask the maker of the product for an ingredients list.

What If Changing to a Gluten-Free Diet Isn't Working?

If you don't improve after starting a gluten-free diet, you may still be eating or using small amounts of gluten. You probably will start responding to the gluten-free diet once you find and cut out all hidden sources of gluten. Hidden sources of gluten include additives made with wheat, such as:

- Modified food starch

- Malt flavoring

- Preservatives

- Stabilizers

If you still have symptoms even after changing your diet, you may have other conditions or disorders that are more common with celiac disease, such as irritable bowel syndrome (IBS), lactose intolerance, microscopic colitis, dysfunction of the pancreas, and small intestinal bacterial overgrowth.

Section 46.3

Chronic Fatigue Syndrome

This section includes text excerpted from "Chronic Fatigue
Syndrome," Office on Women's Health (OWH), U.S. Department of
Health and Human Services (HHS), September 4, 2014

Chronic fatigue syndrome (CFS), also referred to as myalgic enceph-
alomyelitis (ME) or ME/CFS, is a complex, chronic illness that affects
about 1 million Americans. Women are two to four times more likely than
men to be diagnosed with ME/CFS. People with ME/CFS experience a
range of symptoms that makes it hard to do the daily tasks that most of
us do without thinking—like dressing or bathing. Currently, there are no
U.S. Food and Drug Administration (FDA)-approved treatments specific
for ME/CFS. Usually, treatments focus on relieving the symptoms.

Myalgic Encephalomyelitis (ME) / Chronic Fatigue Syndrome (CFS)

ME/CFS is a complex, debilitating illness. ME/CFS may be diagnosed after six months or more of extreme fatigue that is not improved
by bed rest and that may get worse after activities that use physical
or mental energy.

Symptoms affect different parts of the body and can include unre-
freshing sleep, weakness, muscle and joint pain, problems with concentration or memory, and headaches. Symptoms may be mild to severe.
They may come and go, or they may last for weeks, months, or years.
They also can happen over time or come on suddenly.

What Causes ME/CFS?

No one knows for sure what causes ME/CFS. Many people say
it started after a flu-like illness or other infection, such as a cold or
stomach bug. It also can follow infection with the Epstein-Barr virus
(the virus that causes mononucleosis or "mono"). Some people with
ME/CFS report that it started after a time of great physical stress,
such as following surgery.

What Are the Symptoms of ME/CFS?

The symptoms of ME/CFS can come and go or a person may have these symptoms all of the time. At first, one may feel like she has the flu. The main symptoms include:

- Feeling extremely exhausted for more than 24 hours after physical or mental exercise

- Not feeling refreshed after sleeping, or having trouble sleeping

- Having a hard time concentrating, or problems with attention and memory

- Feeling dizzy or faint when sitting up or standing (due to a drop in blood pressure)

- Muscle pain or aches

- Pain or aches in joints without swelling or redness

- Headaches of a new type, pattern, or strength

- Tender lymph nodes in the neck or under the arm

- Sore throat that is constant or goes away and comes back often

Less-common symptoms of ME/CFS include:

- Visual problems (blurring, sensitivity to light, eye pain)

- Psychological symptoms (irritability, mood swings, panic attacks, anxiety)

- Chills and night sweats

- Low grade fever or low body temperature

- Irritable bowel

- Allergies and sensitivities to foods, odors, chemicals, medications, and sound

- Numbness, tingling, or burning sensations in the face, hands, or feet

Symptoms of ME/CFS vary widely from person to person and may be serious or mild. Most symptoms are invisible to others, which can make it hard for friends, family members, and the public to understand the challenges a person with ME/CFS faces. If you think you may have ME/CFS, talk to your doctor.

How Common Is ME/CFS?

Experts think ME/CFS affects about 1 million Americans. Many of these cases have not been diagnosed.

Women are two to four times more likely than men to develop ME/CFS. Children do develop ME/CFS, but not as often as adults or adolescents.

How Is ME/CFS Diagnosed?

Because many symptoms of ME/CFS are also symptoms of other illnesses or side effects of medicine, your doctor will need to do physical exams and tests to help determine if you have ME/CFS. There are no standard lab tests to diagnose ME/CFS.

If you think you may have ME/CFS, see your doctor. Your doctor may:

- Ask you about your physical and mental health.

- Do a physical exam.

- Order lab tests based on your symptoms, such as urine and blood tests, which will tell your doctor if something other than ME/CFS might be causing your symptoms.

- Order tests that check for problems found in people with ME/CFS.

- Classify you as having ME/CFS if:

  - You have the main symptoms of ME/CFS, including extreme fatigue or exhaustion that does not go away and that prevents you from doing the things you want and need to do for you and your family; exhaustion that comes after mental or physical exercise; sleep problems; and pain;

  - You have had the extreme fatigue and other symptoms for 6 months or longer (3 months or longer for children and adolescents);

  - You and your doctor cannot find another explanation for your symptoms.

The process to make a final diagnosis of ME/CFS can take a long time, so try to be patient. It is usually best to develop a relationship—and follow up often—with one doctor so that he or she can get to know you and see how you respond to treatment over time.

While these tests are being done, talk to your doctor about ways to ease your symptoms. Your doctor may also need to learn more about

ME/CFS to help you. If you feel your doctor has doubts about it being a "real" illness, share this document and the links to resources found at the end. If disbelief or doubts continue, consider seeing another doctor for a second opinion.

How Is ME/CFS Treated?

Right now, there is no cure or U.S. Food and Drug Administration (FDA)-approved treatments for ME/CFS. But, there are things you and your doctor can do to help ease your symptoms. Because the symptoms of ME/CFS vary from person to person, the management plan you discuss with your doctor may look very different from the plan of another person with ME/CFS.

Can Complementary or Alternative Medicine Help Manage the Symptoms of ME/CFS?

Some people say that complementary or alternative medicine has helped their ME/CFS symptoms. Keep in mind that many alternative treatments, dietary supplements, and herbal remedies claim to cure ME/CFS, but some might do more harm than good. Talk to your doctor before trying alternative therapies to be sure they're safe.

Section 46.4

Fibromyalgia

This section includes text excerpted from "Questions and Answers about Fibromyalgia," National Institute of Arthritis and Musculoskeletal and Skin Diseases (NIAMS), July 2014.

What Is Fibromyalgia?

Fibromyalgia syndrome is a common and chronic disorder characterized by widespread pain, diffuse tenderness, and a number of other symptoms. The word "fibromyalgia" comes from the Latin term for fibrous tissue (fibro) and the Greek ones for muscle (myo) and pain (algia).

Although fibromyalgia is often considered an arthritis-related condition, it is not truly a form of arthritis (a disease of the joints) because it does not cause inflammation or damage to the joints, muscles, or other tissues. Like arthritis, however, fibromyalgia can cause significant pain and fatigue, and it can interfere with a person's ability to carry on daily activities. Also like arthritis, fibromyalgia is considered a rheumatic condition, a medical condition that impairs the joints and/or soft tissues and causes chronic pain.

In addition to pain and fatigue, people who have fibromyalgia may experience a variety of other symptoms including:

- cognitive and memory problems (sometimes referred to as "fibro fog")

- sleep disturbances

- morning stiffness

- headaches

- irritable bowel syndrome

- painful menstrual periods

- numbness or tingling of the extremities

- restless legs syndrome

- temperature sensitivity

- sensitivity to loud noises or bright lights.

A person may have two or more coexisting chronic pain conditions. Such conditions can include chronic fatigue syndrome, endometriosis, fibromyalgia, inflammatory bowel disease, interstitial cystitis, temporomandibular joint dysfunction, and vulvodynia. It is not known whether these disorders share a common cause.

Who Gets Fibromyalgia?

Scientists estimate that fibromyalgia affects 5 million Americans age 18 or older. For unknown reasons, between 80 and 90 percent of those diagnosed with fibromyalgia are women; however, men and children also can be affected. Most people are diagnosed during middle age, although the symptoms often become present earlier in life.

Several studies indicate that women who have a family member with fibromyalgia are more likely to have fibromyalgia themselves, but the exact reason for this—whether it is heredity, shared environmental factors, or both—is unknown. Researchers are trying to determine whether variations in certain genes cause some people to be more sensitive to stimuli, which lead to pain syndromes.

What Causes Fibromyalgia?

The causes of fibromyalgia are unknown, but there are probably a number of factors involved. Many people associate the development of fibromyalgia with a physically or emotionally stressful or traumatic event, such as an automobile accident. Some connect it to repetitive injuries. Others link it to an illness. For others, fibromyalgia seems to occur spontaneously.

Many researchers are examining other causes, including problems with how the central nervous system (the brain and spinal cord) processes pain.

Some scientists speculate that a person's genes may regulate the way his or her body processes painful stimuli. According to this theory, people with fibromyalgia may have a gene or genes that cause them to react strongly to stimuli that most people would not perceive as painful. There have already been several genes identified that occur more commonly in fibromyalgia patients, and National Institute of Arthritis and Musculoskeletal and Skin Diseases (NIAMS)-supported researchers are currently looking at other possibilities.

How Is Fibromyalgia Diagnosed?

Research shows that people with fibromyalgia typically see many doctors before receiving the diagnosis. One reason for this may be that pain and fatigue, the main symptoms of fibromyalgia, overlap with those of many other conditions. Therefore, doctors often have to rule out other potential causes of these symptoms before making a diagnosis of fibromyalgia. Another reason is that there are currently no diagnostic laboratory tests for fibromyalgia; standard laboratory tests fail to reveal a physiologic reason for pain. Because there is no generally accepted, objective test for fibromyalgia, some doctors unfortunately may conclude a patient's pain is not real, or they may tell the patient there is little they can do.

A doctor familiar with fibromyalgia, however, can make a diagnosis based on criteria established by the American College of Rheumatology (ACR): a history of widespread pain lasting more than 3 months, and other general physical symptoms including fatigue, waking unrefreshed, and cognitive (memory or thought) problems. In making the diagnosis, doctors consider the number of areas throughout the body in which the patient has had pain in the past week.

How Is Fibromyalgia Treated?

Fibromyalgia can be difficult to treat. Not all doctors are familiar with fibromyalgia and its treatment, so it is important to find a doctor who is. Many family physicians, general internists, or rheumatologists (doctors who specialize in arthritis and other conditions that affect the joints or soft tissues) can treat fibromyalgia.

Fibromyalgia treatment often requires a team approach, with your doctor, a physical therapist, possibly other health professionals, and most importantly, yourself, all playing an active role. It can be hard to assemble this team, and you may struggle to find the right professionals to treat you. When you do, however, the combined expertise of these various professionals can help you improve your quality of life.

You may find several members of the treatment team you need at a clinic. There are pain clinics that specialize in pain and rheumatology clinics that specialize in arthritis and other rheumatic diseases, including fibromyalgia.

Only three medications, duloxetine, milnacipran, and pregabalin are approved by the U.S. Food and Drug Administration (FDA) for the treatment of fibromyalgia. Duloxetine was originally developed for and is still used to treat depression. Milnacipran is similar to a drug used to treat depression but is FDA approved only for fibromyalgia. Pregabalin is a medication developed to treat neuropathic pain (chronic pain caused by damage to the nervous system).

Doctors also treat fibromyalgia with a variety of other medications developed and approved for other purposes.

- Analgesics
- Nonsteroidal anti-inflammatory drugs (NSAIDs)
- Complementary and alternative therapies:
  - Massage
  - Movement therapies (such as Pilates and the Feldenkrais method)
  - Chiropractic treatments
  - Acupuncture
  - Various herbs and dietary supplements

Will Fibromyalgia Get Better with Time?

Fibromyalgia is a chronic condition, meaning it lasts a long time—possibly a lifetime. However, it may be comforting to know that fibromyalgia is not a progressive disease. It is never fatal, and it will not cause damage to the joints, muscles, or internal organs. In many people, the condition does improve over time.

What Can I Do to Try to Feel Better?

Besides taking medicine prescribed by your doctor, there are many things you can do to minimize the impact of fibromyalgia on your life. These include:

- Getting enough sleep
- Exercising
- Making changes at work
- Eating well

Section 46.5

Lupus

This section includes text excerpted from "Handout on Health: Systemic Lupus Erythematosus," National Institute of Arthritis and Musculoskeletal and Skin Diseases (NIAMS), June 2016.

What Is Lupus?

Lupus also known as systemic lupus erythematosus (SLE) is one of many disorders of the immune system known as autoimmune diseases. In autoimmune diseases, the immune system turns against parts of the body it is designed to protect. This leads to inflammation and damage to various body tissues. Lupus can affect many parts of the body, including the joints, skin, kidneys, heart, lungs, blood vessels, and brain.

Typically, lupus is characterized by periods of illness, called flares, and periods of wellness, or remission. Understanding how to prevent flares and how to treat them when they do occur helps people with lupus maintain better health.

Who Gets Lupus?

We know that many more women than men have lupus. Lupus is more common in African American women than in Caucasian women and is also more common in women of Hispanic, Asian, and Native American descent. African American and Hispanic women are also more likely to have active disease and serious organ system involvement. In addition, lupus can run in families, but the risk that a child or a brother or sister of a patient will also have lupus is still quite low.

It is difficult to estimate how many people in the United States have the disease, because its symptoms vary widely and its onset is often hard to pinpoint. Although SLE usually first affects people between the ages of 15 and 45 years, it can occur in childhood or later in life as well.

Symptoms of Lupus

Each person with lupus has slightly different symptoms that can range from mild to severe and may come and go over time. However, some of the most common symptoms of lupus include painful or swollen joints (arthritis), unexplained fever, and extreme fatigue. A characteristic red skin rash—the so-called butterfly or malar rash—may appear across the nose and cheeks. Rashes may also occur on the face and ears, upper arms, shoulders, chest, and hands and other areas exposed to the sun. Because many people with lupus are sensitive to sunlight (called photosensitivity), skin rashes often first develop or worsen after sun exposure.

Other symptoms of lupus include chest pain, hair loss, anemia (a decrease in red blood cells), mouth ulcers, and pale or purple fingers and toes from cold and stress. Some people also experience headaches, dizziness, depression, confusion, or seizures. New symptoms may continue to appear years after the initial diagnosis, and different symptoms can occur at different times. In some people with lupus, only one system of the body, such as the skin or joints, is affected. Other people experience symptoms in many parts of their body. Just how seriously a body system is affected varies from person to person.

Diagnosing Lupus

Diagnosing lupus can be difficult. It may take months or even years for doctors to piece together the symptoms to diagnose this complex disease accurately. Making a correct diagnosis of lupus requires knowledge and awareness on the part of the doctor and good communication on the part of the patient. Giving the doctor a complete, accurate medical history (for example, what health problems you have had and for how long) is critical to the process of diagnosis. This information, along with a physical examination and the results of laboratory tests, helps the doctor consider other diseases that may mimic lupus, or determine if you truly have the disease. Reaching a diagnosis may take time as new symptoms appear.

No single test can determine whether a person has lupus, but several laboratory tests may help the doctor to confirm a diagnosis of lupus or rule out other causes for a person's symptoms.

- Medical history
- Complete physical examination
- Laboratory tests:
  - Complete blood count (CBC)
  - Erythrocyte sedimentation rate (ESR)
  - Urinalysis
  - Blood chemistries
  - Complement levels
  - Antinuclear antibody test (ANA)
  - Other autoantibody tests (anti-DNA, anti-Sm, anti-RNP, anti-Ro [SSA], anti-La [SSB])
  - Anticardiolipin antibody test
- Skin biopsy
- Kidney biopsy

Treating Lupus

Diagnosing and treating lupus often require a team effort between the patient and several types of healthcare professionals. Most people will see a rheumatologist for their lupus treatment. Clinical immunologists may also treat people with lupus. As treatment progresses, other professionals often help. These may include nurses, psychologists, social workers, nephrologists, cardiologists, hematologists, endocrinologists, dermatologists, and neurologists. It is also important for people with lupus to have a primary care doctor—usually a family physician or internist—who can coordinate care between their different health providers and treat other problems as they arise.

The range and effectiveness of treatments for lupus have increased dramatically in recent decades, giving doctors more choices in how to manage the disease. Medications used in the treatment of lupus include the following:

- Nonsteroidal anti-inflammatory drugs (NSAIDs) such as ibuprofen and naproxen

- Antimalarials such as hydroxychloroquine

- Corticosteroids such as prednisone, hydrocortisone, methylprednisolone, and dexamethasone

- Immunosuppressives such as cyclophosphamide and mycophenolate mofetil

- B-lymphocyte stimulator (BLyS) protein inhibitor such as belimumab

- Alternative and complementary therapies including special diets, nutritional supplements, fish oils, ointments and creams, chiropractic treatment, and homeopathy

Section 46.6

Rheumatoid Arthritis

This section includes text excerpted from "Handout on Health: Rheumatoid Arthritis," National Institute of Arthritis and Musculoskeletal and Skin Diseases (NIAMS), April 2017.

What Is Rheumatoid Arthritis?

Rheumatoid arthritis (RA) is an inflammatory disease that causes pain, swelling, stiffness, and loss of function in the joints. It occurs when the immune system, which normally defends the body from invading organisms, turns its attack against the membrane lining the joints.

Rheumatoid arthritis has several features that make it different from other kinds of arthritis. For example, rheumatoid arthritis generally occurs in a symmetrical pattern, meaning that if one knee or hand is involved, the other one also is. The disease often affects the wrist joints and the finger joints closest to the hand. It can also affect other parts of the body besides the joints. In addition, people with rheumatoid arthritis may have fatigue, occasional fevers, and a loss of energy.

The course of rheumatoid arthritis can range from mild to severe. In most cases it is chronic, meaning it lasts a long time—often a lifetime. For many people, periods of relatively mild disease activity are punctuated by flares, or times of heightened disease activity. In others, symptoms are constant.

Features of Rheumatoid Arthritis

- Tender, warm, swollen joints.

- Symmetrical pattern of affected joints.

- Joint inflammation often affecting the wrist and finger joints closest to the hand.

- Joint inflammation sometimes affecting other joints, including the neck, shoulders, elbows, hips, knees, ankles, and feet.

- Fatigue, occasional fevers, a loss of energy.

- Pain and stiffness lasting for more than 30 minutes in the morning or after a long rest.

- Symptoms that last for many years.

- Variability of symptoms among people with the disease.

Who Has Rheumatoid Arthritis?

Scientists estimate that about 1.5 million people, or about 0.6 percent of the U.S. adult population, have rheumatoid arthritis. Interestingly, some recent studies have suggested that although the number of new cases of rheumatoid arthritis for older people is increasing, the overall number of new cases may actually be going down.

Rheumatoid arthritis occurs in all races and ethnic groups. Although the disease often begins in middle age and occurs with increased frequency in older people, older teenagers and young adults may also be diagnosed with the disease. (Children and younger teenagers may be diagnosed with juvenile idiopathic arthritis, a condition related to rheumatoid arthritis.) Like some other forms of arthritis, rheumatoid arthritis occurs much more frequently in women than in men. About two to three times as many women as men have the disease.

What Happens in Rheumatoid Arthritis?

Rheumatoid arthritis is primarily a disease of the joints. A joint is the point where two or more bones come together. With a few exceptions (in the skull and pelvis, for example), joints are designed to allow movement between the bones and to absorb shock from movements like walking or repetitive motions. The ends of the bones are covered by a tough, elastic tissue called cartilage. The joint is surrounded by a capsule that protects and supports it. The joint capsule is lined with a type of tissue called synovium, which produces synovial fluid, a clear substance that lubricates and nourishes the cartilage and bones inside the joint capsule.

Like many other rheumatic diseases, rheumatoid arthritis is an autoimmune disease (auto means self), so called because a person's immune system, which normally helps protect the body from infection and disease, attacks joint tissues for unknown reasons. White blood cells, the agents of the immune system, travel to the synovium and cause inflammation (synovitis), characterized by warmth, redness, swelling, and pain—typical symptoms of rheumatoid arthritis. During the inflammation process, the normally thin synovium becomes thick and makes the joint swollen, puffy, and sometimes warm to the touch.

As rheumatoid arthritis progresses, the inflamed synovium invades and destroys the cartilage and bone within the joint. The surrounding muscles, ligaments, and tendons that support and stabilize

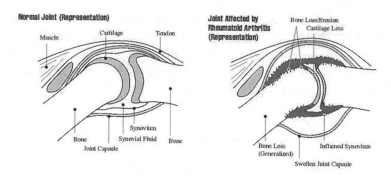

Figure 46.1. *Normal Joint and Joint with Rheumatoid Arthritis*

the joint become weak and unable to work normally. These effects lead to the pain and joint damage often seen in rheumatoid arthritis. Researchers studying rheumatoid arthritis now believe that it begins to damage bones during the first year or two that a person has the disease, which is one reason why early diagnosis and treatment are so important.

Some people with rheumatoid arthritis also have symptoms in places other than their joints. Many people with rheumatoid arthritis develop anemia, or a decrease in the production of red blood cells. Other effects that occur less often include neck pain and dry eyes and mouth. Very rarely, people may have inflammation of the blood vessels (vasculitis), the lining of the lungs (pleurisy), or the sac enclosing the heart (pericarditis).

How Does Rheumatoid Arthritis Affect People's Lives?

Rheumatoid arthritis affects people differently. Some people have mild or moderate forms of the disease, with periods of worsening symptoms, called flares, and periods in which they feel better, called remissions. Others have a severe form of the disease that is active most of the time, lasts for many years or a lifetime, and leads to serious joint damage and disability.

Although rheumatoid arthritis is primarily a disease of the joints, its effects are not just physical. Many people with rheumatoid arthritis also experience issues related to:

- Depression, anxiety.
- Feelings of helplessness.
- Low self-esteem.

Rheumatoid arthritis can affect virtually every area of a person's life from work life to family life. It can also interfere with the joys and responsibilities of family life and may affect the decision to have children.

Fortunately, current treatment strategies allow most people with the disease to lead active and productive lives. These strategies include pain-relieving drugs and medications that slow joint damage, a balance between rest and exercise, and patient education and support programs. In recent years, research has led to a new understanding of rheumatoid arthritis and has increased the likelihood that, in time, researchers will find even better ways to treat the disease.

What Causes Rheumatoid Arthritis?

Scientists still do not know exactly what causes the immune system to turn against the body's own tissues in rheumatoid arthritis, but research over the last few years has begun to piece together the factors involved.

- Genetic (inherited) factors
- Environmental factors
- Other factors:
  - Gender
  - Pregnancy
  - Breastfeeding
  - Contraceptive use
  - Hormonal changes

Even though all the answers are not known, one thing is certain: rheumatoid arthritis develops as a result of an interaction of many factors. Researchers are trying to understand these factors and how they work together.

How Is Rheumatoid Arthritis Diagnosed?

Rheumatoid arthritis can be difficult to diagnose in its early stages for several reasons. First, there is no single test for the disease. In addition, symptoms differ from person to person and can be more severe in some people than in others. Also, symptoms can be similar to those of other types of arthritis and joint conditions, and it may take some time for other conditions to be ruled out. Finally, the full range of symptoms develops over time, and only a few symptoms may be present in the early stages. As a result, doctors use a variety of the following tools to diagnose the disease and to rule out other conditions:

- Medical history
- Physical examination
- Laboratory tests:
  - Rheumatoid factor (RF)
  - Anti-CCP antibodies

- Others:
  - White blood cell count
  - Blood test for anemia
  - Erythrocyte sedimentation rate
  - C-reactive protein
- Imaging tests:
  - X-rays
  - Magnetic resonance imaging (MRI)
  - Ultrasound

How Is Rheumatoid Arthritis Treated?

Doctors use a variety of approaches to treat rheumatoid arthritis. These are used in different combinations and at different times during the course of the disease and are chosen according to the patient's individual situation. No matter what treatment the doctor and patient choose, however, the goals are the same: to relieve pain, reduce inflammation, slow down or stop joint damage, and improve the person's sense of well-being and ability to function.

Good communication between the patient and doctor is necessary for effective treatment. Talking to the doctor can help ensure that exercise and pain management programs are provided as needed, and that drugs are prescribed appropriately. Talking to the doctor can also help people who are making decisions about surgery.

- Health behavior changes: Certain activities can help improve a person's ability to function independently and maintain a positive outlook.
  - Rest and exercise: People with rheumatoid arthritis need a good balance between rest and exercise, with more rest when the disease is active and more exercise when it is not.
  - Joint care: Some people find using a splint for a short time around a painful joint reduces pain and swelling by supporting the joint and letting it rest.
  - Stress reduction: Several techniques can help for coping with stress. Regular rest periods can help, as can relaxation, distraction, or visualization exercises. Exercise programs,

participation in support groups, and good communication with the healthcare team are other ways to reduce stress.

- Healthful diet: An overall nutritious diet with enough—but not an excess of—calories, protein, and calcium is important.

- Climate: Some people notice that their arthritis gets worse when there is a sudden change in the weather. However, there is no evidence that a specific climate can prevent or reduce the effects of rheumatoid arthritis.

- Medications: Most people who have rheumatoid arthritis take medications. Some medications (analgesics) are used only for pain relief; others, such as corticosteroids and nonsteroidal anti-inflammatory drugs (NSAIDs), are used to reduce inflammation. Still others, often called disease-modifying antirheumatic drugs (DMARDs), are used to try to slow the course of the disease.

- Surgery: Several types of surgery are available to patients with severe joint damage. The primary purpose of these procedures is to reduce pain, improve the affected joint's function, and improve the patient's ability to perform daily activities.

- Routine monitoring and ongoing care: Regular medical care is important to monitor the course of the disease, determine the effectiveness and any negative effects of medications, and change therapies as needed. Monitoring typically includes regular visits to the doctor. It also may include blood, urine, and other laboratory tests and X-rays.

- Alternative and complementary therapies: Special diets, vitamin supplements, and other alternative approaches have been suggested for treating rheumatoid arthritis. Research shows that some of these, for example, fish oil supplements, may help reduce arthritis inflammation.

Chapter 47

Cardiovascular Disorders

Chapter Contents

Section 47.1

Heart Disease in Women

This section includes text excerpted from "Heart Disease in Women,"
National Heart, Lung, and Blood Institute (NHLBI), April 21, 2014.

How Does Heart Disease Affect Women?

In the United States, 1 in 4 women dies from heart disease. In
fact, coronary heart disease (CHD)—the most common type of heart
disease—is the #1 killer of both women and men in the United
States.

Other types of heart disease, such as coronary microvascular disease (MVD) and broken heart syndrome, also pose a risk for women.
These disorders, which mainly affect women, are not as well understood as CHD. However, research is ongoing to learn more about coronary MVD and broken heart syndrome.

This section focuses on CHD and its complications. However, it
also includes general information about coronary MVD and broken
heart syndrome.

Coronary Heart Disease

CHD is a disease in which plaque (plak) builds up on the inner
walls of your coronary arteries. These arteries carry oxygen-rich blood
to your heart. When plaque builds up in the arteries, the condition is
called atherosclerosis.

Plaque is made up of fat, cholesterol, calcium, and other substances
found in the blood. Over time, plaque can harden or rupture (break
open).

Hardened plaque narrows the coronary arteries and reduces the
flow of oxygen-rich blood to the heart. This can cause chest pain or
discomfort called angina.

If the plaque ruptures, a blood clot can form on its surface. A large
blood clot can mostly or completely block blood flow through a coronary
artery. This is the most common cause of a heart attack. Over time,
ruptured plaque also hardens and narrows the coronary arteries.

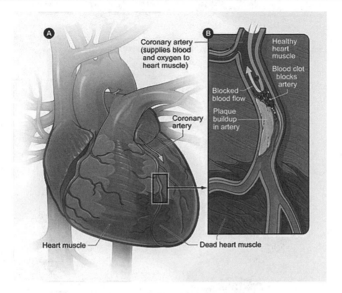

Figure 47.1. *Heart with Muscle Damage and a Blocked Artery*

Figure A is an overview of a heart and coronary artery showing damage (dead heart muscle) caused by a heart attack. Figure B is a cross-section of the coronary artery with plaque buildup and a blood clot resulting from plaque rupture.

Plaque also can develop within the walls of the coronary arteries. Tests that show the insides of the coronary arteries may look normal in people who have this pattern of plaque. Studies are underway to see whether this type of plaque buildup occurs more often in women than in men and why.

In addition to angina and heart attack, CHD can cause other serious heart problems. The disease may lead to heart failure, irregular heartbeats called arrhythmias, and sudden cardiac arrest (SCA).

Coronary Microvascular Disease

Coronary MVD is heart disease that affects the heart's tiny arteries. This disease is also called cardiac syndrome X or nonobstructive CHD. In coronary MVD, the walls of the heart's tiny arteries are damaged or diseased.

Women are more likely than men to have coronary MVD. Many researchers think that a drop in estrogen levels during menopause combined with other heart disease risk factors causes coronary MVD.

Although death rates from heart disease have dropped in the last 30 years, they haven't dropped as much in women as in men. This may be the result of coronary MVD.

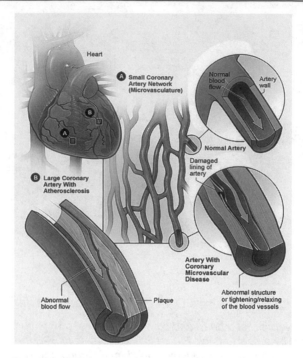

Figure 47.2. *Coronary Microvascular Disease*

Figure A shows the small coronary artery network (microvasculature), containing a normal artery and an artery with coronary MVD. Figure B shows a large coronary artery with plaque buildup.

Standard tests for CHD are not designed to detect coronary MVD. Thus, test results for women who have coronary MVD may show that they are at low risk for heart disease.

Broken Heart Syndrome

Women are also more likely than men to have a condition called broken heart syndrome. In this recently recognized heart problem, extreme emotional stress can lead to severe (but often short term) heart muscle failure.

Broken heart syndrome is also called stress-induced cardiomyopathy or takotsubo cardiomyopathy.

Doctors may misdiagnose broken heart syndrome as a heart attack because it has similar symptoms and test results. However, there's no evidence of blocked heart arteries in broken heart syndrome, and most people have a full and quick recovery.

Researchers are just starting to explore what causes this disorder and how to diagnose and treat it. Often, patients who have broken heart syndrome have previously been healthy.

Other Names for Heart Disease

- Arrhythmia
- Broken heart syndrome, which also is called stress-induced cardiomyopathy or takotsubo cardiomyopathy
- Coronary heart disease, which also is called coronary artery disease
- Coronary microvascular disease, which also is called cardiac syndrome X or nonobstructive coronary heart disease
- Heart failure
- Sudden cardiac arrest

What Causes Heart Disease?

Research suggests that coronary heart disease (CHD) begins with damage to the lining and inner layers of the coronary (heart) arteries. Several factors contribute to this damage. They include:

- Smoking, including secondhand smoke
- High amounts of certain fats and cholesterol in the blood
- High blood pressure
- High amounts of sugar in the blood due to insulin resistance or diabetes
- Blood vessel inflammation

Plaque may begin to buildup where the arteries are damaged. The buildup of plaque in the coronary arteries may start in childhood.

Over time, plaque can harden or rupture (break open). Hardened plaque narrows the coronary arteries and reduces the flow of oxygen-rich blood to the heart. This can cause chest pain or discomfort called angina.

If the plaque ruptures, blood cell fragments called platelets stick to the site of the injury. They may clump together to form blood clots.

Blood clots can further narrow the coronary arteries and worsen angina. If a clot becomes large enough, it can mostly or completely block a coronary artery and cause a heart attack.

In addition to the factors above, low estrogen levels before or after menopause may play a role in causing coronary microvascular disease (MVD). Coronary MVD is heart disease that affects the heart's tiny arteries.

The cause of broken heart syndrome isn't yet known. However, a sudden release of stress hormones may play a role in causing the disorder. Most cases of broken heart syndrome occur in women who have gone through menopause.

Who Is at Risk for Heart Disease?

Certain traits, conditions, or habits may raise your risk for coronary heart disease (CHD). These conditions are known as risk factors. Risk factors also increase the chance that existing CHD will worsen.

Women generally have the same CHD risk factors as men. However, some risk factors may affect women differently than men. For example, diabetes raises the risk of CHD more in women. Also, some risk factors, such as birth control pills and menopause, only affect women.

There are many known CHD risk factors. Your risk for CHD and heart attack rises with the number of risk factors you have and their severity. Risk factors tend to "gang up" and worsen each other's effects.

Having just one risk factor doubles your risk for CHD. Having two risk factors increases your risk for CHD fourfold. Having three or more risk factors increases your risk for CHD more than tenfold.

Also, some risk factors, such as smoking and diabetes, put you at greater risk for CHD and heart attack than others.

More than 75 percent of women aged 40 to 60 have one or more risk factors for CHD. Many risk factors start during childhood; some even develop within the first 10 years of life.

Following are some of the risk factors for heart disease:

- Smoking

- High blood cholesterol and high triglyceride levels

- High blood pressure

- Diabetes and prediabetes

- Overweight and obesity

- Metabolic syndrome

- Birth control pills

- Lack of physical activity

- Unhealthy diet

- Stress or depression

- Anemia

- Sleep apnea

- Aging and menopause

What Are the Signs and Symptoms of Heart Disease?

The signs and symptoms of coronary heart disease (CHD) may differ between women and men. Some women who have CHD have no signs or symptoms. This is called silent CHD.

Silent CHD may not be diagnosed until a woman has signs and symptoms of a heart attack, heart failure, or an arrhythmia (irregular heartbeat).

Other women who have CHD will have signs and symptoms of the disease.

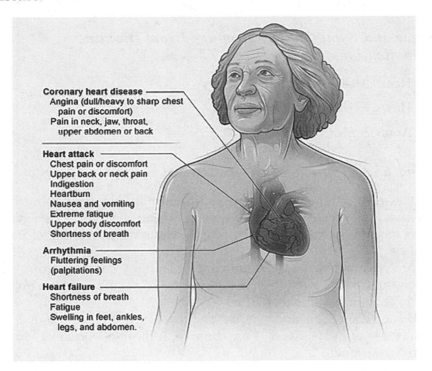

Figure 47.3. *Heart Disease Signs and Symptoms*

The illustration shows the major signs and symptoms of coronary heart disease.

A common symptom of CHD is angina. Angina is chest pain or discomfort that occurs when your heart muscle doesn't get enough oxygen-rich blood.

In men, angina often feels like pressure or squeezing in the chest. This feeling may extend to the arms. Women can also have these angina symptoms. But women also tend to describe a sharp, burning chest pain. Women are more likely to have pain in the neck, jaw, throat, abdomen, or back.

In men, angina tends to worsen with physical activity and go away with rest. Women are more likely than men to have angina while they're resting or sleeping.

In women who have coronary microvascular disease, angina often occurs during routine daily activities, such as shopping or cooking, rather than while exercising. Mental stress also is more likely to trigger angina pain in women than in men.

The severity of angina varies. The pain may get worse or occur more often as the buildup of plaque continues to narrow the coronary (heart) arteries.

Signs and Symptoms of Coronary Heart Disease Complications

- Heart Attack
- Heart Failure
- Arrhythmia

Signs and Symptoms of Broken Heart Syndrome

The most common signs and symptoms of broken heart syndrome are chest pain and shortness of breath. In this disorder, these symptoms tend to occur suddenly in people who have no history of heart disease.

Arrhythmias or cardiogenic shock also may occur. Cardiogenic shock is a condition in which a suddenly weakened heart isn't able to pump enough blood to meet the body's needs.

Some of the signs and symptoms of broken heart syndrome differ from those of heart attack. For example, in people who have broken heart syndrome:

- Symptoms occur suddenly after having extreme emotional or physical stress.

- EKG (electrocardiogram) results don't look the same as the EKG results for a person having a heart attack. (An EKG is a test that records the heart's electrical activity.)

- Blood tests show no signs or mild signs of heart damage.

- Tests show no signs of blockages in the coronary arteries.

- Tests show ballooning and unusual movement of the lower left heart chamber (left ventricle).

- Recovery time is quick, usually within days or weeks (compared with the recovery time of a month or more for a heart attack).

How Is Heart Disease Diagnosed?

Your doctor will diagnose coronary heart disease (CHD) based on your medical and family histories, your risk factors, a physical exam, and the results from tests and procedures.

No single test can diagnose CHD. If your doctor thinks you have CHD, he or she may recommend one or more of the following tests.

- EKG (Electrocardiogram)

- Stress Testing

- Echocardiography

- Chest X-ray

- Blood Tests

- Coronary Angiography and Cardiac Catheterization

Tests Used to Diagnose Broken Heart Syndrome

If your doctor thinks you have broken heart syndrome, he or she may recommend coronary angiography. Other tests are also used to diagnose this disorder, including blood tests, EKG, echo, and cardiac MRI.

How Is Heart Disease Treated?

Treatment for coronary heart disease (CHD) usually is the same for both women and men. Treatment may include lifestyle changes, medicines, medical and surgical procedures, and cardiac rehabilitation (rehab).

The goals of treatment are to:

- Relieve symptoms.

- Reduce risk factors in an effort to slow, stop, or reverse the buildup of plaque.

- Lower the risk of blood clots forming. (Blood clots can cause a heart attack.)

- Widen or bypass plaque-clogged coronary (heart) arteries.

- Prevent CHD complications.

How Can Heart Disease Be Prevented?

Taking action to control your risk factors can help prevent or delay coronary heart disease (CHD). Your risk for CHD increases with the number of CHD risk factors you have.

One step you can take is to adopt a heart healthy lifestyle. A heart healthy lifestyle should be part of a lifelong approach to healthy living.

For example, if you smoke, try to quit. Smoking can raise your risk for CHD and heart attack and worsen other CHD risk factors. Talk with your doctor about programs and products that can help you quit. Also, try to avoid secondhand smoke.

Following a healthy diet also is an important part of a healthy lifestyle. A healthy diet includes a variety of vegetables and fruits. It also includes whole grains, fat-free or low-fat dairy products, and protein foods, such as lean meats, poultry without skin, seafood, processed soy products, nuts, seeds, beans, and peas.

A healthy diet is low in sodium (salt), added sugars, solid fats, and refined grains. Solid fats are saturated fat and trans fatty acids. Refined grains come from processing whole grains, which results in a loss of nutrients (such as dietary fiber).

The National Heart, Lung, and Blood Institute's (NHLBI's) Therapeutic Lifestyle Changes (TLC) and Dietary Approaches to Stop Hypertension (DASH) are two programs that promote healthy eating.

If you're overweight or obese, work with your doctor to create a reasonable weight-loss plan. Controlling your weight helps you control CHD risk factors.

Be as physically active as you can. Physical activity can improve your fitness level and your health. Talk with your doctor about what types of activity are safe for you.

Know your family history of CHD. If you or someone in your family has CHD, be sure to tell your doctor.

If lifestyle changes aren't enough, you also may need medicines to control your CHD risk factors. Take all of your medicines as prescribed.

Living with Heart Disease

If you have coronary heart disease (CHD), you can take steps to control its risk factors and prevent complications. Lifestyle changes and ongoing care can help you manage the disease.

Having CHD raises your risk for a heart attack. Thus, knowing the warning signs of a heart attack is important. If you think you're having a heart attack, call 9–1–1 right away.

Lifestyle Changes

Adopting a heart healthy lifestyle can help you control CHD risk factors. However, making lifestyle changes can be a challenge.

Try to take things one step at a time. Learn about the benefits of lifestyle changes, and make a plan with specific, realistic goals. Reward yourself for your progress.

The good news is that many lifestyle changes help control several CHD risk factors at the same time. For example, physical activity lowers your blood pressure and LDL cholesterol level, helps control diabetes and prediabetes, reduces stress, and helps control your weight.

Ongoing Care

Your CHD risk factors can change over time, so having ongoing care is important. Your doctor will track your blood pressure, blood cholesterol, and blood sugar levels with routine tests. These tests will show whether your doctor needs to adjust your treatment.

Ask your doctor how often you should schedule follow-up visits and blood tests. Between visits, call your doctor if you have any new symptoms or if your symptoms worsen.

You may feel depressed or anxious if you've been diagnosed with CHD. You may worry about heart problems or making lifestyle changes.

Your doctor may recommend medicine, professional counseling, or relaxation therapy if you have depression or anxiety. It's important to treat these conditions because they raise your risk for CHD and heart attack. Depression and anxiety also can make it harder for you to make lifestyle changes.

Heart Attack Warning Signs

If you have CHD, learn the warning signs of a heart attack. Heart attack signs and symptoms include:

- Chest pain or discomfort. This involves uncomfortable pressure, squeezing, fullness, or pain in the center or left side of the chest that can be mild or strong. This pain or discomfort often lasts more than a few minutes or goes away and comes back.

- Upper body discomfort in one or both arms, the back, neck, jaw, or upper part of the stomach.

- Shortness of breath, which may occur with or before chest discomfort.

- Nausea (feeling sick to your stomach), vomiting, light-headedness or fainting, or breaking out in a cold sweat.

- Sleep problems, fatigue (tiredness), and lack of energy.

If you think you're having a heart attack, call 9–1–1 at once. Early treatment can prevent or limit damage to your heart muscle.

If you think you're having a heart attack, do not drive to the hospital or let someone else drive you. Call an ambulance so that medical personnel can begin life-saving treatment on the way to the emergency room.

Let the people you see regularly know you're at risk for a heart attack. They can seek emergency care if you suddenly faint, collapse, or have other severe symptoms.

Living with Broken Heart Syndrome

Most people who have broken heart syndrome make a full recovery within weeks. The risk is low for a repeat episode of this disorder.

To check your heart health, your doctor may recommend echocardiography about a month after you're diagnosed with the syndrome. Talk with your doctor about how often you should schedule follow-up visits.

Section 47.2

Heart Attack and Women

This section includes text excerpted from "Heart Attack and
Women," Office on Women's Health (OWH), U.S. Department of
Health and Human Services (HHS), January 24, 2017.

A heart attack happens when blood flow in an artery to the heart is
blocked by a blood clot or plaque, and the heart muscle begins to die.
Women are more likely than men to die after a heart attack. But if you
get help quickly, treatment can save your life and prevent permanent
damage to your heart.

What Is a Heart Attack?

A heart attack happens when blood flow to your heart muscle is
blocked and the cells in your heart muscle begin to die. Many different
health problems can cause a heart attack, but coronary artery disease
is the most common.

What Are the Symptoms of a Heart Attack in Women?

The most common symptoms of a heart attack for both women
and men are pain and discomfort in the chest and upper body. Other
symptoms, like shortness of breath and nausea, are more common in
women than men.

What Is the Difference between a Heart Attack and Cardiac Arrest?

A heart attack is not the same as cardiac arrest. In a heart attack,
the heart keeps beating. The person has a pulse and usually stays
conscious (awake). During cardiac arrest, the heart stops beating. The
person has no pulse and is unconscious (not awake).

A defibrillator is a machine that sends an electrical shock to the heart to
restore normal rhythm. This treatment must be given as soon as possible.
For cardiac arrest, call 911 and begin CPR (cardiopulmonary resuscitation)

right away. The American Heart Association says that with "hands only" CPR, anyone can give lifesaving treatment to someone having cardiac arrest. Push hard and fast in the center of the chest and keep going until emergency personnel arrive. Do not give CPR for a heart attack.

What Causes a Heart Attack?

Coronary artery disease (CAD) causes most heart attacks. In people with CAD, plaque builds up on the walls of the arteries that supply blood to the heart. This is called atherosclerosis.

Plaque can buildup in fatty clumps or in a thin, smooth layer. Both types are dangerous. The plaque can break open or wear down, causing blood to clump together (clot) in that area. If a clot blocks blood flow to the heart, it can cause a heart attack.

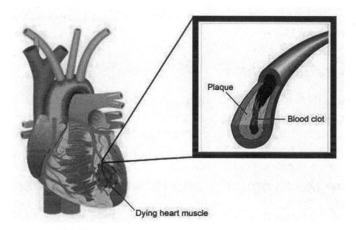

Figure 47.4. *Plaque Buildup in Heart*

This picture shows how CAD causes a heart attack. Plaque builds up in an artery of the heart, and a blood clot forms. The clot blocks blood flow to part of the heart, and the heart muscle begins to die.

A heart attack can also happen if the artery pinches itself closed. This is called a coronary spasm. Coronary spasms are rare. They happen more often in young women than in older women or men.

How Do I Know If I Am at Risk for a Heart Attack?

A heart attack can happen to anyone, woman or man, young or old. Some people are more at risk because of certain health problems, family health history, age, and habits. These are called risk factors.

You can't change some risk factors, like your age, race or ethnicity, or family history. The good news is that you can change or control many risk factors, such as high blood pressure, diabetes, smoking, and unhealthy eating.

Do Women of Color Need to Worry about Heart Attack Risk?

Yes. All women need to be aware of their heart attack risk and take steps to prevent heart disease.

African-American, Hispanic, and American Indian or Alaska Native women often have more heart attack risk factors than white women. These risk factors can include obesity, lack of physical activity, high blood pressure, and diabetes.

African-American women are also more likely to have a heart attack and more likely to die from a heart attack compared with white women.

Do Women Do Worse Than Men after a Heart Attack?

Yes. In all age groups, women do worse than men after a heart attack. Researchers are not sure why this is, especially for younger women.

- **Women between 45 and 65** who have a heart attack are more likely than men of the same age to die within a year of a heart attack. However, heart attack is less common in younger women than in younger men. This is partly because the hormone estrogen protects against heart disease in younger women.

- **Women older than 65** are more likely than men of the same age to die **within a few weeks** of a heart attack. Women usually have heart attacks about 10 years later than men. The average age of a first heart attack for men is 64, but it is 72 for women.

Many women who have had a heart attack go on to lead full, active lives. Know the symptoms of a heart attack and what to do if you have any symptoms. Take steps to recover after a heart attack and prevent another heart attack.

How Is a Heart Attack Diagnosed?

To diagnose a heart attack, a doctor will ask you about your symptoms, your health, and your family health history. The doctor will also order tests.

Doctors often use these types of tests to diagnose a heart attack and choose the best treatment.

- **Blood tests.** During a heart attack, heart muscle cells die and burst open. This process releases proteins into your blood. Heart attack blood tests measure the amount of these protein "markers" of heart damage. Common heart attack blood tests include:

    - Cardiac troponin

    - Creatine Kinase-MB (CKMB)

    - Myoglobin

- **Coronary angiography,** or angiogram. This test takes pictures of a dye flowing through your blood vessels. By watching how smoothly the dye flows, doctors can locate narrowed or blocked coronary arteries that might need to be opened, or find other problems.

Women are more likely than men to have a less-common type of plaque that forms a smooth layer over the arteries instead of a few big lumps. Often, angiograms can't see this thin, smooth plaque, but this type of plaque is still very dangerous. Other tests (such as those described above) might be needed for women who show signs or have symptoms of a heart attack but whose coronary angiography results do not show any problems.

- **Nuclear heart scan.** This test takes pictures to show areas of the heart that may be damaged because they are not getting enough blood. It can also show how well the heart is pumping. Tell your doctor if you are pregnant or breastfeeding. The test uses radioactive material that can harm your baby.

- **Electrocardiogram (ECG or EKG).** This test detects and records your heart's electrical activity. Certain changes in the electrical waves on an ECG can show whether you are having, or have had, a heart attack. An ECG can also be done during physical activity to monitor your heart when it is working hard.

How Is a Heart Attack Treated?

Heart attack is most often treated with medicine or nonsurgical procedures that break up blood clots and restore normal blood flow to the heart. Some treatments will start right away, when the ambulance comes. You will get other treatments later, in the hospital.

Getting treatment right away for a heart attack can help prevent or limit damage to your heart muscle. This is one reason why it is important to call 911 if you think you are having a heart attack, rather than driving yourself to the hospital.

What Medicines Treat a Heart Attack?

Medicines you might receive if you have a heart attack include:

- Clot busters
- Aspirin and blood thinners
- Nitrates
- Beta blockers
- ACE inhibitors

You may also be given other medicines to relieve pain or anxiety or lower your cholesterol.

What Procedures Treat a Heart Attack?

The most common procedures to treat a heart attack include:

- **Angioplasty and stenting.** Angioplasty, also called percutaneous coronary intervention, is a nonsurgical procedure that opens blocked or narrowed coronary arteries. A thin, flexible tube with a medical balloon on the end is threaded through a blood vessel to the narrowed or blocked coronary artery. Once in place, the balloon is inflated to open the artery to allow blood flow to the heart. The balloon is then deflated and removed. A small mesh tube called a stent may be permanently placed in the artery. The stent helps prevent new blockages in the artery.

- **Coronary artery bypass grafting.** The surgeon uses a healthy blood vessel from another part of your body to re-route blood around the blockage in your artery. You may need this surgery if more than one artery is blocked, or if angioplasty and stenting did not work to restore blood flow to the heart.

After a heart attack, you may also need cardiac rehabilitation to recover from the damage the heart attack did to your heart.

How Can I Prevent a Heart Attack?

All women can make changes to help prevent a heart attack. These changes include making healthier food choices, being more physically active, and not smoking. Once you know your heart attack risk factors, you and your doctor can work together to lower your risk.

Even if you had a heart attack before, you can make changes to help prevent another heart attack.

Section 47.3

Stroke in Women

This section includes text excerpted from "Stroke and Women," Office on Women's Health (OWH), U.S. Department of Health and Human Services (HHS), January 24, 2017.

Stroke kills twice as many women as breast cancer each year. In fact, stroke is the fourth leading cause of death for women. Stroke also kills more women than men each year. A stroke can leave you permanently disabled. But many strokes are preventable and treatable. Every woman can take steps to prevent stroke by knowing her risk factors and making healthy changes.

What Is Stroke?

A stroke is sometimes called a "brain attack." Stroke happens when blood flow to a part of the brain stops or is blocked by a blood clot or plaque, and brain cells begin to die.

What Are the Different Types of Stroke?

There are two types of stroke:

- **Stroke caused by a blockage of blood flow to the brain (ischemic stroke).** This is the most common type of stroke. This type of stroke happens most often when an artery is clogged with plaque (atherosclerosis) or a blood clot.

- **Stroke caused by bleeding into the brain (hemorrhagic stroke).** This type of stroke happens when a blood vessel in the brain bursts, and blood bleeds into the brain. This type of stroke can be caused by an aneurysm, which is a thin or weak spot in an artery that can burst.

Both types of stroke can cause brain cells to die. Depending on which part of the brain the stroke affects, you may have problems with your speech, movement, balance, vision, or memory.

If you think you are having a stroke, call 911.

What Is A "Mini-Stroke"?

A "mini-stroke" is also called a transient ischemic attack (TIA, pronounced "T-I-A"). A TIA happens when, for a short time, less blood than normal gets to the brain. You may have some stroke symptoms, or you may not notice any symptoms.

A TIA usually lasts only a few minutes, although it can last up to several hours. Many people do not even know they have had a stroke. A TIA can be a warning sign of a full stroke in the future, or you can have another mini-stroke at a later time.

What Are the Effects of Stroke?

How stroke affects you depends on:

- The type of stroke

- The area of the brain where the stroke happened

- The amount of brain injury

A mild stroke can cause little or no brain damage. A major stroke can cause severe brain damage and even death. Some effects of stroke may improve with time and rehabilitation.

A stroke can happen in different parts of the brain. The brain is divided into four main parts:

- The right hemisphere (or half)

- The left hemisphere (or half)

- The cerebellum, which controls balance and coordination

- The brainstem, which controls all of our body's functions that we don't think about, such as heart rate, blood pressure, sweating, or digestion.

A stroke in the **right half of the brain** can cause:

- Problems moving the left side of your body

- Problems judging distances. You may misjudge distances and fall. Or you might not be able to guide your hands to pick something up.

  - Impaired judgment and behavior. You may misjudge your ability to do things. You may also do things you would not normally do, such as leave your house without getting fully dressed.

  - Short-term memory loss. You may be able to remember events from 30 years ago, but not how to get to the place where you work today.

A stroke in the **left half of the brain** can cause:

- Problems moving the right side of your body.

- Speech and language problems. You may have trouble speaking or understanding others.

- Slow and cautious behavior. You may need a lot of help to complete everyday tasks.

- Memory problems. You may not remember what you did 10 minutes ago. Or you may have a hard time learning new things.

A stroke in the **cerebellum** can cause:

- Stiffness and tightness in the upper body that can cause spasms or jerky movements

- Eye problems, such as blurry or double vision

- Balance problems

- Dizziness, nausea (feeling sick to your stomach), and vomiting

Strokes in the **brain stem** are very harmful. Since impulses that start in the brain must travel through the brainstem on their way to the arms and legs, patients with a brain stem stroke may also develop paralysis.

How Do I Know If I'm at Risk for a Stroke?

A stroke can happen to anyone. Some women are more at risk because of certain health problems, family health history, age, and habits. These are called risk factors.

You can't change some risk factors, like your age, race or ethnicity, or family history. The good news is that you can control many other stroke risk factors, such as high blood pressure, diabetes, smoking, and unhealthy eating.

How Do I Know If I'm Having a Stroke?

Strokes happen fast and are a medical emergency. **If you think you or someone else may be having a stroke, use the F.A.S.T test:**

F—Face: Look in the mirror and smile, or ask the person to smile. Does one side of the face droop?

A—Arms: Raise both arms. Does one arm drift downward?

S—Speech: Repeat a simple phrase, like "Hello, my name is ____." Is the speech slurred or strange?

T—Time: Act fast. If you see any of these signs, **call 911 right away**. Some treatments for stroke work only if given in the first 3 hours after symptoms appear.

Section 47.4

Varicose and Spider Veins

This section includes text excerpted from "Varicose Veins and Spider Veins," Office on Women's Health (OWH), U.S. Department of Health and Human Services (HHS), February 6, 2017.

Varicose veins are enlarged veins that can be blue, red, or flesh-colored. They often look like cords and appear twisted and bulging. Spider veins are like varicose veins, but smaller. Varicose veins and spider veins usually appear in the legs and can cause pain, swelling, or an itchy rash. Varicose veins and spider veins are treatable

What Are Varicose Veins and Spider Veins?

Varicose veins are enlarged veins that can be blue, red, or flesh-colored. They often look like cords and appear twisted and bulging. They can be swollen and raised above the surface of the skin. Varicose veins are often found on the thighs, backs of the calves, or the inside of the leg. During pregnancy, varicose veins can form around the vagina and buttocks.

Spider veins are like varicose veins but smaller. They also are closer to the surface of the skin than varicose veins. Often, they are red or blue. They can look like tree branches or spiderwebs with their short, jagged lines. They can be found on the legs and face and can cover either a very small or very large area of skin.

What Causes Varicose Veins and Spider Veins?

Varicose veins can be caused by weak or damaged valves in the veins. The heart pumps blood filled with oxygen and nutrients to the whole body through the arteries. Veins then carry the blood from the body back to the heart. As your leg muscles squeeze, they push blood back to the heart from your lower body against the flow of gravity. Veins have valves that act as one-way flaps to prevent blood from flowing backwards as it moves up your legs. If the valves become weak, blood can leak back into the veins and collect there. (This problem is called venous insufficiency.) When backed-up blood makes the veins bigger, they can become varicose.

Spider veins can be caused by the backup of blood. They can also be caused by hormone changes, exposure to the sun, and injuries.

How Common Are Abnormal Leg Veins?

About 50 to 55 percent of women and 40 to 45 percent of men in the United States suffer from some type of vein problem. Varicose veins affect half of people 50 years and older.

What Factors Increase My Risk of Varicose Veins and Spider Veins?

Many factors increase a person's chances of developing varicose or spider veins. These include:

- Increasing age
- Medical history
- Hormonal changes
- Pregnancy

- Obesity

- Lack of movement

- Sun exposure

Why Do Varicose Veins and Spider Veins Usually Appear in the Legs?

Most varicose and spider veins appear in the legs due to the pressure of body weight, force of gravity, and task of carrying blood from the bottom of the body up to the heart.

Compared with other veins in the body, leg veins have the toughest job of carrying blood back to the heart. They endure the most pressure. This pressure can be stronger than the one-way valves in the veins.

What Are the Signs of Varicose Veins?

Varicose veins can often be seen on the skin. Some other common symptoms of varicose veins in the legs include:

- Aching pain that may get worse after sitting or standing for a long time

- Throbbing or cramping

- Heaviness

- Swelling

- Rash that's itchy or irritated

- Darkening of the skin (in severe cases)

- Restless legs

Are Varicose Veins and Spider Veins Dangerous?

Spider veins rarely are a serious health problem, but they can cause uncomfortable feelings in the legs. If there are symptoms from spider veins, most often they will be itching or burning. Less often, spider veins can be a sign of blood backup deeper inside that you can't see on the skin. If so, you could have the same symptoms you would have with varicose veins.

Varicose veins may not cause any problems, or they may cause aching pain, throbbing, and discomfort. In some cases, varicose veins can lead to more serious health problems. These include:

- Sores or skin ulcers
- Bleeding
- Superficial thrombophlebitis
- Deep vein thrombosis

Should I See a Doctor about Varicose Veins?

You should see a doctor about varicose veins if:

- The vein has become swollen, red, or very tender or warm to the touch
- There are sores or a rash on the leg or near the ankle
- The skin on the ankle and calf becomes thick and changes color
- One of the varicose veins begins to bleed
- Your leg symptoms are interfering with daily activities
- The appearance of the veins is causing you distress

If you're having pain, even if it's just a dull ache, don't hesitate to get help. Also, even if you don't need to see a doctor about your varicose veins, you should take steps to keep them from getting worse.

How Are Varicose Veins Diagnosed?

Your doctor may diagnose your varicose veins based on a physical exam. Your doctor will look at your legs while you're standing or sitting with your legs dangling. He or she may ask you about your symptoms, including any pain you're having. Sometimes, you may have other tests to find out the extent of the problem and to rule out other disorders.

You might have an ultrasound, which is used to see the veins' structure, check the blood flow in your veins, and look for blood clots. This test uses sound waves to create pictures of structures in your body.

Although less likely, you might have a venogram. This test can be used to get a more detailed look at blood flow through your veins.

If you seek help for your varicose veins, there are several types of doctors you can see, including:

- A phlebologist, which is a vein specialist
- A vascular medicine doctor, who focuses on the blood system

- A vascular surgeon, who can perform surgery and do other procedures

- An interventional radiologist, who specializes in using imaging tools to see inside the body and do treatments with little or no cutting

- A dermatologist, who specializes in skin conditions

Each of these specialists do some or all of the procedures for treating varicose veins. You might start out by asking your regular doctor which specialist he or she recommends. You also might check with your insurance plan to see if it would pay for a particular provider or procedure.

How Are Varicose and Spider Veins Treated?

Varicose veins are treated with lifestyle changes and medical treatments. These can:

- Relieve symptoms

- Prevent complications

- Improve appearance

Your doctor may recommend lifestyle changes if your varicose veins don't cause many symptoms. If symptoms are more severe, your doctor may recommend medical treatments. Some treatment options include:

- Compression stockings

- Sclerotherapy

- Surface laser treatments

- Endovenous techniques (radiofrequency and laser)

Surgery

Surgery is used mostly to treat very large varicose veins. Types of surgery for varicose veins include:

- **Surgical ligation and stripping.** With this treatment, problem veins are tied shut and completely removed from the leg through small cuts in the skin. Removing the veins does not affect the circulation of blood in the leg. Veins deeper in the leg take care of the larger volumes of blood. This surgery requires general anesthesia and must be done in an operating room. It takes between 1 and 4 weeks to recover from the surgery. This surgery is generally safe. Pain in the leg is the most common side effect. Other possible problems include:

- A risk of heart and breathing problems from anesthesia

- Bleeding and congestion of blood. But, the collected blood usually settles on its own and does not require any further treatment.

- Wound infection, inflammation, swelling, and redness

- Permanent scars

- Damage of nerve tissue around the treated vein. It's hard to avoid harming small nerve branches when veins are removed. This damage can cause numbness, burning, or a change in feeling around the scar.

- A deep vein blood clot. These clots can travel to the lungs and heart. The medicine heparin may be used to reduce the chance of these dangerous blood clots. But, heparin also can increase the normal amount of bleeding and bruising after surgery.

- **PIN stripping.** In this treatment, an instrument called a PIN stripper is inserted into a vein. The tip of the PIN stripper is sewn to the end of the vein, and when it is removed, the vein is pulled out. This procedure can be done in an operating room or an outpatient center. General or local anesthesia can be used.

- **Ambulatory phlebectomy.** With ambulatory phlebectomy tiny cuts are made in the skin, and hooks are used to pull the vein out of the leg. Only the parts of your leg that are being pricked will be numbed with anesthesia. The vein is usually removed in 1 treatment. Very large varicose veins can be removed with this treatment while leaving only very small scars. Patients can return to normal activity the day after treatment. Possible side effects of the treatment include slight bruising and temporary numbness.

How Can I Prevent Varicose Veins and Spider Veins?

Not all varicose and spider veins can be prevented. But, there are some steps you can take to reduce your chances of getting new varicose and spider veins. These same things can help ease discomfort from the ones you already have:

- Wear sunscreen to protect your skin from the sun and to limit spider veins on the face.

- Exercise regularly to improve your leg strength, circulation, and vein strength. Focus on exercises that work your legs, such as walking or running.

- Control your weight to avoid placing too much pressure on your legs.

- Don't cross your legs for long times when sitting. It's possible to injure your legs that way, and even a minor injury can increase the risk of varicose veins.

- Elevate your legs when resting as much as possible.

- Don't stand or sit for long periods of time. If you must stand for a long time, shift your weight from one leg to the other every few minutes. If you must sit for long periods of time, stand up and move around or take a short walk every 30 minutes.

- Wear elastic support stockings and avoid tight clothing that constricts your waist, groin, or legs.

- Avoid wearing high heels for long periods of time. Lower-heeled shoes can help tone your calf muscles to help blood move through your veins.

- Eat a low-salt diet rich in high-fiber foods. Eating fiber reduces the chances of constipation, which can contribute to varicose veins. High-fiber foods include fresh fruits and vegetables and whole grains, like bran. Eating less salt can help with the swelling that comes with varicose veins.

Chapter 48

Carpal Tunnel Syndrome in Women

What Is Carpal Tunnel Syndrome?

Carpal tunnel syndrome (CTS) occurs when the median nerve, which runs from the forearm into the palm of the hand, becomes pressed or squeezed at the wrist. The carpal tunnel—a narrow, rigid passageway of ligament and bones at the base of the hand— houses the median nerve and the tendons that bend the fingers. The median nerve provides feeling to the palm side of the thumb and to the index, middle, and part of the ring fingers (although not the little finger). It also controls some small muscles at the base of the thumb.

Sometimes, thickening from the lining of irritated tendons or other swelling narrows the tunnel and causes the median nerve to be compressed. The result may be numbness, weakness, or sometimes pain in the hand and wrist, or occasionally in the forearm and arm. CTS is the most common and widely known of the entrapment neuropathies, in which one of the body's peripheral nerves is pressed upon.

This chapter includes text excerpted from "Carpal Tunnel Syndrome Fact Sheet," National Institute of Neurological Disorders and Stroke (NINDS), January 2017.

What Are the Symptoms of Carpal Tunnel Syndrome?

Symptoms usually start gradually, with frequent burning, tingling, or itching numbness in the palm of the hand and the fingers, especially the thumb and the index and middle fingers. Some carpal tunnel sufferers say their fingers feel useless and swollen, even though little or no swelling is apparent. The symptoms often first appear in one or both hands during the night, since many people sleep with flexed wrists. A person with carpal tunnel syndrome may wake up feeling the need to "shake out" the hand or wrist. As symptoms worsen, people might feel tingling during the day. Decreased grip strength may make it difficult to form a fist, grasp small objects, or perform other manual tasks. In chronic and/or untreated cases, the muscles at the base of the thumb may waste away. Some people are unable to tell between hot and cold by touch.

What Are the Causes of Carpal Tunnel Syndrome?

Carpal tunnel syndrome is often the result of a combination of factors that reduce the available space for the median nerve within the carpal tunnel, rather than a problem with the nerve itself. Contributing factors include trauma or injury to the wrist that cause swelling, such as sprain or fracture; an overactive pituitary gland; an underactive thyroid gland; and rheumatoid arthritis. Mechanical problems in the wrist joint, work stress, repeated use of vibrating hand tools, fluid retention during pregnancy or menopause, or the development of a cyst or tumor in the canal also may contribute to the compression. Often, no single cause can be identified.

Who Is at Risk of Developing Carpal Tunnel Syndrome?

Women are three times more likely than men to develop carpal tunnel syndrome, perhaps because the carpal tunnel itself may be smaller in women than in men. The dominant hand is usually affected first and produces the most severe pain. Persons with diabetes or other metabolic disorders that directly affect the body's nerves and make them more susceptible to compression are also at high risk. Carpal tunnel syndrome usually occurs only in adults.

The risk of developing carpal tunnel syndrome is not confined to people in a single industry or job, but is especially common in those performing assembly line work—manufacturing, sewing, finishing, cleaning, and meat, poultry, or fish packing. In fact, carpal tunnel syndrome is three times more common among assemblers than among data-entry personnel.

How Is Carpal Tunnel Syndrome Diagnosed?

Early diagnosis and treatment are important to avoid permanent damage to the median nerve.

- A medical history and physical examination of the hands, arms, shoulders, and neck can help determine if the person's discomfort is related to daily activities or to an underlying disorder, and can rule out other conditions that cause similar symptoms. The wrist is examined for tenderness, swelling, warmth, and discoloration. Each finger should be tested for sensation and the muscles at the base of the hand should be examined for strength and signs of atrophy.

- Routine laboratory tests and X-rays can reveal fractures, arthritis, and detect diseases that can damage the nerves, such as diabetes.

- Specific tests may reproduce the symptoms of CTS. In the Tinel test, the doctor taps on or presses over the median nerve in the person's wrist. The test is positive when tingling occurs in the affected fingers. Phalen's maneuver (or wrist-flexion test) involves the person pressing the backs of the hands and fingers together with their wrists flexed as far as possible. This test is positive if tingling or numbness occur in the affected fingers within 1–2 minutes. Doctors may also ask individuals to try to make a movement that brings on symptoms.

- Electrodiagnostic tests may help confirm the diagnosis of CTS. A nerve conduction study measures electrical activity of the nerves and muscles by assessing the nerve's ability to send a signal along the nerve or to the muscle. Electromyography is a special recording technique that detects electrical activity of muscle fibers and can determine the severity of damage to the median nerve.

- Ultrasound imaging can show abnormal size of the median nerve. Magnetic resonance imaging (MRI) can show the anatomy of the wrist but to date has not been especially useful in diagnosing carpal tunnel syndrome.

How Is Carpal Tunnel Syndrome Treated?

Treatments for carpal tunnel syndrome should begin as early as possible, under a doctor's direction. Underlying causes such as diabetes or arthritis should be treated first.

Non-Surgical Treatments

- **Splinting.** Initial treatment is usually a splint worn at night.

- **Avoiding daytime activities that may provoke symptoms.** Some people with slight discomfort may wish to take frequent breaks from tasks, to rest the hand. If the wrist is red, warm and swollen, applying cool packs can help.

- **Over-the-counter drugs.** In special circumstances, drugs can ease the pain and swelling associated with carpal tunnel syndrome. Nonsteroidal anti-inflammatory drugs, such as aspirin, ibuprofen, and other nonprescription pain relievers, may provide some short-term relief from discomfort but haven't been shown to treat CTS itself.

- **Prescription medicines.** Corticosteroids (such as prednisone) or the drug lidocaine can be injected directly into the wrist or taken by mouth (in the case of prednisone) to relieve pressure on the median nerve in people with mild or intermittent symptoms. (Caution: Individuals with diabetes and those who may be predisposed to diabetes should note that prolonged use of corticosteroids can make it difficult to regulate insulin levels.)

- **Alternative therapies.** Yoga has been shown to reduce pain and improve grip strength among those with CTS. Some people report relief using acupuncture and chiropractic care but the effectiveness of these therapies remains unproved.

Surgery

Carpal tunnel release is one of the most common surgical procedures in the United States. Generally, surgery involves severing a ligament around the wrist to reduce pressure on the median nerve. Surgery is usually done under local or regional anesthesia (involving some sedation) and does not require an overnight hospital stay. Many people require surgery on both hands. While all carpal tunnel surgery involves cutting the ligament to relieve the pressure on the nerve, there are two different methods used by surgeons to accomplish this.

- **Open release surgery,** the traditional procedure used to correct carpal tunnel syndrome, consists of making an incision up to 2 inches in the wrist and then cutting the carpal ligament to enlarge the carpal tunnel. The procedure is generally done under local anesthesia on an outpatient basis, unless there are unusual medical conditions.

- **Endoscopic surgery** may allow somewhat faster functional recovery and less postoperative discomfort than traditional open release surgery but it may also have a higher risk of complications and the need for additional surgery. The surgeon makes one or two incisions (about ½ inch each) in the wrist and palm, inserts a camera attached to a tube, observes the nerve, ligament, and tendons on a monitor, and cuts the carpal ligament (the tissue that holds joints together) with a small knife that is inserted through the tube.

Following surgery, the ligaments usually grow back together and allow more space than before. Although symptoms may be relieved immediately after surgery, full recovery from carpal tunnel surgery can take months. Almost always there is a decrease in grip strength, which improves over time. Some individuals may develop infections, nerve damage, stiffness, and pain at the scar. Most people need to modify work activity for several weeks following surgery, and some people may need to adjust job duties or even change jobs after recovery from surgery.

Although recurrence of carpal tunnel syndrome following treatment is rare, fewer than half of individuals report their hand(s) feeling completely normal following surgery. Some residual numbness or weakness is common.

How Can Carpal Tunnel Syndrome Be Prevented?

At the workplace, workers can do on-the-job conditioning, perform stretching exercises, take frequent rest breaks, and ensure correct posture and wrist position. Wearing fingerless gloves can help keep hands warm and flexible. Workstations, tools and tool handles, and tasks can be redesigned to enable the worker's wrist to maintain a natural position during work. Jobs can be rotated among workers. Employers can develop programs in ergonomics, the process of adapting workplace conditions and job demands to the capabilities of workers. However, research has not conclusively shown that these workplace changes prevent the occurrence of carpal tunnel syndrome.

Chapter 49

Chronic Pain

Chronic pain is a very real problem and a major concern for those who suffer from it. Unlike acute pain, chronic pain may last long after an injury has healed. For some people, chronic pain can occur even without a prior injury or trauma. Chronic pain is defined as pain lasting 6 months or longer that may limit daily life. For many, chronic pain can last years or even decades. Once pain is chronic, it is not likely that it will ever completely go away. Because of this, treatment strategies should be focused on learning to manage and live a full life with/or in spite of chronic pain.

Chronic pain is common among women Veterans. Chronic pain may include headache, back pain, arthritis, joint problems, fibromyalgia, and pelvic pain, among others.

Whatever the cause, chronic pain can interfere with your life. Specifically, chronic pain can:

- make it difficult to work and perform everyday activities

- contribute to irritability, depressed mood, or anger

- interfere with sleep

- prompt people to withdraw from activities, friends or loved ones, or it may lead to increased conflict

This chapter includes text excerpted from "Chronic Pain," U.S. Department of Veterans Affairs (VA), March 28, 2017.

- make it hard to participate in physical activity, which can contribute to weight gain

- create financial difficulties from lost wages or the high cost of medical treatments

Managing Chronic Pain

Chronic pain can affect many parts of life. Getting through the day may sometimes seem impossible. Many people with pain avoid activity because they fear their pain will worsen. In the case of chronic pain, too much rest can result in muscle loss, which makes pain worse. On the flip side, too much activity can increase pain. Stress, lack of sleep, weight gain and depressed mood can also increase pain.

Understanding how pain interferes with life can help people choose treatments that can reduce pain while improving functioning. Many different types of treatments may be helpful for people with pain. These include things like medications, injections, surgery, implantable nerve stimulators, pain self-management programs, and physical therapy, acupuncture, chiropractic care, yoga, meditation, relaxation, massage, aquatherapy, and biofeedback.

- **Medications** include nonsteroidal antiinflammatory drugs (like ibuprofen), opioids, tramadol, and some antiseizure or antidepressant medications.

- **Injections** like botulinum toxin and cortisone can be used to manage certain types of pain.

- **Cognitive Behavioral Pain Self-Management** programs are usually provided by health psychologists. These programs teach relaxation skills, and other oping strategies to help people manage pain better and to deal with the difficult emotions that can occur when people have pain. They also address sleep problems and are sometimes offered together with physical therapy.

- **Physical Therapy** can help people with chronic pain find a physical activity program that is gentle, moderate, and right for the individual. Types of physical therapy that may help pain include:

  - heat treatment—hot water baths, heating pads, high-frequency sound waves to produce gentle heat deep in your tissues

  - cold treatment—ice packs, ice baths, ice massage

- gentle stretching

- Muscle-strengthening

- body mechanics

- vibration therapy—a probe is applied to a part of your body with moderate pressure and vibrated several thousand times per second

- **Chiropractic care** involves hands-on manipulation of the body as a means to properly align the spine and to restore mobility to joints.

- **Acupuncture** involves the placement of small needles into the skin at various points in the body.

- **Yoga** involves breath control, meditation, and a series of physical poses. Yoga can help strengthen muscles, improve functioning, reduce stress and improve mood.

- **Meditation** teaches awareness techniques to relax the body and quiet the mind. It has been found to help reduce pain, improve mood, and decrease stress.

- **Massage** involves applying pressure to specific points on the body. It can help reduce stress and muscle tension which can reduce pain.

- **Relaxation** treatments come in many forms (imagery, progressive muscle relaxation, deep breathing). These exercises reduce the stress and muscle tension that are common with pain.

- **Aquatherapy** is a water based type of physical therapy. Exercises are done in a pool usually with the help of a specially trained physical therapist.

- **Biofeedback** is used to learn how to control body functions such as muscle tension and other bodily responses to stress. Electrical sensors provide information about physical signals such as increases in heart rate, muscle tension or skin temperature.

Chapter 50

Diabetes in Women

Diabetes is a disease in which blood sugar (glucose) levels in your body are too high. Diabetes can cause serious health problems, including heart attack or stroke, blindness, problems during pregnancy, and kidney failure. More than 13 million women have diabetes, or about one in 10 women ages 20 and older.

What Is Diabetes?

Diabetes is a disease caused by high levels of blood sugar (glucose) in your body. This can happen when your body does not make insulin or does not use insulin correctly.

Insulin is a hormone made in the pancreas, an organ near your stomach. Insulin helps the glucose from food get into your body's cells for energy. If your body does not make enough insulin, or your body does not use the insulin correctly, the glucose stays and builds up in your blood.

Over time, this extra glucose can lead to prediabetes or diabetes. Diabetes puts you at risk for other serious and life-threatening health problems, such as heart disease, stroke, blindness, and kidney damage.

What Are the Different Types of Diabetes?

The three main types of diabetes are:

- **Type 1 diabetes.** Type 1 diabetes is an autoimmune disease, meaning the body's immune (defense) system attacks and

This chapter includes text excerpted from "Diabetes," Office on Women's Health (OWH), U.S. Department of Health and Human Services (HHS), October 29, 2014.

destroys the cells in the pancreas that make insulin. If you have type 1 diabetes, your body does not make insulin, so you must take insulin every day.

- **Type 2 diabetes.** This is the most common type of diabetes. You can get type 2 diabetes at any age, even during childhood. With type 2 diabetes, your body does not make enough insulin or is not able to use its own insulin correctly. When this happens, blood glucose levels rise.

- **Gestational diabetes.** Gestational diabetes is a type of diabetes that happens only during pregnancy. Gestational diabetes can cause health problems for the baby and the mother if not controlled. Although gestational diabetes goes away after your baby is born, having diabetes during pregnancy raises your risk for type 2 diabetes later on.

Am I at Risk for Diabetes?

A risk factor is something that puts you at a higher risk for a disease compared with an average person.

Risk factors for **type 1 diabetes** in women and girls include:

- **Age**: It often develops in childhood.

- **Family health history**: Having a parent or brother or sister with type 1 diabetes

- **Certain viral infections or illnesses**, such as coxsackie virus B (a common cause of hand, foot, and mouth disease), rotavirus (also called stomach flu), and mumps

- **Where you live**: It is more common in people who live in colder climates.

Risk factors for **type 2 diabetes** in women and girls include:

- Overweight or obesity: Body mass index (BMI) of 25 or higher for adults. Find out your BMI. Children and teens weighing above the 85th percentile based on their BMI are at risk for type 2 diabetes.

- Older age: 45 or older. After menopause, women are at higher risk for weight gain, especially more weight around the waist, which raises the risk for type 2 diabetes.

- Family health history: Having a mother, father, brother, or sister with diabetes

- Race/ethnicity: Family background of African-American, American Indian/Alaska Native, Hispanic, Asian-American, and Native Hawaiian/Pacific Islander

- Having a baby that weighed 9 pounds or more at birth

- Having diabetes during pregnancy (gestational diabetes)

- High blood pressure: Taking medicine for high blood pressure or having a blood pressure of 140/90 mmHg or higher. (Both numbers are important. If one or both numbers are usually high, you have high blood pressure.)

- High cholesterol: HDL cholesterol of 35 mg/dL or lower and triglycerides of 250 mg/dL or higher

- Lack of physical activity: Women who are active less than three times a week

- Having polycystic ovary syndrome (PCOS)

- Personal history of heart disease or stroke

If you have any of these risk factors, talk to your doctor about ways to lower your risk for diabetes.

Who Gets Diabetes?

Type 1 diabetes usually develops in childhood, but it can happen at any age. It is more common in whites than in other racial or ethnic groups. About 5 percent of adults with diabetes have type 1 diabetes. Genes you inherit from your parents play an important role in the development of type 1 diabetes. However, where you live may also affect your risk. Type 1 diabetes develops more often in winter and in people who live in colder climates.

Type 2 diabetes is more common in adults, especially in people who are overweight and have a family history of diabetes. About 95 percent of adults with diabetes have type 2 diabetes. Type 2 diabetes is becoming more common in children and teens as more of them become overweight and obese.

Do Women of Color Need to Worry about Diabetes?

Yes. Certain racial and ethnic groups have a higher risk for type 2 diabetes. These groups include:

- **African-Americans.** African-American women are twice as likely to develop diabetes as white women. African-Americans are also more likely to have health problems caused by diabetes and excess weight.

- **Hispanics.** Hispanic women are twice as likely to develop diabetes as white women. Diabetes affects more than one in 10 Hispanics. Among Hispanic women, diabetes affects Mexican-Americans and Puerto Ricans most often.

- **American Indian/Alaskan Native.** Diabetes affects nearly 16 percent of American Indian/Alaskan Native adults.

- **Native Hawaiian/Pacific Islander.** Native Hawaiians/Pacific Islanders are about twice as likely to develop diabetes as whites.

- **Asian-Americans.** Diabetes is the fifth-leading cause of death for Asian-Americans. Asian-American women are also more likely to develop gestational diabetes than white women and usually develop gestational diabetes at a lower body weight.

How Does Diabetes Affect Women Differently than Men?

Diabetes affects women and men in almost equal numbers. However, diabetes affects women differently than men.

Compared with men with diabetes, women with diabetes have:

- A higher risk for heart disease. Heart disease is the most common complication of diabetes.

- Lower survival rates and a poorer quality of life after heart attack

- A higher risk for blindness

- A higher risk for depression. Depression, which affects twice as many women as men, also raises the risk for diabetes in women.

Does Diabetes Raise My Risk for Other Health Problems?

Yes. The longer you have type 2 diabetes, the higher your risk for developing serious medical problems from diabetes. Also, if you smoke and have diabetes, you are even more likely to develop serious medical problems from diabetes, compared with people who have diabetes and do not smoke.

The extra glucose in the blood that leads to diabetes can damage your nerves and blood vessels. Nerve damage from diabetes can lead to pain or a permanent loss of feeling in your hands, feet, and other parts of your body.

Blood vessel damage from diabetes can also lead to:

- Heart disease

- Stroke

- Blindness

- Kidney failure

- Leg or foot amputation

- Hearing loss

Women with diabetes are also at higher risk for:

- Problems getting pregnant

- Problems during pregnancy, including possible health problems for you and your baby

- Repeated urinary and vaginal infections

What Causes Diabetes?

Researchers do not know the exact causes of type 1 and type 2 diabetes. Researchers do know that inheriting certain genes from your family can raise your risk for developing diabetes. Obesity is also a major risk factor for type 2 diabetes. Smoking can also cause type 2 diabetes. And the more you smoke the higher your risk for type 2 diabetes and other serious health problems if you already have diabetes.

Weight loss can help control type 2 diabetes so that you are healthier. Quitting smoking can also help you control your blood sugar levels. Being a healthy weight and not smoking can help all women be healthier.

But, obesity and smoking do not always cause diabetes. Some women who are overweight or obese or smoke never develop diabetes. Also, women who are a normal weight or only slightly overweight can develop diabetes if they have other risk factors, such as a family history of diabetes.

What Are the Signs and Symptoms of Diabetes?

Type 1 diabetes symptoms are usually more severe and may develop suddenly.

Type 2 diabetes may not cause any signs or symptoms at first. Symptoms can develop slowly over time. You may not notice them right away.

Common signs and symptoms of type 1 and type 2 diabetes include:

- Feeling more tired than usual

- Extreme thirst

- Urinating more than usual

- Blurry vision

- Feeling hungrier than usual

- Losing weight without trying

- Sores that are slow to heal

- Dry, itchy skin

- Tingling in the hands or feet

- More infections, such as urinary tract infections and vaginal yeast infections, than usual

Do I Need to Be Tested for Diabetes?

Maybe. You should be tested for diabetes if you are between 40 and 70 years old and are overweight or obese. Your doctor may recommend testing earlier than age 40 if you also have other risk factors for diabetes. Also, talk to your doctor about diabetes testing if you have signs or symptoms of diabetes. Your doctor will use a blood test to see if you have diabetes.

If the testing shows that your blood sugar levels are high, you can begin making healthy changes to your eating habits and getting more physical activity to help prevent diabetes.

What Is Prediabetes?

Prediabetes means your blood sugar (glucose) level is higher than normal, but it is lower than the diabetes range. It also means you are at higher risk of getting type 2 diabetes and heart disease.

As many as 27 million American women have prediabetes. If you have prediabetes, you can make healthy changes, such as doing some type of physical activity on most days, to lower your risk of getting diabetes and return to normal blood sugar levels. Losing 7 percent of your body weight (or 14 pounds if you weigh 200 pounds) can lower your risk for type 2 diabetes by more than half. If you have prediabetes, get your blood glucose checked every year by a doctor or nurse.

How Is Diabetes Treated?

Diabetes treatment includes managing your blood sugar levels to control your symptoms. You can help control your blood sugar levels by eating healthy and getting regular physical activity.

With type 1 diabetes, you also will need to take insulin through shots or an insulin pump. Insulin cannot be taken as a pill.

Type 2 diabetes treatment also may include taking medicine to control your blood sugar. Over time, people with type 2 diabetes make less and less of their own insulin. This may mean that you will need to increase your medicines or start taking insulin shots to keep your diabetes in control.

Is There Anything I Can Do to Prevent Type 1 Diabetes?

Researchers do not know how to prevent type 1 diabetes. Researchers are still looking for ways to prevent type 1 diabetes in women and girls by studying their close relatives who have diabetes.

Is There Anything I Can Do to Prevent Type 2 Diabetes?

Yes. Many studies, including the large Diabetes Prevention Program study, have proven that you can prevent diabetes by losing weight. Weight loss through healthy eating and more physical activity improves the way your body uses insulin and glucose.

- **Weight loss:** Obesity is a leading risk factor for diabetes. Calculate your BMI to see whether you're at a healthy weight. If you're overweight or obese, start making small changes to your eating habits and get more physical activity. Even a small amount of weight loss (7%, or about 14 pounds for a 200-pound woman) can delay or even prevent type 2 diabetes.

- **Eating healthy:** Choose vegetables, whole grains (such as whole wheat or rye bread, whole grain cereal, or brown rice), beans, and fruit. Read food labels to help you choose foods low in saturated fat, trans fat, and sodium. Limit processed foods and sugary foods and drinks.

- **Getting active:** Aim for 30 minutes of physical activity most days of the week and limit the amount of time you spend sitting.

Is It Safe for Women with Diabetes to Get Pregnant?

Yes. If you have type 1 or type 2 diabetes, you can have a healthy pregnancy. If you have diabetes and you want to have a baby, you need to plan ahead, before you get pregnant.

Talk to your doctor before you get pregnant. He or she can talk to you about steps you can take to keep your baby healthy. This may include a diabetes education program to help you better understand your diabetes and how to control it during pregnancy.

Chapter 51

Female Athlete Triad

Do You Exercise a Lot?

Being active is great. In fact, girls should be active at least an hour each day. Sometimes, though, a girl will be very active (such as running every day or playing a competitive sport), but not eat enough to fuel her activity. This can lead to health problems.

The following can happen when girls don't eat enough to fuel their activity:

- A problem called "low energy availability"

- Period (menstrual) problems

- Bone problems

These three sometimes are called the female athlete triad. ("Triad" means a group of three). They sometimes also are called Athletic Performance and Energy Deficit. (This means you have a "deficit," or lack, of the energy your body needs to stay healthy.)

This chapter contains text excerpted from the following sources: Text under the heading "Do You Exercise a Lot?" is excerpted from "Do You Exercise a Lot?" girlshealth.gov, Office on Women's Health (OWH), March 27, 2015; Text under the heading "Amenorrheic Women and the Female Athlete Triad" is excerpted from "Calcium," Office of Dietary Supplements (ODS), National Institutes of Health (NIH), November 17, 2016.

A Problem Called "Low Energy Availability"

Your body needs healthy food to fuel the things it does, like fight infections, heal wounds, and grow. If you exercise, your body needs extra food for your workout. You can get learn how much food to eat based on your activity level using the SuperTracker tool accessible on the Internet at www.choosemyplate.gov/MyPlate-Daily-Checklist.

"Energy availability" means the fuel from food that is not burned up by exercise and so is available for growing, healing, and more. If you exercise a lot and don't get enough nutrition, you may have low energy availability. That means your body won't be as healthy and strong as it should be.

Some female athletes diet to lose weight. They may do this to qualify for their sport or because they think losing weight will help them perform better. But eating enough healthy food is key to having the strength you need to succeed. Also, your body needs good nutrition to make hormones that help with things like healthy periods and strong bones.

Sometimes, girls may exercise too much and eat too little because they have an eating disorder. Eating disorders are serious and can even lead to death, but they are treatable.

Period (Menstrual) Problems

If you are very active, or if you just recently started getting your period (menstruating), you may skip a few periods. But if you work out really hard and do not eat enough, you may skip a lot of periods (or not get your period to begin with) because your body can't make enough of the hormone estrogen.

You may think you wouldn't mind missing your period, but not getting your period should be taken seriously. Not having your period can mean your body is not building enough bone, and the teenage years are the main time for building strong bones.

If you have been getting your period regularly and then miss three periods in a row, see your doctor. Not having your period could be a sign of a serious health problem or of being pregnant. Also see your doctor if you are 15 years old and still have not gotten your period.

Bone Problems

Being physically active helps build strong bones. But you can hurt your bones if you don't eat enough healthy food to fuel all your activity. That's because your body won't be able to make the hormones needed to build strong bones.

One sign that your bones are weak is getting stress fractures, which are tiny cracks in bones. Some places you could get these cracks are your feet, legs, ribs, and spine.

ven if you don't have problems with your bones when you're young, not taking good care of them now can be a problem later in life. Your skeleton is almost completely formed by age 18, so it's important to build strong bones early in life. If you don't, then later on you could wind up with osteoporosis, which is a disease that makes it easier for bones to break.

Signs of Not Eating Enough and Eating Disorders

Sometimes, girls exercise a lot and do not eat enough because they want to lose weight. Sometimes, exercising just lowers a person's appetite. And sometimes limiting food can be a sign that a girl may be developing an eating disorder. Here are some signs that you or a friend may have a problem:

- Worrying about gaining weight if you don't exercise enough
- Trying harder to find time to exercise than to eat
- Chewing gum or drinking water to cope with hunger
- Often wanting to exercise rather than be with friends
- Exercising instead of doing homework or other responsibilities
- Getting very upset if you miss a workout, but not if you miss a meal
- Having people tell you they are worried you are losing too much weight

If you think you or a friend has a problem, talk to a parent, guardian, or trusted adult.

Amenorrheic Women and the Female Athlete Triad

Amenorrhea, the condition in which menstrual periods stop or fail to initiate in women of childbearing age, results from reduced circulating estrogen levels that, in turn, have a negative effect on calcium balance. Amenorrheic women with anorexia nervosa have decreased calcium absorption and higher urinary calcium excretion rates, as well as a lower rate of bone formation than healthy women. The "female athlete triad" refers to the combination of disordered eating, amenorrhea, and osteoporosis. Exercise-induced amenorrhea generally results in decreased bone mass. In female athletes and active women in the military, low bone-mineral density, menstrual irregularities, certain dietary patterns, and a history of prior stress fractures are associated with an increased risk of future stress fractures. Such women should be advised to consume adequate amounts of calcium and vitamin D. Supplements of these nutrients have been shown to reduce the risk of stress fractures in female Navy recruits during basic training.

Chapter 52

Gastrointestinal and Digestive Disorders Common in Women

Chapter Contents

Section 52.1

Irritable Bowel Syndrome (IBS)

This section includes text excerpted from "Irritable
Bowel Syndrome (IBS)," National Institute of Diabetes and
Digestive and Kidney Diseases (NIDDK), February 2015.

What Is Irritable Bowel Syndrome (IBS)?

Irritable bowel syndrome (IBS) is a group of symptoms—including
pain or discomfort in your abdomen and changes in your bowel movement patterns—that occur together. Doctors call IBS a functional
gastrointestinal (GI) disorder. Functional GI disorders happen when
your GI tract behaves in an abnormal way without evidence of damage
due to a disease

What Are the Four Types of IBS?

Doctors often classify IBS into one of four types based on your usual
stool consistency. These types are important because they affect the
types of treatment that are most likely to improve your symptoms.

The four types of IBS are:

- IBS with constipation, or IBS-C
  - hard or lumpy stools at least 25 percent of the time
  - loose or watery stools less than 25 percent of the time
- IBS with diarrhea, or IBS-D
  - loose or watery stools at least 25 percent of the time
  - hard or lumpy stools less than 25 percent of the time
- Mixed IBS, or IBS-M
  - hard or lumpy stools at least 25 percent of the time
  - loose or watery stools at least 25 percent of the time
- Unsubtyped IBS, or IBS-U
  - hard or lumpy stools less than 25 percent of the time
  - loose or watery stools less than 25 percent of the time

Who Is More Likely to Develop IBS?

IBS affects about twice as many women as men and most often occurs in people younger than age 45.

What Are the Symptoms of IBS?

The most common symptoms of irritable bowel syndrome (IBS) include pain or discomfort in your abdomen and changes in how often you have bowel movements or how your stools look. The pain or discomfort of IBS may feel like cramping and have at least two of the following:

- Your pain or discomfort improves after a bowel movement.
- You notice a change in how often you have a bowel movement.
- You notice a change in the way your stools look.

IBS is a chronic disorder, meaning it lasts a long time, often years. However, the symptoms may come and go. You may have IBS if:

- You've had symptoms at least three times a month for the past 3 months.
- Your symptoms first started at least 6 months ago.

People with IBS may have diarrhea, constipation, or both. Some people with IBS have only diarrhea or only constipation. Some people have symptoms of both or have diarrhea sometimes and constipation other times. People often have symptoms soon after eating a meal.

Other symptoms of IBS are:

- bloating
- the feeling that you haven't finished a bowel movement
- whitish mucus in your stool

Women with IBS often have more symptoms during their menstrual periods.

While IBS can be painful, IBS doesn't lead to other health problems or damage your gastrointestinal (GI) tract.

What Causes IBS?

Doctors aren't sure what causes IBS. Experts think that a combination of problems can lead to IBS.

Physical Problems

Brain-Gut Signal Problems

Signals between your brain and the nerves of your gut, or small and large intestines, control how your gut works. Problems with brain-gut signals may cause IBS symptoms.

GI Motility Problems

If you have IBS, you may not have normal motility in your colon. Slow motility can lead to constipation and fast motility can lead to diarrhea. Spasms can cause abdominal pain. If you have IBS, you may also experience hyperreactivity—a dramatic increase in bowel contractions when you feel stress or after you eat.

Pain Sensitivity

If you have IBS, the nerves in your gut may be extra sensitive, causing you to feel more pain or discomfort than normal when gas or stool is in your gut. Your brain may process pain signals from your bowel differently if you have IBS.

Infections

A bacterial infection in the GI tract may cause some people to develop IBS. Researchers don't know why infections in the GI tract lead to IBS in some people and not others, although abnormalities of the GI tract lining and mental health problems may play a role.

Small Intestinal Bacterial Overgrowth

Normally, few bacteria live in your small intestine. Small intestinal bacterial overgrowth is an increase in the number or a change in the type of bacteria in your small intestine. These bacteria can produce extra gas and may also cause diarrhea and weight loss. Some experts think small intestinal bacterial overgrowth may lead to IBS. Research continues to explore a possible link between the two conditions.

Neurotransmitters (Body Chemicals)

People with IBS have altered levels of neurotransmitters—chemicals in the body that transmit nerve signals—and GI hormones. The role these chemicals play in IBS is unclear.

Younger women with IBS often have more symptoms during their menstrual periods. Postmenopausal women have fewer symptoms compared with women who are still menstruating. These findings suggest that reproductive hormones can worsen IBS problems.

Genetics

Whether IBS has a genetic cause, meaning it runs in families, is unclear. Studies have shown IBS is more common in people with family members who have a history of GI problems.

Food Sensitivity

Many people with IBS report that foods rich in carbohydrates, spicy or fatty foods, coffee, and alcohol trigger their symptoms. However, people with food sensitivity typically don't have signs of a food allergy. Researchers think that poor absorption of sugars or bile acids may cause symptoms.

Mental Health Problems

Psychological, or mental health, problems such as panic disorder, anxiety, depression, and posttraumatic stress disorder are common in people with IBS. The link between mental health and IBS is unclear. GI disorders, including IBS, are sometimes present in people who have reported past physical or sexual abuse. Experts think people who have been abused tend to express psychological stress through physical symptoms.

If you have IBS, your colon may respond too much to even slight conflict or stress. Stress makes your mind more aware of the sensations in your colon. IBS symptoms can also increase your stress level.

How Do Doctors Diagnose IBS?

Your doctor may be able to diagnose irritable bowel syndrome (IBS) based on a review of your medical history, symptoms, and physical exam. Your doctor may also order tests.

To diagnose IBS, your doctor will take a complete medical history and perform a physical exam.

Medical History

The medical history will include questions about:

- your symptoms

- family history of gastrointestinal (GI) tract disorders
- recent infections
- medicines
- stressful events related to the start of your symptoms

Your doctor will look for a certain pattern in your symptoms. Your doctor may diagnose IBS if

- your symptoms started at least 6 months ago
- you've had pain or discomfort in your abdomen at least three times a month for the past 3 months
- your abdominal pain or discomfort has two or three of the following features:
  - Your pain or discomfort improves after a bowel movement.
  - You notice a change in how often you have a bowel movement.
  - You notice a change in the way your stools look.

Physical Exam

During a physical exam, your doctor usually:

- checks for abdominal bloating
- listens to sounds within your abdomen using a stethoscope
- taps on your abdomen checking for tenderness or pain

What Tests Do Doctors Use to Diagnose IBS?

In most cases, doctors don't need to perform tests to diagnose IBS. Your doctor may perform a blood test to check for other conditions or problems. Your doctor may perform more tests based on the results of the blood test and if you have:

- a family history of celiac disease, colon cancer, or inflammatory bowel disease
- a fever
- anemia
- bleeding from your rectum
- weight loss

How Do Doctors Treat IBS?

Though irritable bowel syndrome (IBS) doesn't have a cure, your doctor can manage the symptoms with a combination of diet, medicines, probiotics, and therapies for mental health problems. You may have to try a few treatments to see what works best for you. Your doctor can help you find the right treatment plan.

How Can My Diet Treat the Symptoms of IBS?

Eating smaller meals more often, or eating smaller portions, may help your irritable bowel syndrome (IBS) symptoms. Large meals can cause cramping and diarrhea if you have IBS.

Eating foods that are low in fat and high in carbohydrates, such as pasta, rice, whole-grain breads and cereals, fruits, and vegetables, may help.

Fiber may improve constipation symptoms caused by IBS because it makes stool soft and easier to pass. Fiber is a part of foods such as whole-grain breads and cereals, beans, fruits, and vegetables. The U.S. Department of Agriculture (USDA) and U.S. Department of Health and Human Services (HHS) state in its *Dietary Guidelines for Americans,* 2010 that adults should get 22 to 34 grams of fiber a day.

While fiber may help constipation, it may not reduce the abdominal discomfort or pain of IBS. In fact, some people with IBS may feel a bit more abdominal discomfort after adding more fiber to their diet. Add foods with fiber to your diet a little at a time to let your body get used to them. Too much fiber at once can cause gas, which can trigger symptoms in people with IBS. Adding fiber to your diet slowly, by 2 to 3 grams a day, may help prevent gas and bloating.

Section 52.2

Inflammatory Bowel Disease (IBD)

This section includes text excerpted from "Inflammatory Bowel
Disease (IBD)," Centers for Disease Control and Prevention (CDC),
March 14, 2017.

Inflammatory bowel disease (IBD) is a broad term that describes
conditions characterized by chronic inflammation of the gastrointestinal tract. The two most common inflammatory bowel diseases are
ulcerative colitis and Crohn's disease. Inflammation affects the entire
digestive tract in Crohn's disease and only the large intestine (also
called the colon) in ulcerative colitis. Both illnesses involved an abnormal response to the body's immune system.

What Is Inflammatory Bowel Disease (IBD)?

Inflammatory bowel disease (IBD) is a term for two conditions
(Crohn's disease and ulcerative colitis) that are characterized by
chronic inflammation of the gastrointestinal (GI) tract. Prolonged
inflammation results in damage to the GI tract.

Table 52.1. Differences between Crohn's Disease and Ulcerative
Colitis

Crohn's Disease	Ulcerative Colitis
Can affect any part of the GI tract (from the mouth to the anus)—Most often it affects the portion of the small intestine before the large intestine/colon.	Occurs in the large intestine (colon) and the rectum
Damaged areas appear in patches that are next to areas of healthy tissue	Damaged areas are continuous (not patchy)—usually starting at the rectum and spreading further into the colon
Inflammation may reach through the multiple layers of the walls of the GI tract	Inflammation is present only in the innermost layer of the lining of the colon

What Are the Symptoms of IBD?

Some common symptoms are:

- Persistent diarrhea
- Abdominal pain
- Rectal bleeding/bloody stools
- Weight loss
- Fatigue

What Causes IBD?

The exact cause of IBD is unknown, but IBD is the result of a defective immune system. A properly functioning immune system attacks foreign organisms, such as viruses and bacteria, to protect the body. In IBD, the immune system responds incorrectly to environmental triggers, which causes inflammation of the gastrointestinal tract. There also appears to be a genetic component—someone with a family history of IBD is more likely to develop this inappropriate immune response.

How Is IBD Diagnosed?

IBD is diagnosed using a combination of endoscopy (for Crohn's disease) or colonoscopy (for ulcerative colitis) and imaging studies, such as contrast radiography, magnetic resonance imaging (MRI), or computed tomography (CT). Physicians may also check stool samples to make sure symptoms are not being caused by an infection or run blood tests to help confirm the diagnosis.

How Is IBD Treated?

Several types of medications may be used to treat IBD: aminosalicylates, corticosteroids (such as prednisone), immunomodulators, and the newest class approved for IBD—the "biologics." Several vaccinations for patients with IBD are recommended to prevent infections. Severe IBD may require surgery to remove damaged portions of the gastrointestinal tract, but advances in treatment with medications mean that surgery is less common than it was a few decades ago. Since Crohn's disease and ulcerative colitis affect different parts of the GI tract, the surgical procedures are different for the two conditions.

Section 52.3

Gallstones

This section includes text excerpted from "Dieting & Gallstones,"
National Institute of Diabetes and Digestive and Kidney Diseases
(NIDDK), February 2015.

According to estimates, as many as 20 million Americans have gallstones—solid deposits that may form in the gallbladder. Most people
with gallstones do not know that they have them and experience no
symptoms (signs that a disease is present). Others may have symptoms
like pain and nausea in the abdomen (the part of the body that holds
the stomach, intestines, and other organs), often after meals. In some
cases, gallstones may cause serious health problems that require the
gallbladder to be removed.

Although it is not clear what causes gallstones, many factors may
increase your chances of having problems related to gallstones. These
factors include having too much body fat, especially around your waist,
and losing weight very quickly. This section will tell you more about
gallstones, how they are linked to obesity and dieting, and how you
may help prevent this very common health problem.

What Are Gallstones?

Gallstones are hard crystals that may form in the gallbladder, a
small pear-shaped organ located on the right side of the abdomen,
under the liver. The gallbladder helps the body digest foods by storing
and releasing bile into the small intestine. Bile, a liquid made in the
liver, has bile salts and other substances that help break down fats
so they can be digested.

Gallstones form when substances in the bile join together to form
crystals. These crystals lodge in the inner lining of the gallbladder,
growing into gallstones over time. Gallstones can vary from the size
of little pebbles to as large as golf balls. The gallbladder may have one
or more gallstones of different sizes.

In the United States, most gallstones are made of cholesterol, a type
of fat that is created in the liver and is also found in foods from animal

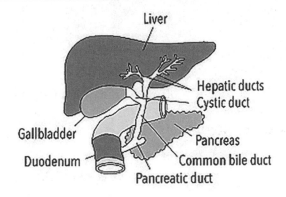

Figure 52.1. *Gallbladder*

sources, such as dairy products, eggs, meat, and poultry. Cholesterol gallstones are yellow in color. Other types of gallstones, called pigment stones, are made up of other substances in the bile.

How Can I Tell If I Have Gallstones?

Most people who have gallstones have no signs. These gallstones are called "silent gallstones" and do not need to be treated.

In some people, a gallstone may become stuck in the narrow canal, or duct, that carries bile from the gallbladder to the small intestine. The blockage may cause the gallbladder, ducts, or more rarely, the liver or pancreas to become inflamed.

Signs of gallstones or a gallstone attack include these:

- severe pain in the upper-right side of the abdomen that starts suddenly and lasts from 30 minutes to many hours

- pain under the right shoulder or in the right shoulder blade

- indigestion after eating foods high in fat or protein, including desserts and fried foods

Gallstone attacks often take place during the night.

Symptoms of a Serious Gallbladder Attack

You may want to seek help right away if you have any of these symptoms:

- abdominal pain that lasts more than 5 hours

- clay-colored stools

- fever or chills

- nausea and vomiting

- yellowish color of the skin or of the whites of the eyes

What Causes Gallstones?

What causes gallstones is not clear. Most gallstones are made up of cholesterol, a type of fat made in the liver and obtained from some foods.

Gallstones may form when:

- the liver releases too much cholesterol into the bile

- there are not enough bile salts in the bile to dissolve the cholesterol

- there are other substances in the bile that cause the cholesterol to form crystals

- the gallbladder does not empty completely or often enough, which concentrates the bile

Gallstones are more common among women and adults ages 40 and older than among other groups. The female sex hormone estrogen may help explain why gallstones are more common among women than among men. Estrogen may increase the amount of cholesterol in the bile and decrease gallbladder movement, which may lead to gallstones.

Other factors that may increase your chances of developing gallstones are these:

- diabetes

- family history of gallstones

- high triglycerides (a type of fat in the blood)

- lack of physical activity

- low HDL (good) cholesterol

- obesity, particularly a large waist size

- pregnancy

- rapid weight loss

Some drugs may also increase your chances of getting gallstones. Among them are drugs that have estrogen, such as birth control pills and hormone replacement therapy (medicine that may be given to some women to address problems related to menopause). Taking drugs that lower cholesterol levels in the blood may also make it more likely that you will develop gallstones, as some of these drugs may make the liver release more cholesterol into the bile.

How May Obesity Increase My Chances of Getting Gallstones?

Being overweight or obese may increase your chances of having gallstones, especially among female. Researchers have found that people who are obese may produce high levels of cholesterol. This may produce bile having more cholesterol than it can dissolve. When this happens, gallstones can form.

People who are obese may also have large gallbladders that do not work well. Some studies have shown that women and men who carry large amounts of fat around their waist may be more likely to develop gallstones than those who carry fat around their hips and thighs.

Although rapid weight loss may increase your chances of developing gallstones, obesity may be a bigger problem. In addition to gallstones, obesity is linked to many serious health problems, including diabetes, heart disease, stroke, and certain types of cancer.

For those who are overweight or obese, even a small weight loss of 10 percent of body weight over a period of 6 months can improve health. In addition, weight loss may bring other benefits such as better mood, increased energy, and positive self-image.

How May Rapid Weight Loss Increase My Chances of Getting Gallstones?

Losing weight very quickly may increase your chances of forming gallstones. If you have silent gallstones, you may also be more likely to develop symptoms. People who lose more than 3 pounds per week may have a greater chance of getting gallstones than those who lose weight more slowly.

Some ways of treating obesity, such as weight-loss surgery and very low-calorie diets (VLCDs), may increase your chances of developing gallstones by promoting rapid weight loss.

Weight-loss surgery is an operation on the stomach and/or intestines to help people lose weight by limiting food intake and/or by affecting how food is digested.

A very low-calorie diet is a very restrictive diet that uses a commercially prepared formula providing about 800 calories per day. A healthcare provider closely supervises these types of diets.

Several factors may increase your chances of having problems with gallstones after weight-loss surgery or a VLCD. They include:

- existing gallstones before your surgery or VLCD, especially if they are causing symptoms

- a large amount of excess weight before the surgery or VLCD

- very rapid weight loss after the surgery or VLCD

Your chances of developing gallstones may vary by type of treatment. Diets or surgeries that cause very rapid weight loss may be more likely to lead to gallstone problems than diets or surgeries that lead to slower weight loss.

If you are starting a VLCD or having weight-loss surgery, talk to your healthcare provider about how to reduce your chances of getting gallstones.

Is Weight Cycling a Problem?

Weight cycling, or losing and regaining weight repeatedly, may also lead to gallstones. The more weight you lose and regain during a cycle, the greater your chances of developing gallstones.

When trying to lose weight on your own, stay away from "crash diets" that promise to help you drop the pounds quickly. Aim for losing weight at a slower pace and keeping it off over time.

How May I Safely Lose Weight and Reduce My Chances of Getting Gallstones?

Losing weight at a slow pace may make it less likely that you will develop gallstones. Depending on your starting weight, experts recommend losing about 1/2 to 2 pounds per week.

When making healthy food choices to help you lose weight, you can choose food that may also lower your chances of developing gallstones.

Experts recommend the following:

- Eat more foods high in fiber, like brown rice, oats, and whole wheat bread.

- Eat fewer refined grains and less sugar.

- Eat healthy fats, like fish oil and olive oil, to help your gallbladder contract and empty on a regular basis.

Regular physical activity, which may improve your health, is also related to a reduced chance of developing gallstones. To lose weight or prevent weight gain, aim for 300 minutes (5 hours) of moderately intense aerobic activity each week. Aerobic activity uses your large muscles (back, chest, and legs), increases your heart rate, and may make you breathe harder. To sustain weight loss, you may need at least 60 to 90 minutes a day.

If you are thinking about starting an eating and physical activity plan to lose weight, talk with your healthcare provider first. Together, you can discuss various eating and physical activity programs, your medical history, and the benefits and risks of losing weight, including the chances of developing gallstones.

How Are Gallstones Treated?

Silent gallstones are usually left alone and sometimes disappear on their own. Gallstones that are causing symptoms are usually treated.

The most common way to treat gallstones that are causing symptoms is to remove the organ. This operation is called a cholecystectomy. In most cases, surgeons can use a laparoscope, a thin, lighted tube that shows them what is inside your abdomen. The surgery is done while you are under general anesthesia (asleep and pain-free). The surgeon makes small cuts in your abdomen to insert the surgical tools and take out the gallbladder.

Most people go home on the same day or the day after this surgery. If there were problems during your surgery, or if you have bleeding, a lot of pain, or a fever, you may need to stay in the hospital longer. In general, you can expect to go home once you are able to eat and drink without pain and are able to walk without help. It may take about a week for you to fully recover.

Chapter 53

Lung Disease in Women

What Is Lung Disease?

Lung disease refers to disorders that affect the lungs, the organs that allow us to breathe. Breathing problems caused by lung disease may prevent the body from getting enough oxygen. Examples of lung diseases are:

- Asthma, chronic bronchitis, and emphysema
- Infections, such as influenza and pneumonia
- Lung cancer
- Sarcoidosis and pulmonary fibrosis

Lung disease is a major concern for women. The number of U.S. women diagnosed with lung disease is on the rise. More women are also dying from lung disease.

What Types of Lung Disease Are Most Common in Women?

Three of the most common lung diseases in women are asthma, chronic obstructive pulmonary disease (COPD), and lung cancer.

This chapter includes text excerpted from "Lung Disease," Office on Women's Health (OWH), U.S. Department of Health and Human Services (HHS), June 12, 2017.

Asthma

Asthma is a chronic (ongoing) disease of the airways in the lungs called bronchial tubes. Bronchial tubes carry air into and out of the lungs. In people with asthma, the walls of these airways become inflamed (swollen) and oversensitive. The airways overreact to things like smoke, air pollution, mold, and many chemical sprays. They also can be irritated by allergens (like pollen and dust mites) and by respiratory infections (like a cold). When the airways overreact, they get narrower. This limits the flow of air into and out of the lungs and causes trouble breathing. Asthma symptoms include wheezing, coughing, and tightness in the chest.

Women are more likely than men to have asthma and are more likely to die from it. The percentage of women, especially young women, with asthma is rising in the United States. Researchers are not sure why. Many experts think that air pollution and allergens play a role in this increase. Breathing tobacco smoke also is linked to an increased risk of asthma.

Chronic Obstructive Pulmonary Disease

Chronic obstructive pulmonary disease (COPD) refers to chronic obstructive bronchitis and emphysema. These conditions often occur together. Both diseases limit airflow into and out of the lungs and make breathing difficult. COPD usually gets worse with time.

A person with COPD has ongoing inflammation of the bronchial tubes, which carry air into and out of the lungs. This irritation causes the growth of cells that make mucus. The extra mucus leads to a lot of coughing. Over time, the irritation causes the walls of the airways to thicken and develop scars. The airways may become thickened enough to limit airflow to and from the lungs. If that happens, the condition is called chronic obstructive bronchitis.

In emphysema, the lung tissue gets weak, and the walls of the air sacs (alveoli) break down. Normally, oxygen from the air goes into the blood through these air sac walls. In a person with emphysema, the ruined air sac walls means less oxygen can pass into the blood. This causes shortness of breath, coughing, and wheezing.

More than twice as many women as men are now diagnosed with chronic bronchitis. The rate of emphysema among women has increased by 5 percent in recent years but has decreased among men. And more women have died from COPD than men every year since 2000. Researchers are trying to understand why. Cigarette smoking, a main cause of COPD, has increased among women.

One theory is that cigarette smoke is more damaging to women than to men.

Lung Cancer

Lung cancer is a disease in which abnormal (malignant) lung cells multiply and grow without control. These cancerous cells can invade nearby tissues, spread to other parts of the body, or both. The two major kinds of lung cancer are named for the way the cells look under a microscope. They are:

- **Small cell lung cancer.** This kind of lung cancer tends to spread quickly.

- **Non-small cell lung cancer.** This is a term for several types of lung cancers that act in a similar way. Most lung cancers are non-small cell. This kind of lung cancer tends to spread more slowly than small cell lung cancer.

In the United States, more women now die from lung cancer than from any other type of cancer. Tobacco use is the major cause of lung cancer.

Other Lung Diseases

Less common lung problems that affect women include:

- **Pulmonary emboli.** These are blood clots that travel to the lungs from other parts of the body and plug up blood vessels in the lungs. Some factors that increase your risk include being pregnant, having recently given birth, and taking birth control pills or menopausal hormone therapy. Pulmonary emboli can affect blood flow in the lungs and can reduce oxygen flow into the blood. Very large emboli can cause sudden death.

- **Pulmonary hypertension.** This is high blood pressure in the arteries that bring blood to the lungs. It can affect blood flow in the lungs and can reduce oxygen flow into the blood.

- **Sarcoidosis and pulmonary fibrosis.** These inflammatory diseases cause stiffening and scarring in the lungs.

- **LAM (lymphangioleiomyomatosis).** This is a rare lung disease that mostly affects women in their mid-30s and 40s. Muscle-like cells grow out of control in certain organs, including the lungs.

- **Influenza (the flu) and pneumonia.** Flu is a respiratory infection that is caused by a virus and can damage the lungs. Usually, people recover well from the flu, but it can be dangerous and even deadly for some people. Those at greater risk include older people, young children, pregnant women, and people with certain health conditions like asthma. Pneumonia is a severe inflammation of the lungs that can be caused by bacteria, viruses, and fungi. Fluid builds up in the lungs and may lower the amount of oxygen that the blood can get from air that's breathed in. People most at risk are older than 65 or younger than 2, or already have health problems. Vaccines are the best protection against flu and pneumonia.

What Causes Lung Disease?

Experts don't know the causes of all types of lung disease, but they do know the causes of some. These include:

- **Smoking.** Smoke from cigarettes, cigars, and pipes is the number one cause of lung disease. Don't start smoking, or quit if you already smoke. If you live or work with a smoker, avoid secondhand smoke. Ask smokers to smoke outdoors. Secondhand smoke is especially bad for babies and young children.

- **Radon.** This colorless, odorless gas is present in many homes and is a recognized cause of lung cancer. You can check for radon with a kit bought at many hardware stores. Radon can be reduced in your home if you find out there are high levels.

- **Asbestos.** This is natural mineral fiber that is used in insulation, fireproofing materials, car brakes, and other products. Asbestos can give off small fibers that are too small to be seen and can be inhaled. Asbestos harms lung cells, causing lung scarring and lung cancer. It can cause mesothelioma, which is a cancer that forms in the tissue covering the lungs and many other organs of the body.

- **Air pollution.** Recent studies suggest that some air pollutants like car exhaust may contribute to asthma, COPD, lung cancer, and other lung diseases.

Some diseases that affect the lungs, like the flu, are caused by germs (bacteria, viruses, and fungi).

How Would I Know If I Have a Lung Disease?

Early signs of lung disease are easy to overlook. Often, an early sign of lung disease is not having your usual level of energy.

The signs and symptoms can differ by the type of lung disease. Common signs are:

- Trouble breathing

- Shortness of breath

- Feeling like you're not getting enough air

- Decreased ability to exercise

- A cough that won't go away

- Coughing up blood or mucus

- Pain or discomfort when breathing in or out

Make sure to call your doctor if you have any of these symptoms.

How Can I Find Out If I Have Asthma?

Asthma can be hard to diagnose. The signs of asthma can seem like the signs of COPD, pneumonia, bronchitis, pulmonary embolism, anxiety, and heart disease.

Common symptoms of asthma are:

- Coughing

- Wheezing

- Chest tightness

- Shortness of breath

To diagnose asthma, the doctor asks about your symptoms and what seems to trigger them, reviews your health history, and does a physical exam.

To confirm the diagnosis, the doctor may do other tests, such as:

- Spirometry

- Bronchoprovocation

- Chest X-ray or EKG (electrocardiogram)

- Other tests:

  - The doctor may want to test for other problems that might be causing the symptoms. These include stomach acid backing up into the throat, vocal cord problems, or sleep apnea.

How Is Asthma Treated?

Asthma is a chronic disease. Medicines can be used to treat asthma, but they cannot cure it. You can help control your symptoms by working with your doctor to set up and then follow a personal asthma action plan. The plan will include possible medications and ways to avoid things that trigger your asthma.

Following an Asthma Action Plan

Your asthma action plan will show:

- The kinds of medicines you should take

- When to take your medicines

- How to regularly monitor your asthma

- Ways to avoid what triggers your asthma

- When to call your doctor or go to the emergency room

Taking medicines

Asthma medicines work by opening the lung airways. The medicines used to treat asthma fall into two groups: long-term control and quick relief.

Long-term control medicines are to be taken every day, usually over a long period of time. They help prevent symptoms from starting. Once symptoms occur, they do not give quick relief. These medicines include:

- **Inhaled corticosteroids.** These are the preferred medicines for long-term asthma control. They relieve airway inflammation and swelling.

- **Long-acting beta2-agonists.** These inhaled medicines are often added to low-dose inhaled corticosteroids to improve long-term asthma control.

- **Leukotriene modifiers.** These pills help block the chain reaction that causes inflammation in the airways.

- **Cromolyn and nedocromil**. These inhaled medicines can help keep airways from reacting in response to an asthma trigger.

- **Theophylline**. This is a pill that helps open the airways.

Quick-relief medicines are used only when needed. These include short-acting inhaled beta2-agonists and short-acting bronchodilators, like albuterol and pirbuteral. Quick-relief medicines often relieve symptoms in minutes. They do this by quickly relaxing tightened muscles around the airways. They are taken when symptoms worsen to prevent a full-blown asthma attack and to stop attacks once they have started.

Avoiding Asthma Triggers

Avoid things that make your asthma worse. Common asthma triggers are tobacco smoke, animal dander, dust mites, air pollution, mold, and pollens. You can try "fragrance-free" products if your asthma is triggered by fragrances. Talk to your doctor about allergy shots if your asthma symptoms are linked to allergens that you cannot avoid. The shots may lessen or prevent the symptoms but will not cure the asthma. You can reduce your exposure to air pollution by limiting your outdoor activities on days when the air quality in your neighborhood is poor.

What about Pregnancy and Asthma?

People with COPD have symptoms that develop very slowly over many years. As a result, many people ignore these symptoms until their disease has reached an advanced stage. COPD can be easily diagnosed and can be managed.

The symptoms of COPD include:

- An ongoing cough that often produces large amounts of mucus

- Shortness of breath, especially during physical activity

- Wheezing

- Chest tightness

If you have some or all of these symptoms, make sure to talk to your doctor.

To find out if you have COPD, the doctor will:

- Ask about your symptoms

- Ask about your medical history, including family history

- Ask about your history of exposure to things that can cause COPD, such as tobacco smoke, air pollution, or chemicals

- Do a physical exam, including using a stethoscope to listen for wheezing or other abnormal chest sounds

The main test to check for COPD is spirometry. For this test, you will be asked to take a deep breath and blow as hard as you can into a tube that is connected to a spirometer. This machine measures how much air you breathe out and how fast.

Other tests can include:

- Chest X-ray or chest computed tomography (CT) scan

- Arterial blood gas test

How Is COPD Treated?

Damage to the lungs cannot be repaired. The disease can be slowed by avoiding certain exposures, though. For smokers, the best approach is to stop smoking. You should also limit your exposure to smoke, dust, fumes, and irritating vapors at home and work. Also limit outdoor activities during air pollution alerts. Treatment can relieve symptoms. Common medicines are:

- **Bronchodilators** to open up air passages in the lungs

- **Inhaled steroids** to relieve symptoms by reducing inflammation in the lungs

- **Antibiotics** to clear up infections in the lungs

For patients with COPD, doctors may also recommend:

- **Flu shots.** Influenza (flu) can cause serious problems for people with COPD.

- **Pneumonia shots.** The pneumococcal vaccine reduces the risk of some kinds of pneumonia.

- **Pulmonary rehabilitation.** This treatment helps people cope physically and mentally with COPD. It can include exercise, training to manage the disease, diet advice, and counseling.

- **Oxygen therapy.** The patient receives extra oxygen, either through a tube or mask.

- **Surgery.** Sometimes surgery can help people with severe COPD feel better. Lung transplant surgery is becoming more common for people with severe emphysema. Another procedure called lung volume reduction surgery is also used to treat some patients with severe COPD of the emphysema type. In this surgery, the most damaged part of each lung is removed.

How Do I Find Out If I Have Lung Cancer?

Usually there are no warning signs of early lung cancer. By the time most people with lung cancer have symptoms, the cancer has become more serious.

Symptoms of lung cancer may include:

- A cough that doesn't go away or gets worse
- Breathing trouble, like shortness of breath
- Coughing up blood
- Chest pain
- Hoarseness or wheezing
- Pneumonia that doesn't go away or that goes away and comes back

In addition, you may feel very tired, have a loss of appetite, or unexplained weight loss. If you have symptoms of lung cancer, it's important to talk to your doctor. The doctor will ask about your health history, smoking history, and exposure to harmful substances. He or she will also do a physical exam and may suggest some tests.

Common tests for diagnosis of lung cancer include:

- Chest X-rays
- Sputum cytology
- Bronchoscopy
- Fine-needle aspiration
- Thoracotomy

If I Smoke, Should I Get Tested for Lung Cancer?

Testing for cancer before a person has any symptoms is called screening. Screening may help find cancers early, when they may be easier to treat.

Many studies show that screening smokers with X-rays or sputum cytology does not save lives. But recently a major study showed that CT scans of older people who smoke a lot (or used to smoke a lot) can save lives. Experts are still working to figure out who should get CT screening. There are risks and benefits to screening for lung cancer.

For now, the U.S. Preventive Services Task Force (USPSTF) makes no recommendation either for or against routine screening for lung cancer. If you're concerned about your lung cancer risk, talk to your doctor about whether screening is right for you. Of course, the best way to reduce your risk of lung cancer is not to smoke.

How Is Lung Cancer Treated?

Sometimes lung cancer treatments are used to try to cure the cancer. Other times, treatments are used to stop the cancer from spreading and to relieve symptoms.

Your specific treatment will depend on:

- The type of lung cancer

- Where the cancer is and if it has spread to other parts of the body

- Your age and overall health

Your doctor may recommend one treatment or a combination of treatments.

- Surgery

- Radiation therapy

- Chemotherapy

- Targeted therapy

Can I Lower My Risk for Lung Disease?

Things you can do to reduce your risk of lung diseases include:

- **Stop smoking.** If you smoke, the most important thing you can do is stop. Talk to your doctor about the best way to quit. All kinds of smoking (cigarettes, cigars, pipes, and marijuana) can boost the chances of lung disease.

- **Avoid secondhand smoke.** If you live or work with people who smoke cigarettes, pipes, or cigars, ask them to smoke outside. Non-smokers have the right to a smoke-free workplace.

- **Test for radon.** Find out if there are high levels of the gas radon in your home or workplace. You can buy a radon test kit at most hardware stores. The U.S. Environmental Protection Agency (EPA) offers information on how to deal with radon.

- **Avoid asbestos.** Exposure to asbestos can cause scarring of the lungs, lung cancer, and other serious lung disease. Asbestos can be a particular concern for those whose jobs put them in contact with it. This includes people who maintain buildings that have insulation or other materials that contain asbestos and people who repair car brakes or clutches. Employers of those who work with asbestos should offer training about asbestos safety and should regularly check levels of exposure. They also should provide ways to limit exposure, such as special breathing masks that filter asbestos dust from the air.

- **Protect yourself from dust and chemical fumes.** Working in dusty conditions and with chemicals can increase your risk of lung disease. And the risk is not just from industrial chemicals. Many products used at home, like paints and solvents, can cause or aggravate lung disease. Read labels and carefully follow instructions for use. If possible, avoid using products that cause eye, nose, or throat irritation. If you can't avoid them, use them as little as possible and only in a well-ventilated area. Wear protective equipment such as a special mask. Make sure you know which type of equipment you need and how to wear it.

- **Eat a healthy diet.** The National Cancer Institute notes that studies show that eating a lot of fruits or vegetables may help lower the risk of lung cancer. Of course, diet can't undo the damage caused by unhealthy behaviors like smoking.

- **Ask your doctor if you should have a spirometry test.** Some groups recommend routine spirometry testing of at-risk people, such as people who are over 45 and smoke and those who are exposed to lung-damaging substances at work.

- **Ask your doctor about protecting yourself from flu and pneumonia with vaccinations.**

- **See your doctor** if you have a cough that won't go away, trouble breathing, pain or discomfort in your chest, or any of the other symptoms described here.

709

Chapter 54

Mental Health Concerns among Women

Chapter Contents

Section 54.1

Anxiety Disorders

This section includes text excerpted from "Anxiety
Disorders," Office on Women's Health (OWH), U.S. Department of
Health and Human Services (HHS), February 12, 2015.

Anxiety is a normal response to stress. But when it becomes hard
to control and affects your day-to-day life, it can be disabling. Anxiety
disorders affect nearly one in five adults in the United States. Women
are more than twice as likely as men to get an anxiety disorder in
their lifetime. Anxiety disorders are often treated with counseling,
medicine, or a combination of both. Some women also find that yoga
or meditation helps with anxiety disorders.

What Is Anxiety?

Anxiety is a feeling of worry, nervousness, or fear about an event
or situation. It is a normal reaction to stress. It helps you stay alert
for a challenging situation at work, study harder for an exam, or
remain focused on an important speech. In general, it helps you
cope.

But anxiety can be disabling if it interferes with daily life, such as
making you dread nonthreatening day-to-day activities like riding the
bus or talking to a coworker. Anxiety can also be a sudden attack of
terror when there is no threat.

What Are Anxiety Disorders?

Anxiety disorders happen when excessive anxiety interferes with
your everyday activities such as going to work or school or spending
time with friends or family. Anxiety disorders are serious mental illnesses. They are the most common mental disorders in the United
States. Anxiety disorders are more than twice as common in women
as in men.

What Are the Major Types of Anxiety Disorder?

The major types of anxiety disorder are:

- **Generalized anxiety disorder (GAD).** People with GAD worry excessively about ordinary, day-to-day issues, such as health, money, work, and family. With GAD, the mind often jumps to the worst-case scenario, even when there is little or no reason to worry. Women with GAD may be anxious about just getting through the day. They may have muscle tension and other stress-related physical symptoms, such as trouble sleeping or upset stomach. At times, worrying keeps people with GAD from doing everyday tasks. Women with GAD have a higher risk of depression and other anxiety disorders than men with GAD. They also are more likely to have a family history of depression.

- **Panic disorder.** Panic disorders are twice as common in women as in men. People with panic disorder have sudden attacks of terror when there is no actual danger. Panic attacks may cause a sense of unreality, a fear of impending doom, or a fear of losing control. A fear of one's own unexplained physical symptoms is also a sign of panic disorder. People having panic attacks sometimes believe they are having heart attacks, losing their minds, or dying.

- **Social phobia.** Social phobia, also called social anxiety disorder, is diagnosed when people become very anxious and self-conscious in everyday social situations. People with social phobia have a strong fear of being watched and judged by others. They may get embarrassed easily and often have panic attack symptoms.

- **Specific phobia.** A specific phobia is an intense fear of something that poses little or no actual danger. Specific phobias could be fears of closed-in spaces, heights, water, objects, animals, or specific situations. People with specific phobias often find that facing, or even thinking about facing, the feared object or situation brings on a panic attack or severe anxiety.

Some other conditions that are not considered anxiety disorders but are similar include:

- **Obsessive-compulsive disorder (OCD).** People with OCD have unwanted thoughts (obsessions) or behaviors (compulsions) that

713

cause anxiety. They may check the oven or iron again and again or perform the same routine over and over to control the anxiety these thoughts cause. Often, the rituals end up controlling the person.

- **Posttraumatic stress disorder (PTSD).** PTSD starts after a scary event that involved physical harm or the threat of physical harm. The person who gets PTSD may have been the one who was harmed, or the harm may have happened to a loved one or even a stranger.

Who Gets Anxiety Disorders?

Anxiety disorders affect about 40 million American adults every year. Anxiety disorders also affect children and teens. About 8 percent of teens ages 13 to 18 have an anxiety disorder, with symptoms starting around age 6.

Women are more than twice as likely as men to get an anxiety disorder in their lifetime. Also, some types of anxiety disorders affect some women more than others:

- **Generalized anxiety disorder (GAD)** affects more American Indian/Alaskan Native women than women of other races and ethnicities. GAD also affects more white women and Hispanic women than Asian or African-American women.

- **Social phobia** and **panic disorder** affect more white women than women of other races and ethnicities.

What Causes Anxiety Disorders?

Researchers think anxiety disorders are caused by a combination of factors, which may include:

- Hormonal changes during the menstrual cycle

- Genetics. Anxiety disorders may run in families.

- Traumatic events. Experiencing abuse, an attack, or sexual assault can lead to serious health problems, including anxiety, posttraumatic stress disorder, and depression.

What Are the Signs and Symptoms of an Anxiety Disorder?

Women with anxiety disorders experience a combination of anxious thoughts or beliefs, physical symptoms, and changes in behavior, including avoiding everyday activities they used to do. Each anxiety disorder has different symptoms. They all involve a fear and dread about things that may happen now or in the future.

Physical symptoms may include:

- Weakness

- Shortness of breath

- Rapid heart rate

- Nausea

- Upset stomach

- Hot flashes

- Dizziness

Physical symptoms of anxiety disorders often happen along with other mental or physical illnesses. This can cover up your anxiety symptoms or make them worse.

How Are Anxiety Disorders Diagnosed?

Your doctor or nurse will ask you questions about your symptoms and your medical history. Your doctor may also do a physical exam or other tests to rule out other health problems that could be causing your symptoms.

Anxiety disorders are diagnosed when fear and dread of nonthreatening situations, events, places, or objects become excessive and are uncontrollable. Anxiety disorders are also diagnosed if the anxiety has lasted for at least six months and it interferes with social, work, family, or other aspects of daily life.

How Are Anxiety Disorders Treated?

Treatment for anxiety disorders depends on the type of anxiety disorder you have and your personal history of health problems, violence, or abuse.

Often, treatment may include:

- Counseling (called psychotherapy)

- Medicine

- A combination of counseling and medicine

How Does Counseling Help Treat Anxiety Disorders?

Your doctor may refer you for a type of counseling for anxiety disorders called cognitive behavioral therapy (CBT). You can talk to a trained mental health professional about what caused your anxiety disorder and how to deal with the symptoms.

For example, you can talk to a psychiatrist, psychologist, social worker, or counselor. CBT can help you change the thinking patterns around your fears. It may help you change the way you react to situations that may create anxiety. You may also learn ways to reduce feelings of anxiety and improve specific behaviors caused by chronic anxiety. These strategies may include relaxation therapy and problem solving.

What Types of Medicine Treat Anxiety Disorders?

Several types of medicine treat anxiety disorders. These include:

- Antianxiety (benzodiazepines)
- Beta blockers
- Selective serotonin reuptake inhibitors (SSRIs)
- Tricyclics
- Monoamine oxidase inhibitors (MAOIs)

All medicines have risks. You should talk to your doctor about the benefits and risks of all medicines.

What If My Anxiety Disorder Treatment Is Not Working?

Sometimes, you may need to work with your doctor to try several different treatments or combinations of treatments before you find one that works for you.

If you are having trouble with side effects from medicines, talk to your doctor or nurse. Do not stop taking your medicine without talking to a doctor or nurse. Your doctor may adjust how much medicine you take and when you take it.

What If My Anxiety Disorder Comes Back?

Sometimes symptoms of an anxiety disorder come back after you have finished treatment. This may happen during or after a stressful event. It may also happen without any warning.

Many people with anxiety disorders do get better with treatment. But, if your symptoms come back, your doctor will work with you to change or adjust your medicine or treatment plan.

You can also talk to your doctor about ways to identify and prevent anxiety from coming back. This may include writing down your feelings or meeting with your counselor if you think your anxiety is uncontrollable.

Can Complementary or Alternative Medicine Help Manage Anxiety Disorders?

Maybe. Some women say that complementary or alternative medicine (CAM) therapies helped lower their anxiety.

CAM therapies that may help anxiety include:

- **Physical activity.** Regular physical activity raises the level of brain chemicals that control mood and affect anxiety and depression. Many studies show that all types of physical activity, including yoga and Tai Chi, help reduce anxiety.

- **Meditation.** Studies show meditation may improve anxiety. Regular meditation may help by boosting activity in the area of your brain responsible for feelings of serenity and joy.

Will My Anxiety Disorder Treatment Affect My Pregnancy?

If your treatment is counseling, it will not affect your pregnancy.

If you are on medicine to treat your anxiety disorder, talk to your doctor. Some medicines used to treat anxiety can affect your unborn baby.

If I Take Medicine to Treat My Anxiety Disorder, Can I Breastfeed My Baby?

It depends. Some medicines used to treat anxiety can pass through breastmilk. Certain antidepressants, such as some selective serotonin reuptake inhibitors (SSRIs), are safe to take during breastfeeding.

Do not stop taking your medicine too quickly. Talk to your doctor to find out what medicine is best for you and your baby.

How Do Anxiety Disorders Affect Other Health Conditions?

Anxiety disorders may affect other health problems that are common in women. These include:

- Depression

- Irritable bowel syndrome (IBS)

- Chronic pain

- Cardiovascular disease

- Asthma

Section 54.2

Depression in Women

This section includes text excerpted from "Depression,"
Office on Women's Health (OWH), U.S. Department of
Health and Human Services (HHS), February 12, 2016.

When a person has a depressive disorder, it hurts their daily life, normal functioning, and causes pain for both the person with the disorder and those who care about him or her. Depression is a common but serious illness, and most who have it need treatment to get better. Different kinds of depression include:

- **Major depressive disorder.** Also called major depression, this is a combination of symptoms that interfere with a person's ability to work, sleep, study, eat, and enjoy once-pleasurable activities.

- **Dysthymic disorder.** Also called dysthymia, this kind of depression lasts for a long time (two years or longer). The symptoms are less severe than major depression but can prevent one from living normally or feeling well.

Some forms of depressive disorder exhibit slightly different characteristics than those described above, or they may develop under unique circumstances. However, not all scientists agree on how to characterize and define these forms of depression. They include:

- **Psychotic depression**, which occurs when a severe depressive illness is accompanied by some form of psychosis, such as a break with reality, hallucinations, and delusions.

- **Postpartum depression**, which is diagnosed if a new mother develops a major depressive episode within one month after delivery.

- **Seasonal affective disorder (SAD)**, which is a depression during the winter months, when there is less natural sunlight.

The U.S. Preventive Services Task Force (USPSTF) recommends screening for depression for everyone, including women who are pregnant or recently had a baby.

Symptoms of depression include:

- Persistent sad, anxious, or "empty" feelings

- Feelings of hopelessness and/or pessimism

- Feelings of guilt, worthlessness, and/or helplessness

- Irritability, restlessness

- Loss of interest in activities or hobbies once pleasurable, including sex

- Fatigue and decreased energy

- Difficulty concentrating, remembering details and making decisions

- Insomnia, early-morning wakefulness, or excessive sleeping

- Overeating, or appetite loss

- Thoughts of suicide, suicide attempts

- Persistent aches or pains, headaches, cramps or digestive problems that do not get better, even with treatment

Treatment

Depression, even the most severe cases, can be treated. The sooner treatment begins, the more effective it is.

The first step to getting appropriate treatment is to visit a doctor. Certain medications, and some medical conditions (such as viruses or a thyroid disorder), can cause the same symptoms as depression. A doctor can rule out these possibilities with a physical exam, by asking questions, and lab tests. If the doctor can rule out a medical condition as a cause, he or she should conduct a psychological exam or refer the patient to a mental health professional.

The doctor or mental health professional will conduct a complete diagnostic exam. He or she should discuss any family history of depression, and get a complete history of symptoms. He or she should also ask if the patient is using alcohol or drugs, and whether the patient is thinking about death or suicide.

The most common treatments for depression are medication (antidepressants) and psychotherapy.

Section 54.3

Eating Disorders

This section includes text excerpted from "Eating Disorders: About More Than Food," National Institute of Mental Health (NIMH), September 2015.

What Are Eating Disorders?

The eating disorders anorexia nervosa, bulimia nervosa, and binge-eating disorder, and their variants, all feature serious disturbances in eating behavior and weight regulation. They are associated with a wide range of adverse psychological, physical, and social consequences. A person with an eating disorder may start out just eating smaller or larger amounts of food, but at some point, their urge to eat less or more spirals out of control. Severe distress or concern about body weight or shape, or extreme efforts to manage weight or food intake, also may characterize an eating disorder.

Eating disorders are real, treatable medical illnesses. They frequently coexist with other illnesses such as depression, substance abuse, or anxiety disorders. Other symptoms can become life-threatening if a person does not receive treatment, which is reflected by anorexia being associated with the highest mortality rate of any psychiatric disorder.

Eating disorders affect both genders, although rates among women and girls are 2½ times greater than among men and boys. Eating disorders frequently appear during the teen years or young adulthood but also may develop during childhood or later in life.

What Are the Different Types of Eating Disorders?

Anorexia Nervosa

Many people with anorexia nervosa see themselves as overweight, even when they are clearly underweight. Eating, food, and weight control become obsessions. People with anorexia nervosa typically weigh themselves repeatedly, portion food carefully, and eat very small quantities of only certain foods. Some people with anorexia nervosa also may engage in binge eating followed by extreme dieting, excessive exercise, self-induced vomiting, or misuse of laxatives, diuretics, or enemas.

Symptoms of anorexia nervosa include:

- Extremely low body weight

- Severe food restriction

- Relentless pursuit of thinness and unwillingness to maintain a normal or healthy weight

- Intense fear of gaining weight

- Distorted body image and self-esteem that is heavily influenced by perceptions of body weight and shape, or a denial of the seriousness of low body weight

- Lack of menstruation among girls and women.

Some who have anorexia nervosa recover with treatment after only one episode. Others get well but have relapses. Still others have a more chronic, or long-lasting, form of anorexia nervosa, in which their health declines as they battle the illness.

Other symptoms and medical complications may develop over time, including:

- Thinning of the bones (osteopenia or osteoporosis)

- Brittle hair and nails

- Dry and yellowish skin

- Growth of fine hair all over the body (lanugo)

- Mild anemia, muscle wasting, and weakness
- Severe constipation
- Low blood pressure, or slowed breathing and pulse
- Damage to the structure and function of the heart
- Brain damage
- Multi-organ failure
- Drop in internal body temperature, causing a person to feel cold all the time
- Lethargy, sluggishness, or feeling tired all the time
- Infertility

Bulimia Nervosa

People with bulimia nervosa have recurrent and frequent episodes of eating unusually large amounts of food and feel a lack of control over these episodes. This binge eating is followed by behavior that compensates for the overeating such as forced vomiting, excessive use of laxatives or diuretics, fasting, excessive exercise, or a combination of these behaviors.

Unlike anorexia nervosa, people with bulimia nervosa usually maintain what is considered a healthy or normal weight, while some are slightly overweight. But like people with anorexia nervosa, they often fear gaining weight, want desperately to lose weight, and are intensely unhappy with their body size and shape. Usually, bulimic behavior is done secretly because it is often accompanied by feelings of disgust or shame. The binge eating and purging cycle can happen anywhere from several times a week to many times a day.

Other symptoms include:

- Chronically inflamed and sore throat
- Swollen salivary glands in the neck and jaw area
- Worn tooth enamel, and increasingly sensitive and decaying teeth as a result of exposure to stomach acid
- Acid reflux disorder and other gastrointestinal problems
- Intestinal distress and irritation from laxative abuse
- Severe dehydration from purging of fluids

- Electrolyte imbalance—too low or too high levels of sodium, calcium, potassium, and other minerals that can lead to a heart attack or stroke

Binge-Eating Disorder

People with binge-eating disorder lose control over their eating. Unlike bulimia nervosa, periods of binge eating are not followed by compensatory behaviors like purging, excessive exercise, or fasting. As a result, people with binge-eating disorder often are overweight or obese. People with binge-eating disorder who are obese are at higher risk for developing cardiovascular disease and high blood pressure. They also experience guilt, shame, and distress about their binge eating, which can lead to more binge eating.

How Are Eating Disorders Treated?

Typical treatment goals include restoring adequate nutrition, bringing weight to a healthy level, reducing excessive exercise, and stopping binging and purging behaviors. Specific forms of psychotherapy, or talk therapy—including a family-based therapy called the Maudsley approach and cognitive behavioral approaches—have been shown to be useful for treating specific eating disorders. Evidence also suggests that antidepressant medications approved by the U.S. Food and Drug Administration (FDA) may help for bulimia nervosa and also may be effective for treating co-occurring anxiety or depression for other eating disorders.

Treatment plans often are tailored to individual needs and may include one or more of the following:

- Individual, group, or family psychotherapy
- Medical care and monitoring
- Nutritional counseling
- Medications (for example, antidepressants)

Some patients also may need to be hospitalized to treat problems caused by malnutrition or to ensure they eat enough if they are very underweight. Complete recovery is possible.

Section 54.4

Seasonal Affective Disorder

This section includes text excerpted from
"Seasonal Affective Disorder," National Institute of
Mental Health (NIMH), March 2016.

Seasonal affective disorder (SAD) is a type of depression that comes and goes with the seasons, typically starting in the late fall and early winter and going away during the spring and summer. Depressive episodes linked to the summer can occur, but are much less common than winter episodes of SAD.

Signs and Symptoms

Seasonal affective disorder (SAD) is not considered as a separate disorder. It is a type of depression displaying a recurring seasonal pattern. To be diagnosed with SAD, people must meet full criteria for major depression coinciding with specific seasons (appearing in the winter or summer months) for at least 2 years. Seasonal depressions must be much more frequent than any non-seasonal depressions.

Symptoms of Major Depression

- Feeling depressed most of the day, nearly every day
- Feeling hopeless or worthless
- Having low energy
- Losing interest in activities you once enjoyed
- Having problems with sleep
- Experiencing changes in your appetite or weight
- Feeling sluggish or agitated
- Having difficulty concentrating
- Having frequent thoughts of death or suicide

Symptoms of the winter pattern of SAD include:

- Having low energy
- Hypersomnia
- Overeating
- Weight gain
- Craving for carbohydrates
- Social withdrawal (feel like "hibernating")

Symptoms of the less frequently occurring summer SAD include:

- Poor appetite with associated weight loss
- Insomnia
- Agitation
- Restlessness
- Anxiety
- Episodes of violent behavior

Risk Factors

Attributes that may increase your risk of SAD include:

- **Being female**
- **Living far from the equator.** SAD is more frequent in people who live far north or south of the equator. For example, 1 percent of those who live in Florida and 9 percent of those who live in New England or Alaska suffer from SAD.
- **Family history.** People with a family history of other types of depression are more likely to develop SAD than people who do not have a family history of depression.
- **Having depression or bipolar disorder.** The symptoms of depression may worsen with the seasons if you have one of these conditions (but SAD is diagnosed only if seasonal depressions are the most common).
- **Younger age**. Younger adults have a higher risk of SAD than older adults. SAD has been reported even in children and teens.

Causes

The causes of SAD are unknown, but research has found some biological clues:

- People with SAD may have trouble regulating one of the key neurotransmitters involved in mood, serotonin. One study found that people with SAD have 5 percent more serotonin transporter protein in winter months than summer months. Higher serotonin transporter protein leaves less serotonin available at the synapse because the function of the transporter is to recycle neurotransmitter back into the presynaptic neuron.

- People with SAD may overproduce the hormone melatonin. Darkness increases production of melatonin, which regulates sleep. As winter days become shorter, melatonin production increases, leaving people with SAD to feel sleepier and more lethargic, often with delayed circadian rhythms.

- People with SAD also may produce less Vitamin D. Vitamin D is believed to play a role in serotonin activity. Vitamin D insufficiency may be associated with clinically significant depression symptoms.

Treatments and Therapies

There are four major types of treatment for SAD:

- Medication: Selective serotonin reuptake inhibitors (SSRIs) are used to treat SAD. The U.S. Food and Drug Administration (FDA) has also approved the use of bupropion, another type of antidepressant, for treating SAD.

- Light therapy: The idea behind light therapy is to replace the diminished sunshine of the fall and winter months using daily exposure to bright, artificial light. Symptoms of SAD may be relieved by sitting in front of a light box first thing in the morning, on a daily basis from the early fall until spring.

- Psychotherapy: Cognitive behavioral therapy (CBT) is type of psychotherapy that is effective for SAD (CBT-SAD). CBT-SAD relies on basic techniques of CBT such as identifying negative thoughts and replacing them with more positive thoughts along with a technique called behavioral activation.

- Vitamin D: At present, vitamin D supplementation by itself is not regarded as an effective SAD treatment. The reason behind its use is that low blood levels of vitamin D were found in people with SAD. The low levels are usually due to insufficient dietary intake or insufficient exposure to sunshine. However, the evidence for its use has been mixed.

These may be used alone or in combination.

Chapter 55

Migraine Headaches in Women

What Is Migraine?

Migraine is a medical condition. Most people who suffer from migraines get headaches that can be quite severe. A migraine headache is usually an intense, throbbing pain on one, or sometimes, both sides of the head. Most people with migraine headache feel the pain in the temples or behind one eye or ear, although any part of the head can be involved. Besides pain, migraine also can cause nausea and vomiting and sensitivity to light and sound. Some people also may see spots or flashing lights or have a temporary loss of vision.

Migraine can occur any time of the day, though it often starts in the morning. The pain can last a few hours or up to one or two days. Some people get migraines once or twice a week. Others, only once or twice a year. Most of the time, migraines are not a threat to your overall health. But migraine attacks can interfere with your day-to-day life.

We don't know what causes migraine, but some things are more common in people who have them:

- Most often, migraine affects people between the ages of 15 and 55.

This chapter includes text excerpted from "Migraine," Office on Women's Health (OWH), U.S. Department of Health and Human Services (HHS), June 12, 2017.

- Most people have a family history of migraine or of disabling headache.

- They are more common in women.

- Migraine often becomes less severe and less frequent with age.

How Common Are Migraines?

Migraine pain and symptoms affect 29.5 million Americans. Migraine is the most common form of disabling headache that sends patients to see their doctors.

What Causes Migraines?

The exact cause of migraine is not fully understood. Most researchers think that migraine is due to abnormal changes in levels of substances that are naturally produced in the brain. When the levels of these substances increase, they can cause inflammation. This inflammation then causes blood vessels in the brain to swell and press on nearby nerves, causing pain.

Genes also have been linked to migraine. People who get migraines may have abnormal genes that control the functions of certain brain cells.

Experts do know that people with migraines react to a variety of factors and events, called triggers. These triggers can vary from person to person and don't always lead to migraine. A combination of triggers—not a single thing or event—is more likely to set off an attack. A person's response to triggers also can vary from migraine to migraine. Many women with migraine tend to have attacks triggered by:

- Lack of or too much sleep

- Skipped meals

- Bright lights, loud noises, or strong odors

- Hormone changes during the menstrual cycle

- Stress and anxiety, or relaxation after stress

- Weather changes

- Alcohol (often red wine)

- Caffeine (too much or withdrawal)

- Foods that contain *nitrates,* such as hot dogs and lunch meats

- Foods that contain MSG (monosodium glutamate), a flavor enhancer found in fast foods, broths, seasonings, and spices

- Foods that contain *tyramine,* such as aged cheeses, soy products, fava beans, hard sausages, smoked fish, and Chianti wine

- Aspartame (NutraSweet® and Equal®)

To pinpoint your migraine triggers, keep a headache diary. Each day you have a migraine headache, put that in your diary. Also write down the:

- The time of day your headache started

- Where you were and what you were doing when the migraine started

- What you ate or drank 24 hours before the attack

- Each day you have your period, not just the first day (This can allow you and your doctor to see if your headaches occur at the same or similar time as your period.)

Talk with your doctor about what sets off your headaches to help find the right treatment for you.

Are There Different Kinds of Migraine?

Yes, there are many forms of migraine. The two forms seen most often are migraine with aura and migraine without aura.

Migraine with aura (previously called classical migraine). With a migraine with aura, a person might have these sensory symptoms (the so-called "aura") 10 to 30 minutes before an attack:

- Seeing flashing lights, zigzag lines, or blind spots

- Numbness or tingling in the face or hands

- Disturbed sense of smell, taste, or touch

- Feeling mentally "fuzzy"

Only one in five people who get migraine experience an aura. Women have this form of migraine less often than men.

Migraine without aura (previously called common migraine). With this form of migraine, a person does not have an aura but has all the other features of an attack.

How Can I Tell If I Have a Migraine or Just a Bad Tension-Type Headache?

Compared with migraine, tension-type headache is generally less severe and rarely disabling. Compare your symptoms with those in this chart to see what type of headache you might be having.

Table 55.1. Migraine versus Bad Tension-Type Headache

Symptom	Tension Headache	Migraine Headache
Intensity of pain: Mild-to-moderate	x	x
Intensity of pain: Moderate-to-severe		x
Quality of pain: Intense pounding or throbbing and/or debilitating		x
Quality of pain: Distracting, but not debilitating	x	
Quality of pain: Steady ache	x	x
Location of pain: One side of head		x
Location of pain: Both sides of head	x	x
Nausea, vomiting		x
Sensitivity to light and/or sounds	rare	x
Aura before onset of headache		x

Although fatigue and stress can bring on both tension and migraine headaches, migraines can be triggered by certain foods, changes in the body's hormone levels, and even changes in the weather.

There also are differences in how types of headaches respond to treatment with medicines. Although some over-the-counter drugs used to treat tension-type headaches sometimes help migraine headaches, the drugs used to treat migraine attacks do not work for tension-type headaches for most people.

You can't tell the difference between a migraine and a tension-type headache by how often they occur. Both can occur at irregular intervals. Also, in rare cases, both can occur daily or almost daily.

How Can I Tell If I Have a Migraine or a Sinus Headache?

Many people confuse a sinus headache with a migraine because pain and pressure in the sinuses, nasal congestion, and watery eyes often occur with migraine. To find out if your headache is sinus or migraine, ask yourself these questions:

In addition to my sinus symptoms, do I have:

- Moderate-to-severe headache

- Nausea

- Sensitivity to light

If you answer "yes" to two or three of these questions, then most likely you have migraine with sinus symptoms. A true sinus headache is rare and usually occurs due to sinus infection. In a sinus infection, you would also likely have a fever and thick nasal secretions that are yellow, green, or blood-tinged. A sinus headache should go away with treatment of the sinus infection.

When Should I Seek Help for My Headaches?

Sometimes, headache can signal a more serious problem. You should talk to your doctor about your headaches if:

- You have several headaches per month and each lasts for several hours or days

- Your headaches disrupt your home, work, or school life

- You have nausea, vomiting, vision, or other sensory problems (such as numbness or tingling)

- You have pain around the eye or ear

- You have a severe headache with a stiff neck

- You have a headache with confusion or loss of alertness

- You have a headache with convulsions

- You have a headache after a blow to the head

- You used to be headache-free, but now have headaches a lot

What Tests Are Used to Find Out If I Have Migraine?

If you think you get migraine headaches, talk with your doctor. Before your appointment, write down:

- How often you have headaches

- Where the pain is

- How long the headaches last

- When the headaches happen, such as during your period

- Other symptoms, such as nausea or blind spots

- Any family history of migraine

- All the medicines that you are taking for all your medical problems, even the over-the-counter medicines (better still, bring the medicines in their containers to the doctor)

- All the medicines you have taken in the past that you can recall and, if possible, the doses you took and any side effects you had

Your doctor may also do an exam and ask more questions about your health history. This could include past head injury and sinus or dental problems. Your doctor may be able to diagnose migraine just from the information you provide.

You may get a blood test or other tests, such as computerized tomography (CT) scan or magnetic resonance imaging (MRI), if your doctor thinks that something else is causing your headaches. Work with your doctor to decide on the best tests for you.

Are Migraine Headaches More Common In Women than Men?

Yes. About three out of four people who have migraines are women. Migraines are most common in women between the ages of 20 and 45. At this time of life women often have more job, family, and social duties. Women tend to report more painful and longer lasting headaches and more symptoms, such as nausea and vomiting. All these factors make it hard for a woman to fulfill her roles at work and at home when migraine strikes.

I Get Migraines Right before My Period. Could They Be Related to My Menstrual Cycle?

More than half of migraines in women occur right before, during, or after a woman has her period. This often is called "menstrual migraine." But, just a small fraction of women who have migraine around their period only have migraine at this time. Most have migraine headaches at other times of the month as well.

How the menstrual cycle and migraine are linked is still unclear. We know that just before the cycle begins, levels of the female hormones, estrogen and progesterone, go down sharply. This drop in hormones may trigger a migraine, because estrogen controls chemicals in the brain that affect a woman's pain sensation.

Talk with your doctor if you think you have menstrual migraine. You may find that medicines, making lifestyle changes, and home treatment methods can prevent or reduce the pain.

Can Migraine Be Worse during Menopause?

If your migraine headaches are closely linked to your menstrual cycle, menopause may make them less severe. As you get older, the nausea and vomiting may decrease as well. About two-thirds of women with migraines report that their symptoms improve with menopause.

But for some women, menopause worsens migraine or triggers them to start. It is not clear why this happens. Menopausal hormone therapy, which is prescribed for some women during menopause, may be linked to migraines during this time. In general, though, the worsening of migraine symptoms goes away once menopause is complete.

Can Using Birth Control Pills Make My Migraines Worse?

In some women, birth control pills improve migraine. The pills may help reduce the number of attacks and their attacks may become less severe. But in other women, the pills may worsen their migraines. In still other women, taking birth control pills has no effect on their migraines.

The reason for these different responses is not well understood. For women whose migraines get worse when they take birth control pills, their attacks seem to occur during the last week of the cycle. This is because the last seven pills in most monthly pill packs don't have hormones; they are there to keep you in the habit of taking your birth control daily. Without the hormones, your body's estrogen levels drop sharply. This may trigger migraine in some women.

Talk with your doctor if you think birth control pills are making your migraines worse. Switching to a pill pack in which all the pills for the entire month contain hormones and using that for three months in a row can improve headaches. Lifestyle changes, such as getting on a regular sleep pattern and eating healthy foods, can help too.

Can Stress Cause Migraines?

Yes. Stress can trigger both migraine and tension-type headache. Events like getting married, moving to a new home, or having a baby can cause stress. But studies show that everyday stresses—not major life changes—cause most headaches. Juggling many roles, such as being a mother and wife, having a career, and financial pressures, can be daily stresses for women.

Making time for yourself and finding healthy ways to deal with stress are important. Some things you can do to help prevent or reduce stress include:

- Eating healthy foods

- Being active (at least 30 minutes most days of the week is best)

- Doing relaxation exercises

- Getting enough sleep

Try to figure out what causes you to feel stressed. You may be able to cut out some of these stressors. For example, if driving to work is stressful, try taking the bus or subway. You can take this time to read or listen to music, rather than deal with traffic. For stressors you can't avoid, keeping organized and doing as much as you can ahead of time will help you to feel in control.

What Are Rebound Migraines?

Women who use acute pain-relief medicine more than two or three times a week or more than 10 days out of the month can set off a cycle called rebound. As each dose of medicine wears off, the pain comes back, leading the patient to take even more. This overuse causes your medicine to stop helping your pain and actually start causing headaches. Rebound headaches can occur with both over-the-counter and prescription pain-relief medicines. They can also occur whether you take them for headache or for another type of pain. Talk to your doctor if you're caught in a rebound cycle.

How Are Migraines Treated?

Migraine has no cure. But your migraines can be managed with your doctor's help. Together, you will find ways to treat migraine symptoms when they happen, as well as ways to help make your migraines less frequent and severe. Your treatment plan may include some or all of these methods.

- **Medicine.** There are two ways to approach the treatment of migraines with drugs: stopping a migraine in progress (called "abortive" or "acute" treatment) and prevention. Many people with migraine use both forms of treatment.

- **Acute treatment.** Over-the-counter pain-relief drugs such as aspirin, acetaminophen, or NSAIDs (nonsteroidal anti-inflammatory drugs) like ibuprofen relieve mild migraine pain for some people. If these drugs don't work for you, your doctor might want you to try a prescription drug. Two classes of drugs that doctors often try first are:

  - Triptans, which work by balancing the chemicals in the brain. Examples include sumatriptan (Imitrex®), rizatriptan (Maxalt®), zolmitriptan (Zomig®), almotriptan (Axert®), eletriptan (Relpax®), naratriptan (Amerge®), and frovatriptan (Frova®). Triptans can come as tablets that you swallow, tablets that dissolve on your tongue, nasal sprays, and as a shot. They should not be used if you have heart disease or high blood pressure.

  - Ergot derivatives (ergotamine tartrate and dihydoergotamine), which work in the same way as triptans. They should not be used if you have heart disease or high blood pressure.

Most acute drugs for migraine work best when taken right away, when symptoms first begin. Always carry your migraine medicine with you in case of an attack. For people with extreme migraine pain, a powerful "rescue" drug might be prescribed, too. Because not everyone responds the same way to migraine drugs, you will need to work with your doctor to find the treatment that works best for you.

How Can Migraines Be Prevented?

Some medicines used daily can help prevent attacks. Many of these drugs were designed to treat other health conditions, such as epilepsy and depression. Some examples are:

- Antidepressants, such as amitriptyline (Elavil®) or venlafaxine (Effexor®)

- Anticonvulsants, such as divalproex sodium (Depakote®) or topiramate (Topamax®)

- Beta-blockers, such as propranolol (Inderal®) or timolol (Blocadren®)

- Calcium channel blockers, such as verapamil

These drugs may not prevent all migraines, but they can help a lot. Hormone therapy may help prevent attacks in women whose migraines seem to be linked to their menstrual cycle. Ask your doctor about prevention drugs if:

- Your migraines do not respond to drugs for symptom relief
- Your migraines are disabling or cause you to miss work, family activities, or social events
- You are using pain-relief drugs more than two times a week

Lifestyle changes. Practicing these habits can reduce the number of migraine attacks:

- Avoid or limit triggers.
- Get up and go to bed the same time every day.
- Eat healthy foods and do not skip meals.
- Engage in regular physical activity.
- Limit alcohol and caffeine intake.
- Learn ways to reduce and cope with stress.

Alternative methods. Biofeedback has been shown to help some people with migraine. It involves learning how to monitor and control your body's responses to stress, such as lowering heart rate and easing muscle tension. Other methods, such as acupuncture and relaxation, may help relieve stress. Counseling also can help if you think your migraines may be related to depression or anxiety. Talk with your doctor about these treatment methods.

Chapter 56

Osteoporosis

Osteoporosis, or porous bone, is a disease characterized by low bone mass and structural deterioration of bone tissue, leading to bone fragility and an increased risk of fractures of the hip, spine, and wrist. Men as well as women are affected by osteoporosis, a disease that can be prevented and treated. In the United States, more than 53 million people either already have osteoporosis or are at high risk due to low bone mass.

For women, bone loss is fastest in the first few years after menopause, and it continues into the postmenopausal years. Osteoporosis—which mainly affects women but may also affect men—will develop when bone resorption occurs too quickly or when replacement occurs too slowly. Osteoporosis is more likely to develop if you did not reach optimal peak bone mass during your bone-building years.

Risk Factors

Certain risk factors are linked to the development of osteoporosis and contribute to an individual's likelihood of developing the disease. Many people with osteoporosis have several risk factors, but others who develop the disease have no known risk factors. Some risk factors cannot be changed, but you can change others.

This chapter includes text excerpted from "Osteoporosis Overview," National Institute of Arthritis and Musculoskeletal and Skin Diseases (NIAMS), June 2015.

Risk Factors You Cannot Change

- **Gender.** Your chances of developing osteoporosis are greater if you are a woman. Women have less bone tissue and lose bone faster than men because of the changes that happen with menopause.

- **Age.** The older you are, the greater your risk of osteoporosis. Your bones become thinner and weaker as you age.

- **Body size.** Small, thin-boned women are at greater risk.

- **Ethnicity.** Caucasian and Asian women are at highest risk. African American and Hispanic women have a lower but significant risk.

- **Family history.** Fracture risk may be due, in part, to heredity. People whose parents have a history of fractures also seem to have reduced bone mass and may be at risk for fractures.

Risk Factors You Can Change

- **Sex hormones.** Abnormal absence of menstrual periods (amenorrhea), low estrogen level (menopause), and low testosterone level in men can bring on osteoporosis.

- **Anorexia nervosa.** Characterized by an irrational fear of weight gain, this eating disorder increases your risk for osteoporosis.

- **Calcium and vitamin D intake.** A lifetime diet low in calcium and vitamin D makes you more prone to bone loss.

- **Medication use.** Long-term use of certain medications, such as glucocorticoids and some anticonvulsants can lead to loss of bone density and fractures.

- **Lifestyle.** An inactive lifestyle or extended bed rest tends to weaken bones.

- **Cigarette smoking.** Smoking is bad for bones as well as the heart and lungs.

- **Alcohol intake.** Excessive consumption of alcohol increases the risk of bone loss and fractures.

Symptoms

Osteoporosis is often called a silent disease because bone loss occurs without symptoms. People may not know that they have osteoporosis until their bones become so weak that a sudden strain, bump, or fall causes a hip to fracture or a vertebra to collapse. Collapsed vertebrae may initially be felt or seen in the form of severe back pain, loss of height, or spinal deformities such as kyphosis (severely stooped posture).

Detection

Following a comprehensive medical assessment, your doctor may recommend that you have your bone mass measured. A bone mineral density (BMD) test is an important measure of your bone health. BMD tests can identify osteoporosis, determine your risk for fractures (broken bones), and measure your response to osteoporosis treatment. The most widely recognized BMD test is a central dual-energy X-ray absorptiometry, or central DXA test. It is painless—a bit like having an X-ray, but with much less exposure to radiation. It can measure bone density at your hip and spine. BMD tests can:

- Detect low bone density before a fracture occurs.

- Confirm a diagnosis of osteoporosis if you already have one or more fractures.

- Predict your chances of fracturing in the future.

- Determine your rate of bone loss, and monitor the effects of treatment if the test is conducted at intervals of a year or more.

Treatment

A comprehensive osteoporosis treatment program includes a focus on proper nutrition, exercise, and safety issues to prevent falls that may result in fractures. In addition, your doctor may prescribe a medication to slow or stop bone loss, increase bone density, and reduce fracture risk.

Nutrition: The foods we eat contain a variety of vitamins, minerals, and other important nutrients that help keep our bodies healthy. All of these nutrients are needed in balanced proportion. In particular, calcium and vitamin D are needed for strong bones and for your heart, muscles, and nerves to function properly.

Exercise: Exercise is an important component of an osteoporosis prevention and treatment program. Exercise not only improves your bone health, but it increases muscle strength, coordination, and balance, and leads to better overall health. Although exercise is good for someone with osteoporosis, it should not put any sudden or excessive strain on your bones. As extra insurance against fractures, your doctor can recommend specific exercises to strengthen and support your back.

Therapeutic medications: Several medications are available for the prevention and/or treatment of osteoporosis, including: bisphosphonates; estrogen agonists/antagonists (also called selective estrogen receptor modulators or SERMS); calcitonin; parathyroid hormone; estrogen therapy; hormone therapy; and a recently approved RANK ligand (RANKL) inhibitor.

Prevention

To reach optimal peak bone mass and continue building new bone tissue as you age, you should consider several factors.

Calcium: An inadequate supply of calcium over a lifetime contributes to the development of osteoporosis. Many published studies show that low calcium intake appears to be associated with low bone mass, rapid bone loss, and high fracture rates. National nutrition surveys show that many people consume less than half the amount of calcium recommended to build and maintain healthy bones. Food sources of calcium include low-fat dairy products, such as milk, yogurt, cheese, and ice cream; dark green, leafy vegetables, such as broccoli, collard greens, bok choy, and spinach; sardines and salmon with bones; tofu; almonds; and foods fortified with calcium, such as orange juice, cereals, and breads. Depending on how much calcium you get each day from food, you may need to take a calcium supplement.

Calcium needs change during one's lifetime. The body's demand for calcium is greater during childhood and adolescence, when the skeleton is growing rapidly, and during pregnancy and breastfeeding. Postmenopausal women and older men also need to consume more calcium. Also, as you age, your body becomes less efficient at absorbing calcium and other nutrients. Older adults also are more likely to have chronic medical problems and to use medications that may impair calcium absorption.

Vitamin D: Vitamin D plays an important role in calcium absorption and bone health. Food sources of vitamin D include egg yolks, saltwater fish, and liver. Many people obtain enough vitamin D naturally; however, studies show that vitamin D production decreases in the elderly, in people who are housebound, and for people in general during the winter. Adults should have vitamin D intakes of 600 IU (International Units) daily up to age 70. Women and men over age 70 should increase their uptake to 800 IU daily.

Exercise: Like muscle, bone is living tissue that responds to exercise by becoming stronger. Weight-bearing exercise is the best for your bones because it forces you to work against gravity. Examples include walking, hiking, jogging, climbing stairs, weight training, tennis, and dancing.

Smoking: Smoking is bad for your bones as well as your heart and lungs. Women who smoke have lower levels of estrogen compared with nonsmokers, and they often go through menopause earlier. Smokers also may absorb less calcium from their diets.

Alcohol: Regular consumption of 2 to 3 ounces a day of alcohol may be damaging to the skeleton, even in young women and men. Those who drink heavily are more prone to bone loss and fracture, because of both poor nutrition and increased risk of falling.

Medications that cause bone loss: Several medications can contribute to bone loss. For example, the long-term use of glucocorticoids (medications prescribed for a wide range of diseases, including arthritis, asthma, Crohn's disease, lupus, and other diseases of the lungs, kidneys, and liver) can lead to a loss of bone density and fracture. Bone loss also can result from long-term treatment with certain antiseizure drugs, such as phenytoin and barbiturates; gonadotropin-releasing hormone (GnRH) drugs used to treat endometriosis; excessive use of aluminum-containing antacids; certain cancer treatments; and excessive thyroid hormone. It is important to discuss the use of these drugs with your doctor and not to stop or change your medication dose on your own.

Chapter 57

Thyroid Disorders in Women

Your thyroid produces thyroid hormone, which controls many activities in your body, including how fast you burn calories and how fast your heart beats. Diseases of the thyroid cause it to make either too much or too little of the hormone. Depending on how much or how little hormone your thyroid makes, you may often feel restless or tired, or you may lose or gain weight. Women are more likely than men to have thyroid diseases, especially right after pregnancy and after menopause.

What Is the Thyroid?

Your thyroid is a small butterfly-shaped gland found at the base of your neck, just below your Adam's apple. This gland makes thyroid hormone that travels in your blood to all parts of your body. The thyroid hormone controls your body's metabolism in many ways, including how fast you burn calories and how fast your heart beats.

This chapter includes text excerpted from "Thyroid Disease," Office on Women's Health (OWH), U.S. Department of Health and Human Services (HHS), February 6, 2017.

How Do Thyroid Problems Affect Women?

Women are more likely than men to have thyroid disease. One in eight women will develop thyroid problems during her lifetime. In women, thyroid diseases can cause:

- **Problems with your menstrual period.** Your thyroid helps control your menstrual cycle. Too much or too little thyroid hormone can make your periods very light, heavy, or irregular. Thyroid disease also can cause your periods to stop for several months or longer, a condition called amenorrhea. If your body's immune system causes thyroid disease, other glands, including your ovaries, may be involved. This can lead to early menopause (before age 40).

- **Problems getting pregnant.** When thyroid disease affects the menstrual cycle, it also affects ovulation. This can make it harder for you to get pregnant.

- **Problems during pregnancy.** Thyroid problems during pregnancy can cause health problems for the mother and the baby.

Sometimes, symptoms of thyroid problems are mistaken for menopause symptoms. Thyroid disease, especially hypothyroidism, is more likely to develop after menopause.

Are Some Women More at Risk for Thyroid Disease?

Yes. You may want to talk to your doctor about getting tested if you:

- Had a thyroid problem in the past
- Had surgery or radiotherapy affecting the thyroid gland
- Have a condition such as goiter, anemia, or type 1 diabetes

Screening for thyroid disease is not recommended for most women.

What Kinds of Thyroid Disease Affect Women?

These thyroid diseases affect more women than men:

- Disorders that cause hypothyroidism
- Disorders that cause hyperthyroidism
- Thyroiditis, especially postpartum thyroiditis
- Goiter

- Thyroid nodules

- Thyroid cancer

What Is Hypothyroidism?

Hypothyroidism is when your thyroid does not make enough thyroid hormones. It is also called underactive thyroid. This slows down many of your body's functions, like your metabolism.

The most common cause of hypothyroidism in the United States is Hashimoto disease. In people with Hashimoto disease, the immune system mistakenly attacks the thyroid. This attack damages the thyroid so that it does not make enough hormones.

Hypothyroidism also can be caused by:

- Hyperthyroidism treatment (radioiodine)

- Radiation treatment of certain cancers

- Thyroid removal

What Are the Signs and Symptoms of Hypothyroidism?

Symptoms of hypothyroidism develop slowly, often over several years. At first, you may feel tired and sluggish. Later, you may develop other signs and symptoms of a slowed-down metabolism, including:

- Feeling cold when other people do not

- Constipation

- Muscle weakness

- Weight gain, even though you are not eating more food

- Joint or muscle pain

- Feeling sad or depressed

- Feeling very tired

- Pale, dry skin

- Dry, thinning hair

- Slow heart rate

- Less sweating than usual

- A puffy face

- A hoarse voice

- More than usual menstrual bleeding

You also may have high low-density lipoprotein (LDL) or "bad" cholesterol, which can raise your risk for heart disease.

How Is Hypothyroidism Treated?

Hypothyroidism is treated with medicine that gives your body the thyroid hormone it needs to work normally. The most common medicines are man-made forms of the hormone that your thyroid makes. You will likely need to take thyroid hormone pills for the rest of your life. When you take the pills as your doctor tells you to, the pills are very safe.

What Is Hyperthyroidism?

Hyperthyroidism, or overactive thyroid, causes your thyroid to make more thyroid hormone than your body needs. This speeds up many of your body's functions, like your metabolism and heart rate.

The most common cause of hyperthyroidism is Graves disease. Graves disease is a problem with the immune system.

What Are the Signs and Symptoms of Hyperthyroidism?

At first, you might not notice the signs or symptoms of hyperthyroidism. Symptoms usually begin slowly. But, over time, a faster metabolism can cause symptoms such as:

- Weight loss, even if you eat the same or more food (most but not all people lose weight)

- Eating more than usual

- Rapid or irregular heartbeat or pounding of your heart

- Feeling nervous or anxious

- Feeling irritable

- Trouble sleeping

- Trembling in your hands and fingers

- Increased sweating

- Feeling hot when other people do not

- Muscle weakness

- Diarrhea or more bowel movements than normal

- Fewer and lighter menstrual periods than normal

- Changes in your eyes that can include bulging of the eyes, redness, or irritation

Hyperthyroidism raises your risk for osteoporosis, a condition that causes weak bones that break easily. In fact, hyperthyroidism might affect your bones before you have any of the other symptoms of the condition. This is especially true of women who have gone through menopause or who are already at high risk of osteoporosis.

How Is Hyperthyroidism Treated?

Your doctor's choice of treatment will depend on your symptoms and the cause of your hyperthyroidism. Treatments include:

- Medicine
    - Antithyroid medicines
    - Beta blockers
- Radioiodine
- Surgery

What Is Thyroiditis?

Thyroiditis is inflammation of the thyroid. It happens when the body's immune system makes antibodies that attack the thyroid. Causes of thyroiditis include:

- Autoimmune diseases, like type 1 diabetes and rheumatoid arthritis

- Genetics

- Viral or bacterial infection

- Certain types of medicines

Two common types of thyroiditis are Hashimoto disease and postpartum thyroiditis.

What Is Postpartum Thyroiditis?

Postpartum thyroiditis, or inflammation of the thyroid after giving birth, affects 10 percent of women. It often goes undiagnosed because symptoms are much like the "baby blues" that may follow delivery. Women with postpartum thyroiditis may feel very tired and moody.

Postpartum thyroiditis typically happens in two phases, though not everyone with the condition goes through both phases:

- The first phase starts 1 to 4 months after giving birth and typically last 1 to 2 months. In this phase, you may have signs and symptoms of hyperthyroidism because the damaged thyroid leaks thyroid hormones out into the bloodstream.

- The second phase starts about 4 to 8 months after delivery and lasts 6 to 12 months. In this phase, you may have signs and symptoms of hypothyroidism because the thyroid has lost most of its hormones or because the immune attack is over and the thyroid may recover later.

Who Is at Risk for Postpartum Thyroiditis?

Your immune system may cause postpartum thyroiditis. If you have an autoimmune disease, like type 1 diabetes, your risk is higher. Your risk is also higher if:

- Have a personal history or family history of thyroid disorders
- Had postpartum thyroiditis after a previous pregnancy
- Have chronic viral hepatitis

How Is Postpartum Thyroiditis Treated?

Treatment for postpartum thyroiditis depends on the phase of the disease and what symptoms you have. For example, if you get symptoms of hyperthyroidism in the first phase, your treatment may include medicines to slow down the heart rate.

In most women who have postpartum thyroiditis, the thyroid returns to normal within 12 to 18 months after symptoms start. But if you have a history of postpartum thyroiditis, your risk is higher for developing permanent hypothyroidism within 5 to 10 years.

What Is a Goiter?

A goiter is an unusually enlarged thyroid gland. It may happen only for a short time and may go away on its own without treatment. Or it could be a symptom of another thyroid disease that requires treatment. Goiter is more common in women than in men and especially in women before menopause.

Some common causes of goiter include:

- Hashimoto disease

- Graves disease

- Thyroid nodules

- Thyroiditis

- Thyroid cancer

Usually, the only symptom of a goiter is a swelling in your neck. It may be large enough that you can see it or feel the lump with your hand. A very large goiter can also cause a tight feeling in your throat, coughing, or problems swallowing or breathing.

Your doctor will do tests to see if it is caused by another thyroid disease.

How Is Goiter Treated?

You may not need treatment if your thyroid works normally and the symptoms do not bother you.

If you do need treatment, medicine should make the thyroid shrink back to near normal size. You may need surgery to take out part or most of the thyroid.

What Are Thyroid Nodules?

A thyroid nodule is a swelling in one section of the thyroid gland. The nodule may be solid or filled with fluid or blood. You may have just one thyroid nodule or many.

Thyroid nodules are common and affect four times as many women as men. Researchers do not know why nodules form in otherwise normal thyroids.

What Are the Signs and Symptoms of Thyroid Nodules?

Most thyroid nodules do not cause symptoms and are not cancerous. Some thyroid nodules make too much thyroid hormone, causing hyperthyroidism. Sometimes, nodules grow so big that they cause problems with swallowing or breathing. About one-third of nodules are found by the patient, another third by the doctor, and the other third through an imaging test of the neck.

You can sometimes see or feel a thyroid nodule yourself. Stand in front of a mirror and raise your chin slightly. Look for a bump on either side of your windpipe below your Adam's apple. If the bump moves up and down when you swallow, it may be a thyroid nodule. Ask your doctor to look at it.

How Are Thyroid Nodules Treated?

Treatment depends on the type of nodule or nodules that you have. Treatments include:

- **Watchful waiting.** If your nodule is not cancerous, your doctor may decide to just watch your condition. You will get regular physical exams, blood tests, and perhaps thyroid ultrasound tests. If your nodule does not change, you may not need further treatment.

- **Surgery.** Surgery may be necessary to take out nodules that may be cancerous or large nodules that cause problems breathing or swallowing.

- **Radioiodine.** This type of treatment is helpful if you have nodules that make too much thyroid hormone. Radioiodine causes nodules to shrink and make smaller amounts of thyroid hormone.

What Is Thyroid Cancer?

Thyroid cancer happens when cancer cells form from the tissues of the thyroid gland.

Most people with thyroid cancer have a thyroid nodule that does not cause any symptoms. If you do have symptoms, you may have swelling or a lump in your neck. The lump may cause problems swallowing. Some people get a hoarse voice.

To tell if the lump or nodule is cancerous, your doctor will order certain tests. Most thyroid nodules are not cancerous.

Who Is at Risk for Thyroid Cancer?

About three times as many women get thyroid cancer as men. The number of women with thyroid cancer is also going up. By 2020, the number of women with thyroid cancer is expected to double, from 34,000 women to more than 70,000 women.

Thyroid cancer is more common in women who:

- Are between the ages of 25 and 65

- Had radiation therapy to the head or neck, especially in child-hood, to treat cancer

- Have a history of goiter

- Have a family history of thyroid cancer

How Is Thyroid Cancer Treated?

The main treatment for thyroid cancer is surgery to take out the whole thyroid gland or as much of it as can be safely removed. Surgery alone can cure thyroid cancer if the cancer is small and has not yet spread to lymph nodes.

Your doctor may also use radioiodine therapy after surgery. Radio-iodine therapy destroys any thyroid cancer cells that were not removed during surgery or that have spread to other parts of the body.

Your doctor may also talk with you about other treatments for thyroid cancer.

How Are Thyroid Diseases Diagnosed?

It can be hard to tell if you have a thyroid disease. The symptoms are the same as many other health problems. Your doctor may start by asking about your health history and if any of your family members has had thyroid disease. Your doctor may also give you a physical exam and check your neck for thyroid nodules.

Depending on your symptoms, your doctor may also do other tests, such as:

- Blood tests

- Radioactive iodine uptake test

High levels of radioiodine mean that your thyroid makes too much of the thyroid hormone. Low levels mean that your thyroid does not make enough thyroid hormone.

- **Thyroid scan.** A thyroid scan uses the same radioiodine dose that was given by mouth for your uptake test. You lie on a table while a special camera makes an image of your thyroid on a computer screen. This test shows the pattern of iodine uptake in the thyroid.

Three types of nodules show up in this test:

- "Hot" nodules
- "Warm" nodules
- "Cold" nodules

- **Thyroid ultrasound.** The thyroid ultrasound uses sound waves to make a picture of the thyroid on a computer screen. This test can help your doctor tell what type of nodule you have and how large it is. You may need more thyroid ultrasounds over time to see if your nodule is growing or shrinking.

Ultrasound may also be helpful in finding thyroid cancer, although by itself it cannot be used to diagnose thyroid cancer.

- **Thyroid fine needle biopsy.** This test tells whether thyroid nodules have normal cells in them. Your doctor may numb an area on your neck. Your doctor will then stick a very thin needle into the thyroid to take out some cells and fluid. A doctor will then look at the cells under a microscope to see if they are normal. Cells that are not normal could mean thyroid cancer.

Can Thyroid Disease Cause Problems Getting Pregnant?

Both hyperthyroidism and hypothyroidism can make it harder for you to get pregnant. This is because problems with the thyroid hormone can upset the balance of the hormones that cause ovulation. Hypothyroidism can also cause your body to make more prolactin, the hormone that tells your body to make breast milk. Too much prolactin can prevent ovulation.

Thyroid problems can also affect the menstrual cycle. Your periods may be heavier or irregular, or you may not have any periods at all for several months or longer (called amenorrhea).

How Does Thyroid Disease Affect Pregnancy?

Pregnancy-related hormones raise the level of thyroid hormones in the blood. Thyroid hormones are necessary for the baby's brain development while in the womb.

It can be harder to diagnose thyroid problems during pregnancy because of the change in hormone levels that normally happen during pregnancy. But it is especially important to check for problems before getting pregnant and during pregnancy. Uncontrolled hyperthyroidism and hypothyroidism can cause problems for both mother and baby.

Hyperthyroidism that is not treated with medicine during pregnancy can cause:

- Premature birth (birth of the baby before 39 to 40 weeks, or full-term)
- Preeclampsia, a serious condition starting after 20 weeks of pregnancy.
- Preeclampsia causes high blood pressure and problems with the kidneys and other
- organs. The only cure for preeclampsia is childbirth.
- Thyroid storm (sudden, severe worsening of symptoms)
- Fast heart rate in the newborn, which can lead to heart failure, poor weight gain, or an enlarged thyroid that can make it hard to breathe
- Low birth weight (smaller than 5 pounds)
- Miscarriage

Hypothyroidism that is not treated with medicine during pregnancy can cause:

- Anemia (lower than normal number of healthy red blood cells)
- Preeclampsia
- Low birth weight (smaller than 5 pounds)
- Miscarriage
- Stillbirth
- Problems with the baby's growth and brain development

Chapter 58

Urinary Tract Disorders

Chapter Contents

Section 58.1

Interstitial Cystitis (Painful Bladder Syndrome)

This section includes text excerpted from "Interstitial Cystitis (Painful Bladder Syndrome)," National Institute of Diabetes and Digestive and Kidney Diseases (NIDDK), January 2017.

What Is Interstitial Cystitis (IC)?

Interstitial cystitis (IC), also called bladder pain syndrome, is a chronic, or long-lasting, condition that causes painful urinary symptoms. Symptoms of IC may be different from person to person. For example, some people feel mild discomfort, pressure, or tenderness in the pelvic area. Other people may have intense pain in the bladder or struggle with urinary urgency, the sudden need to urinate, or frequency, the need to urinate more often.

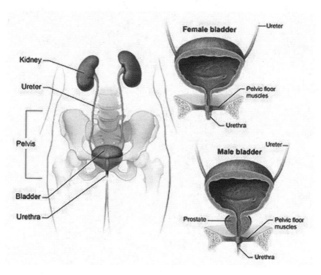

Figure 58.1. *Interstitial Cystitis*

Interstitial cystitis (IC) can cause pain in your bladder and pelvic area.

Healthcare professionals diagnose IC by ruling out other conditions with similar symptoms.

Researchers don't know the exact cause of IC. Some researchers believe IC may result from conditions that cause inflammation in various organs and parts of the body.

Severe IC symptoms can affect your quality of life. You may feel like you can't exercise or leave your home because you have to use the bathroom too often, or perhaps your relationship is suffering because sex is painful.

Working with healthcare professionals, including a urologist or urogynecologist, along with a pain specialist, may help improve your IC symptoms.

How Common Is IC?

IC is common. The condition may affect between 3 million and 8 million women and between 1 million and 4 million men in the United States.

Who Is More Likely to Develop IC?

IC can occur at any age, including during childhood, but is most common in adult women and men. About twice as many women are affected as men. However, more men may struggle with IC than researchers originally thought.

Some research suggests that women are more likely to develop IC if they have a history of being sexually abused or physically traumatized.

What Other Health Problems Do People with IC Have?

Many women with IC are more likely to have other conditions such as irritable bowel syndrome, fibromyalgia, and chronic fatigue syndrome. Allergies and some autoimmune diseases are also associated with IC.

Vulvodynia, which is chronic pain in the vulva that often causes a burning or stinging feeling, or rawness, is commonly associated with IC. Vulvodynia has symptoms that overlap with IC.

What Are the Complications of IC?

The symptoms of IC—such as urgency, frequency, and pain—may lead you to decrease your physical and social activity and negatively affect your quality of life.

Women with pelvic pain or vulvodynia often have pain during sexual intercourse, which can damage your relationships and self-image. Men also can experience pelvic pain that causes uncomfortable or painful sex. Sometimes sex can increase bladder pain attacks, also called symptom flares.

Sexual complications may cause people to avoid further intimacy, possibly leading to depression and guilt. Like many people who deal with chronic pain, people with IC are more likely to struggle with sleep loss due to the frequent need to urinate, and with anxiety and depression.

Medical tests such as pelvic exams and Pap tests often are painful for women with IC symptoms, especially those who may have pelvic floor muscle spasm. Don't avoid these tests. Talk with a healthcare professional about how to make pelvic exams and Pap tests more comfortable and how often you should have them.

What Are the Symptoms of IC?

People with interstitial cystitis (IC) have repeat discomfort, pressure, tenderness or pain in the bladder, lower abdomen, and pelvic area. Symptoms vary from person to person, may be mild or severe, and can even change in each person as time goes on.

Symptoms may include a combination of these symptoms:

Urgency

Urgency is the feeling that you need to urinate right now. A strong urge is normal if you haven't urinated for a few hours or if you have been drinking a lot of liquids. With IC, you may feel pain or burning along with an urgent need to urinate before your bladder has had time to fill.

Frequency

Frequency is urinating more often than you think you should need to, given the amount of liquid you are drinking. Most people urinate between four and seven times a day. Drinking large amounts of liquid can cause more frequent urinating. Taking blood pressure medicines called diuretics, or water pills, can also cause more frequent urinating. Some people with IC feel a strong, painful urge to urinate many times a day.

Pain

As your bladder starts to fill, you may feel pain—rather than just discomfort—that gets worse until you urinate. The pain usually improves for a while once you empty your bladder. People with IC rarely have constant bladder pain. The pain may go away for weeks or months and then return. People with IC sometimes refer to an attack of bladder pain as a symptom flare.

Some people may have pain without urgency or frequency. This pain may come from a spasm in the pelvic floor muscles, the group of muscles that is attached to your pelvic bones and supports your bladder, bowel, and uterus or prostate. Pain from pelvic floor muscle spasm may get worse during sex.

What Causes IC?

Researchers don't know the exact cause of IC. Researchers are working to understand the causes of IC and to find effective treatments.

How Do Healthcare Professionals Diagnose IC?

Healthcare professionals will use your medical history, a physical exam, and lab tests to diagnose IC.

A healthcare professional will ask if you have a history of health problems related to IC. He or she will ask questions about your symptoms and other questions to help find the cause of your bladder problems.

If you are a woman who has IC symptoms, a healthcare professional may also perform a pelvic exam. During the pelvic exam, the healthcare professional will check your pelvic floor muscles to see if any of your painful symptoms are related to spasm in your pelvic floor muscles.

For men, a healthcare professional may perform a digital rectal exam to check for prostate problems and to check your pelvic floor muscles.

Doctors diagnose IC based on:

- pain in or near the bladder, usually with urinary frequency and urgency

- the absence of other diseases and conditions that could cause similar symptoms, such as urinary tract infections (UTIs), bladder cancer, endometriosis in women.

What Tests Do Doctors Use to Diagnose IC?

A healthcare professional may use the following tests to look inside your urethra and bladder, and may even take a tissue sample from inside your bladder. The healthcare professional will use tests to rule out certain diseases and conditions, such as UTI and bladder cancer. If the test results are normal and all other diseases and conditions are ruled out, your doctor may diagnose IC.

How Do Doctors Treat IC?

Researchers have not found one treatment for interstitial cystitis (IC) that works for everyone. Doctors aim current treatments at relieving symptoms in each person on an individual basis.

A healthcare professional will work with you to find a treatment plan that meets your needs. Your plan may include:

- lifestyle changes

- bladder training

- physical therapy

- medicines

- bladder procedures

Some treatments may work better for you than others. You also may need to use a combination of these treatments to relieve your symptoms.

A healthcare professional may ask you to fill out a form, called a symptom scale, with questions about how you feel. The symptom scale may allow a healthcare professional to better understand how you are responding to treatment.

You may have to try several different treatments before you find one that works for you. Your symptoms may disappear with treatment, a change in what you eat, or without a clear reason. Even when your symptoms go away, they may return after days, weeks, months, or even years. Researchers do not know why. With time, you and your doctor should be able to find a treatment that gives you some relief and helps you cope with IC.

Can What I Eat or Drink Relieve or Prevent IC?

No research consistently links certain foods or drinks to IC. However, some research strongly suggests a relationship between diet and symptoms. Healthy eating and staying hydrated are important for your overall health, including bladder health.

Some people with IC find that certain foods or drinks trigger or worsen their symptoms, such as alcohol, tomatoes, spices, chocolate, caffeinated and citrus beverages, and high-acid foods. Some people also note that their symptoms get worse after eating or drinking products with artificial sweeteners, or sweeteners that are not found naturally in foods and beverages.

Learning which foods trigger or worsen symptoms may take some effort. Keep a food diary and note the times you have bladder pain. For example, the diary might reveal that your symptom flares always happen after you eat tomatoes or oranges.

Stopping certain foods and drinks—and then adding them back to what you normally eat and drink one at a time—may help you figure out which foods or drinks, if any, affect your symptoms. Talk with your healthcare professional about how much liquid you should drink to prevent dehydration based on your health, how active you are, and where you live. Water is the best liquid for bladder health.

Some doctors recommend taking an antacid with meals. This medicine reduces the amount of acid that gets into the urine.

Section 58.2

Urinary Incontinence in Women

This section includes text excerpted from "Urinary Incontinence," Office on Women's Health (OWH), U.S. Department of Health and Human Services (HHS), June 12, 2017.

What Is Urinary Incontinence (UI)?

Urinary incontinence (UI) is also known as "loss of bladder control" or "urinary leakage." UI is when urine leaks out before you can get to a bathroom. If you have UI, you are not alone. Millions of women have this problem, especially as they get older.

Some women may lose a few drops of urine when they cough or laugh. Others may feel a sudden urge to urinate and cannot control it. Urine loss can also occur during sexual activity and can cause great emotional distress.

What Causes UI?

UI is also known as "loss of bladder control" or "urinary leakage." UI is when urine leaks out before you can get to a bathroom. If you have UI, you are not alone. Millions of women have this problem, especially as they get older.

Some women may lose a few drops of urine when they cough or laugh. Others may feel a sudden urge to urinate and cannot control it. Urine loss can also occur during sexual activity and can cause great emotional distress.

UI is usually caused by problems with muscles and nerves that help to hold or pass urine.

Urine is stored in the bladder. It leaves the body through a tube that is connected to the bladder called the urethra. Look at the images below to see how this process works.

Muscles in the wall of the bladder contract to force urine out through the urethra. At the same time, sphincter muscles around the urethra relax to let the urine pass out of the body.

Incontinence happens if the bladder muscles suddenly contract or the sphincter muscles are not strong enough to hold back urine.

UI is twice as common in women as in men. Pregnancy, childbirth, and menopause are major reasons why. But both women and men can become incontinent from brain injury, birth defects, stroke, diabetes, multiple sclerosis, and physical changes associated with aging.

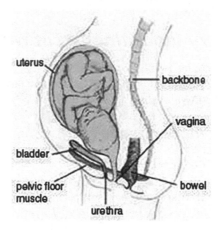

Figure 58.2. *Urinary Incontinence*

- **Pregnancy**—Unborn babies push down on the bladder, urethra (tube that you urinate from), and pelvic floor muscles. This pressure may weaken the pelvic floor support and lead to leaks or problems passing urine.

- **Childbirth**—Many women leak urine after giving birth. Labor and vaginal birth can weaken pelvic floor support and damage nerves that control the bladder. Most problems with bladder control during pregnancy and childbirth go away after the muscles have time to heal. Talk to your doctor if you still have bladder problems 6 weeks after childbirth.

- **Menopause**—Some women have bladder control problems after they stop having periods. After menopause, the body stops making the female hormone estrogen. Some experts think this loss of estrogen weakens the urethral tissue.

Other causes of UI that can affect women and men are:

- **Constipation**—Problems with bladder control can happen to people with chronic (long-term) constipation.

- **Medicines**—UI may be a side effect of medicines such as diuretics ("water pills" used to treat heart failure, liver cirrhosis, hypertension, and certain kidney diseases). Hormone replacement has been shown to cause worsening UI.

- **Caffeine and alcohol**—Drinks with caffeine, such as coffee or soda, cause the bladder to fill quickly and sometimes leak.

- **Infection**—Infections of the urinary tract and bladder may cause incontinence for a short time. Bladder control returns when the illness goes away.

- **Nerve damage**—Damaged nerves may send signals to the bladder at the wrong time, or not at all. Trauma or diseases such as diabetes and multiple sclerosis can cause nerve damage. Nerves may also become damaged during childbirth.

- **Excess weight**—Being overweight is also known to put pressure on the bladder and make incontinence worse.

What Are the Types of UI?

- **Stress incontinence**—Leakage happens with coughing, sneezing, exercising, laughing, lifting heavy things, and other movements that put pressure on the bladder. This is the most common type of incontinence in women. It is often caused by physical changes from pregnancy, childbirth, and menopause. It can be treated and sometimes cured.

- **Urge incontinence**—This is sometimes called "overactive bladder." Leakage usually happens after a strong, sudden urge to urinate. This may occur when you don't expect it, such as during sleep, after drinking water, or when you hear or touch running water.

- **Functional incontinence**—People with this type of incontinence may have problems thinking, moving, or speaking that keep them from reaching a toilet. For example, a person with Alzheimer disease may not plan a trip to the bathroom in time to urinate. A person in a wheelchair may be unable to get to a toilet in time.

- **Overflow incontinence**—Urine leakage happens because the bladder doesn't empty completely. Overflow incontinence is less common in women.

- **Mixed incontinence**—This is 2 or more types of incontinence together (usually stress and urge incontinence).

- **Transient incontinence**—Urine leakage happens for a short time due to an illness (such as a bladder infection or pregnancy). The leaking stops when the illness is treated.

How Do I Talk to My Doctor about UI?

Many women do not want to talk to their doctor about such a personal topic. But UI is a common medical problem. Millions of women have the same problem. Many have been treated successfully. Your doctor has probably heard many stories like yours.

Even if you feel shy, it is up to you to take the first step. Some doctors don't treat bladder control problems, so they may not think to ask about it. They might expect you to bring up the subject.

Family practitioners and internists can treat bladder problems. If your doctor does not treat such problems, ask for help finding a doctor who does, such as a urologist, OB/GYN, or urogynecologist.

Here are some questions to ask your doctor:

- Could what I eat or drink cause bladder problems?

- Could my medicines (prescription and over-the-counter) cause bladder problems?

- Could other medical conditions cause loss of bladder control?

- What are the treatments to regain bladder control? Which one is best for me?

- What can I do about the odor and rash caused by urine?

It also helps to keep a bladder diary. This means you write down when you leak urine. Be sure to note what you were doing at the time, such as sneezing, coughing, laughing, stepping off a curb, or sleeping. Take this log with you when you visit your doctor.

How Do I Find out If I Have UI?

Schedule a visit with your doctor. Your doctor will ask you about your symptoms and take a medical history, including:

- How often you empty your bladder

- How and when you leak urine

- How much urine you leak

Your doctor will do a physical exam to look for signs of health problems that can cause incontinence. Your doctor also will do a test to figure out how well your bladder works and how much it can hold. For this test, you will drink water and urinate into a measuring pan. The doctor will then measure any urine still in the bladder. Your doctor also may order other tests such as:

- **Bladder stress test**—During this test, you will cough or bear down as the doctor watches for loss of urine.

- **Urinalysis**—A urinalysis tests your urine for signs of infection or other causes of incontinence.

- **Ultrasound**—Sound waves are used to take a picture of the kidneys, bladder, and urethra.

- **Cystoscopy**—A doctor places a thin tube connected to a tiny camera in the urethra to look at the inside of the urethra and bladder.

- **Urodynamics**—A doctor places a thin tube into your bladder and your bladder is filled with water. The doctor then measures the pressure in the bladder.

Your doctor may ask you to write down when you empty your bladder and how much urine you produce for a day or a week.

How Is UI Treated?

There are many ways to treat UI. Your doctor will work with you to find the best treatment for you.

Types of treatments include:

- **Behavioral treatments:** By changing some basic behaviors, you may be able to improve your UI. Behavioral treatments include:

  - Pelvic muscle exercises (Kegel exercises): Exercising your pelvic floor muscles regularly can help reduce or cure stress leakage.

  - Bladder retraining: You may regain bladder control by going to the bathroom at set times, before you get the urge to urinate. You can slowly increase the time between set bathroom trips as you gain control.

- **Weight loss:** Extra weight puts more pressure on your bladder and nearby muscles. This can cause bladder control problems. Work with your doctor to plan a diet and exercise program if you are overweight.

- **Dietary changes:** Some foods and beverages are thought to contribute to bladder leakage. Avoid:

  - Alcoholic beverages

  - Carbonated beverages (with or without caffeine)

  - Coffee or tea (with or without caffeine)

  - Other changes include drinking fewer fluids after dinner and eating enough fiber to avoid constipation. Also avoid drinking too much. Six 8-ounce glasses of fluid a day is enough for most people.

- **Quitting smoking:** Studies show that smokers have more frequent and severe urine leaks.

- **Medicines for bladder control:** Medications can reduce some types of leakage. Some medicines, for example, help relax the bladder muscles and prevent bladder spasms.

- **Devices:** A pessary is the most common device used to treat stress incontinence.

- **Nerve stimulation:** Some people with urge incontinence may not respond to behavioral treatments or medicine. In this case, electrical stimulation of the nerves that control the bladder may help.

- **Biofeedback:** Biofeedback helps you learn how your body works. A therapist puts an electrical patch over your bladder and urethral muscles. A wire connected to the patch is linked to a TV screen. You and your therapist watch the screen to see when these muscles contract, so you can learn to control these muscles.

- **Surgery:** Surgery is most effective for people with stress UI who have not been helped by other treatments.

- **Catheterization:** The doctor may suggest a catheter if you are incontinent because your bladder never empties completely (overflow incontinence). This is also an option if your bladder cannot empty because of poor muscle tone, past surgery, or a spinal cord injury.

Section 58.3

Urinary Tract Infections in Women

This section includes text excerpted from "Urinary Tract Infections," Office on Women's Health (OWH), U.S. Department of Health and Human Services (HHS), December 23, 2014.

What Is a Urinary Tract Infection (UTI)?

A urinary tract infection (UTI) is an infection anywhere in the urinary tract. The urinary tract makes and stores urine and removes it from the body. Parts of the urinary tract include:

- **Kidneys**—collect waste from blood to make urine

- **Ureters**—carry the urine from the kidneys to the bladder

- **Bladder**—stores urine until it is full

- **Urethra**—a short tube that carries urine from the bladder out of your body when you pass urine

What Causes UTIs?

Bacteria, a type of germ that gets into your urinary tract, cause a UTI. This can happen in many ways:

- Wiping from back to front after a bowel movement (BM). Germs can get into your urethra, which has its opening in front of the vagina.

- Having sexual intercourse. Germs in the vagina can be pushed into the urethra.

- Waiting too long to pass urine. When urine stays in the bladder for a long time, more germs are made, and the worse a UTI can become.

- Using a diaphragm for birth control, or spermicides (creams that kill sperm) with a diaphragm or on a condom.

- Anything that makes it hard to completely empty your bladder, like a kidney stone.

- Having diabetes, which makes it harder for your body to fight other health problems.

- Loss of estrogen (a hormone) and changes in the vagina after menopause. Menopause is when you stop getting your period.

- Having had a catheter in place. A catheter is a thin tube put through the urethra into the bladder. It's used to drain urine during a medical test and for people who cannot pass urine on their own.

What Are the Signs of a UTI?

If you have an infection, you may have some or all of these signs:

- Pain or stinging when you pass urine.

- An urge to pass urine a lot, but not much comes out when you go.

- Pressure in your lower belly.

- Urine that smells bad or looks milky, cloudy, or reddish in color. If you see blood in your urine, tell a doctor right away.

- Feeling tired or shaky or having a fever.

How Does a Doctor Find out If I Have a Urinary Tract Infection (UTI)?

To find out if you have a UTI, your doctor will need to test a clean sample of your urine. The doctor or nurse will give you a clean plastic cup and a special wipe. Wash your hands before opening the cup. When you open the cup, don't touch the inside of the lid or inside of the cup. Put the cup in easy reach. Separate the labia, the outer lips of the vagina, with one hand. With your other hand, clean the genital area with the wipe. Wipe from front to back. Do not touch or wipe the anus. While still holding the labia open, pass a little bit of urine into the toilet. Then, catch the rest in the cup. This is called a "clean-catch" sample. Let the rest of the urine fall into the toilet.

If you are prone to UTIs, your doctor may want to take pictures of your urinary tract with an X-ray or ultrasound. These pictures can show swelling, stones, or blockage. Your doctor also may want to look inside your bladder using a cystoscope. It is a small tube that's put into the urethra to see inside of the urethra and bladder.

How Is a UTI Treated?

UTIs are treated with antibiotics, medicines that kill the bacteria that cause the infection. Your doctor will tell you how long you need to take the medicine. Make sure you take all of your medicine, even if you feel better! Many women feel better in one or two days.

If you don't take medicine for a UTI, the UTI can hurt other parts of your body. Also, if you're pregnant and have signs of a UTI, see your doctor right away. A UTI could cause problems in your pregnancy, such as having your baby too early or getting high blood pressure. Also, UTIs in pregnant women are more likely to travel to the kidneys.

Will a UTI Hurt My Kidneys?

If treated right away, a UTI is not likely to damage your kidneys or urinary tract. But UTIs that are not treated can cause serious problems in your kidneys and the rest of your body.

How Can I Keep from Getting UTIs?

These are steps you can take to try to prevent a UTI. But you may follow these steps and still get a UTI. If you have symptoms of a UTI, call your doctor.

- Urinate when you need to. Don't hold it. Pass urine before and after sex. After you pass urine or have a bowel movement (BM), wipe from front to back.

- Drink water every day and after sex. Try for 6 to 8 glasses a day.

- Clean the outer lips of your vagina and anus each day. The anus is the place where a bowel movement leaves your body, located between the buttocks.

- Don't use douches or feminine hygiene sprays.

- If you get a lot of UTIs and use spermicides, or creams that kill sperm, talk to your doctor about using other forms of birth control.

- Wear underpants with a cotton crotch. Don't wear tight-fitting pants, which can trap in moisture.

- Take showers instead of tub baths.

I Get UTIs a Lot. Can My Doctor Do Something to Help?

About one in five women who get UTIs will get another one. Some women get three or more UTIs a year. If you are prone to UTIs, ask your doctor about your treatment options. Your doctor may ask you to take a small dose of medicine every day to prevent infection. Or, your doctor might give you a supply of antibiotics to take after sex or at the first sign of infection. "Dipsticks" can help test for UTIs at home. They are useful for some women with repeat UTIs. Ask your doctor if you should use dipsticks at home to test for UTI. Your doctor may also want to do special tests to see what is causing repeat infections.

Part Seven

Additional Help and Information

Chapter 59

Glossary of Women's Health Terms

allergies: Allergies are disorders that involve an immune response in the body. Allergies are reactions to allergens such as plant pollen, other grasses and weeds, certain foods, rubber latex, insect bites, or certain drugs.

Alzheimer disease: Alzheimer disease is a brain disease that cripples the brain's nerve cells over time and destroys memory and learning.

anemia: Anemia occurs when the amount of red blood cells or hemoglobin becomes reduced, causing fatigue that can be severe.

bacterial vaginosis: A vaginal infection that develops when there is an increase in harmful bacteria in the vagina.

blood pressure: Blood pressure is the force of blood against the walls of arteries. Blood pressure is noted as two numbers—the systolic pressure (as the heart beats) over the diastolic pressure (as the heart relaxes between beats). The numbers are written one above or before the other, with the systolic number on top and the diastolic number on the bottom. For example, a blood pressure reading of 120/80 mmHg (millimeters of mercury) is called 120 over 80.

This glossary contains terms excerpted from documents produced by several sources deemed reliable.

diabetes: Diabetes is a disease in which blood glucose (blood sugar) levels are above normal.

eating disorder: Eating disorders, such as anorexia nervosa, bulimia nervosa, and binge-eating disorder, involve serious problems with eating. This could include an extreme decrease of food or severe over-eating, as well as feelings of distress and concern about body shape or weight.

ectopic pregnancy: This is a pregnancy that is not in the uterus. It happens when a fertilized egg settles and grows in a place other than the inner lining of the uterus. Most happen in the fallopian tube but can happen in the ovary, cervix, or abdominal cavity.

endometriosis: Endometriosis is a condition in which tissue that normally lines the uterus grows in other areas of the body, usually inside the abdominal cavity, but acts as if it were inside the uterus.

estrogen: Estrogen is a group of female hormones that are responsible for the development of breasts and other secondary sex characteristics in women.

fallopian tubes: Tubes on each side of ovaries to the uterus.

genetic counseling: This type of counseling is a communication process between a specially trained health professional and a person concerned about the genetic risk of disease. The person's family and personal medical history may be discussed, and counseling may lead to genetic testing.

heart disease: Heart disease involves a number of abnormal conditions affecting the heart and the blood vessels in the heart. The most common type of heart disease is coronary artery disease, which is the gradual buildup of plaques in the coronary arteries, the blood vessels that bring blood to the heart.

hormone: A hormone is a substance produced by one tissue and conveyed by the bloodstream to another to effect a function of the body, such as growth or metabolism.

immune system: The immune system is a complex system in the body that recognizes and responds to potentially harmful substances, like infections, in order to protect the body.

immunization: Also called vaccination, an immunization is a shot that contains germs that have been killed or weakened. When given to a healthy person, it triggers the immune system to respond and build immunity to a disease.

infertility: Infertility refers to a condition in which a couple has problems conceiving, or getting pregnant, after one year of regular sexual intercourse without using any birth control methods.

inflammation: This term is used to describe an area on the body that is swollen, red, hot, and in pain.

inflammatory bowel disease (IBD): IBD is a long-lasting problems that cause irritation and ulcers in the gastrointestinal tract.

influenza: Also called the flu, influenza is a respiratory infection caused by multiple viruses. The viruses pass through the air and enter the body through the nose or mouth.

lactation: The production and secretion of milk by the breast glands.

menopausal hormone therapy (MHT): MHT replaces the hormones that a woman's ovaries stop making at the time of menopause, easing symptoms like hot flashes and vaginal dryness.

menopause: The time of life when a woman's ovaries stop working and menstrual periods stop. A woman is said to be in menopause when she hasn't had a period for 12 months in a row.

menstrual cycle: The menstrual cycle is a recurring cycle in which the lining of the uterus thickens in preparation for pregnancy and then is shed if pregnancy does not occur.

migraine: Migraine is a medical condition that usually involves a very painful headache, usually felt on one side of the head. Besides intense pain, migraine also can cause nausea and vomiting and sensitivity to light and sound.

nerves: Nerves are cells in the human body that are the building blocks of the nervous system (the system that records and transmits information chemically and electrically within a person).

obesity: Obesity means having too much body fat. People with a body mass index (BMI) of 30 or higher are obese.

osteoarthritis (OA): OA is a joint disease that mostly affects cartilage, the slippery tissue that covers the ends of bones in a joint. The top layer of cartilage breaks down and wears away. This allows bones under the cartilage to rub together, which causes pain, swelling, and loss of motion of the joint.

osteoporosis: Osteoporosis is a bone disease that is characterized by progressive loss of bone density and thinning of bone tissue, causing bones to break easily.

ovarian cancer: This is cancer of the ovary or ovaries, which are organs in the female reproductive system that make eggs and hormones. Most ovarian cancers develop from the cells that cover the outer surface of the ovary, called epithelial cells.

ovary (ovaries): Part of a woman's reproductive system, the ovaries produce her eggs. Each month, through the process called ovulation, the ovaries release eggs into the fallopian tubes, where they travel to the uterus, or womb. If an egg is fertilized by a man's sperm, a woman becomes pregnant and the egg grows and develops inside the uterus.

ovulation: Ovulation is the release of a single egg from a follicle that developed in the ovary. It usually occurs regularly, around day 14 of a 28-day menstrual cycle.

Pap test: A procedure in which cells and secretions are collected from inside and around the cervix for examination under a microscope.

pelvic exam: During this exam, the doctor or nurse practitioner looks for redness, swelling, discharge, or sores on the outside and inside of the vagina. A Pap test tests for cell changes on the cervix.

pelvic inflammatory disease: Pelvic inflammatory disease is an infection of the female reproductive organs that are above the cervix, such as the fallopian tubes and ovaries. It is the most common and serious problem caused by sexually transmitted diseases.

perimenopause: This is the phase in a woman's reproductive life-cycle leading up to menopause. During perimenopause, a woman's body slowly makes less of the hormones estrogen and progesterone. This causes some women to have symptoms such as hot flashes and changes in their periods.

perinatal asphyxia: This condition occurs when the baby does not get enough oxygen in the uterus or during labor and delivery.

polycystic ovary syndrome (PCOS): PCOS is a health problem that can affect a woman's menstrual cycle, ability to have children, hormones, heart, blood vessels, and appearance. With PCOS, women typically have high levels of androgens or male hormones, missed or irregular periods, and many small cysts in their ovaries.

postpartum depression (PPD): Postpartum depression is a serious condition that requires treatment from a healthcare provider. With this condition, feelings of the baby blues (feeling sad, anxious, afraid, or confused after having a baby) do not go away or get worse.

preconception health: This involves a woman's health before she becomes pregnant. It involves knowing how health conditions and risk factors could affect a woman or her unborn baby if she becomes pregnant.

preeclampsia: Also known as toxemia, preeclampsia is a syndrome occurring in a pregnant woman after her 20th week of pregnancy that causes high blood pressure and problems with the kidneys and other organs.

premenstrual syndrome (PMS): PMS is a group of symptoms linked to the menstrual cycle that occur in the week or two weeks before menstruation. The symptoms usually go away after menstruation begins and can include acne, breast swelling and tenderness, feeling tired, having trouble sleeping, upset stomach, bloating, constipation or diarrhea, headache or backache, appetite changes or food cravings, joint or muscle pain, trouble concentrating or remembering, tension, irritability, mood swings or crying spells, and anxiety or depression.

preterm birth: Also called premature birth, it is a birth that occurs before the 37th week of pregnancy.

progesterone: Progesterone is a female hormone produced by the ovaries. Progesterone, along with estrogen, prepares the uterus (womb) for a possible pregnancy each month and supports the fertilized egg if conception occurs. Progesterone also helps prepare the breasts for milk production and breastfeeding.

progestin: Progestin is a hormone that works by causing changes in the uterus. When taken with the hormone estrogen, progestin works to prevent thickening of the lining of the uterus.

psychosis: A mental disorder characterized by delusional or disordered thinking detached from reality; symptoms often include hallucinations.

puberty: Puberty is the time when the body is changing from the body of a child to the body of an adult. This process begins earlier in girls than in boys, usually between ages 8 and 13.

radical mastectomy: Surgery for breast cancer in which the breast, chest muscles, and all of the lymph nodes under the arm are removed.

sexually transmitted disease: An infectious disease that spreads from person to person during sexual contact.

tamoxifen: A drug used to treat certain types of breast cancer in women. It is also used to prevent breast cancer in women who have had ductal carcinoma in situ and in women who are at a high risk of developing breast cancer.

thyroid: The thyroid is a small gland in the neck that makes and stores hormones that help regulate heart rate, blood pressure, body temperature, and the rate at which food is converted into energy.

tumor: A tumor is an abnormal mass of tissue that results when cells divide more than they should or do not die when they should.

ultrasound: This is a painless, harmless test that uses sound waves to produce images of the organs and structures of the body on a screen.

urinary tract infection (UTI): A UTI is an infection anywhere in the urinary tract, or organs that collect and store urine and release it from your body (the kidneys, ureters, bladder, and urethra). An infection occurs when microorganisms, usually bacteria from the digestive tract, cling to the urethra (opening to the urinary tract) and begin to multiply.

uterine fibroids: Fibroids are common, benign tumors that grow in the muscle of the uterus, or womb.

uterus: The uterus is a woman's womb, or the hollow, pear-shaped organ located in a woman's lower abdomen between the bladder and the rectum.

yeast infections: Yeast infections are common infections in women caused by an overgrowth of the fungus *Candida*. It is normal to have some yeast in your vagina, but sometimes it can overgrow because of hormonal changes in your body, such as during pregnancy, or from taking certain medications, such as antibiotics.

weight control: This refers to achieving and maintaining a healthy weight with healthy eating and physical activity.

Chapter 60

Directory of Women's Health Resources and Organizations

General Women's Health Resources

Agency for Healthcare Research and Quality (AHRQ)
Office of Communications and Knowledge Transfer
5600 Fishers Ln.
Seventh Fl.
Rockville, MD 20857
Toll-Free: 800-358-9295
Phone: 301-427-1104
Toll-Free TDD: 888-586-6340
Website: www.ahrq.gov/contact/index.html

American Academy of Family Physicians (AAFP)
P.O. Box 11210
Shawnee Mission, KS 66207-1210
Toll-Free: 800-274-2237
Phone: 913-906-6000
Fax: 913-906-6075
Website: www.nf.aafp.org/myacademy/contactus

Resources in this chapter were compiled from several sources deemed reliable; all contact information was verified and updated in August 2017.

American College of Obstetricians and Gynecologists (ACOG)
409 12th St. S.W.
P.O. Box 70620
Washington, DC 20024-9998
Toll-Free: 800-673-8444
Phone: 202-638-5577
Website: www.acog.org/
About-ACOG/Contact-Us
E-mail: resources@acog.org

Centers for Disease Control and Prevention (CDC)
1600 Clifton Rd.
Atlanta, GA 30329-4027
Toll-Free: 800-CDC-INFO
(800-232-4636)
Toll-Free TTY: 888-232-6348
Website: www.cdc.gov/women
E-mail: cdcinfo@cdc.gov

Healthfinder.gov
U.S. Department of Health and
Human Services (HHS)
1101 Wootton Pkwy
Rockville, MD 20852
Website: www.healthfinder.gov/
aboutus/contactus.aspx
E-mail: healthfinder@hhs.gov

HealthyWomen
National Women's Health
Resource Center (NWHRC)
P.O. Box 430
Red Bank, NJ 07701
Toll-Free: 877-986-9472
Phone: 732-530-3425
Fax: 732-865-7225
Website: www.healthywomen.
org/about-us/contact-us
E-mail: info@healthywomen.org

MedlinePlus
Website: www.medlineplus.gov

National Center for Complementary and Integrative Health (NCCIH)
NCCIH Clearinghouse
P.O. Box 7923
Gaithersburg, MD 20898-7923
Toll-Free: 888-644-6226
Toll-Free TTY: 866-464-3615
Toll-Free Fax: 866-464-3616
Website: www.nccih.nih.
gov/research/camonpubmed/
background.htm
E-mail: info@nccih.nih.gov

National Institute of Allergy and Infectious Diseases (NIAID)
Office of Communications and
Government Relations
5601 Fishers Ln.
MSC 9806
Bethesda, MD 20892-9806
Toll-Free: 866-284-4107
Phone: 301-496-5717
TDD: 800-877-8339
Fax: 301-402-3573
Website: www.niaid.nih.gov/
global/contact-us
E-mail: ocpostoffice@niaid.nih.gov

National Institute of Diabetes and Digestive and Kidney Diseases (NIDDK)
Office of Communications and
Public Liaison NIDDK, NIH
Bldg. 31 Rm. 9A06
31 Center Dr. MSC 2560
Bethesda, MD 20892-2560
Phone: 301-435-8115
Website: www.niddk.nih.gov

National Institute on Aging (NIA)
Bldg. 31 Rm. 5C27
31 Center Dr. MSC 2292
Bethesda, MD 20892
Toll-Free: 800-222-2225
Phone: 301-496-1752
Toll-Free TTY: 800-222-4225
Fax: 301-496-1072
Website: www.nia.nih.gov
E-mail: info@niapublications.org

National Women's Health Network (NWHN)
1413 K St. N.W.
Fourth Fl.
Washington, D.C. 20005
Phone: 202-628-2640
Fax: 202-682-2648
Website: www.nwhn.org/
contact-us
E-mail: nwhn@nwhn.org

Office of Minority Health (OMH) Resource Center
P.O. Box 37337
Washington, DC 20013-7337
Toll Free: 800-444-6472
Phone: 240-453-2882
TDD: 301-251-1432
Fax: 301-251-2160
Website: www.minorityhealth.
hhs.gov/omh/content.
aspx?lvl=1&lvlid=1&ID=10116
E-mail: info@minorityhealth.
hhs.gov

Office of Research on Women's Health (ORWH)
National Institutes of Health (NIH)
6707 Democracy Blvd.
Bethesda, MD 20817
Phone: 301-402-1770
Fax: 301-402-0005
Website: www.orwh.od.nih.gov/
about/contact

Office on Women's Health (OWH)
200 Independence Ave. S.W.
Rm. 712E
Washington, DC 20201
Toll-Free: 800-994-9662
Phone: 202-690-7650
Fax: 202-205-2631
Website: www.womenshealth.
gov/contact-us

Society for Women's Health Research (SWHR)
1025 Connecticut Ave. N.W.
Ste. 601
Washington, DC 20036
Phone: 202-223-8224
Fax: 202-833-3472
Website: www.swhr.org/about/
contact-us
E-mail: info@swhr.org

U.S. Food and Drug Administration (FDA)
10903 New Hampshire Ave.
WO32-2333
Silver Spring, MD 20993
Toll-Free: 888-INFO-FDA
(888-463-6332)
Phone: 301-796-9440
Website: www.fda.gov

Weight-Control Information Network (WIN)
National Institute of Diabetes and Digestive and Kidney Diseases (NIDDK)
1 WIN Way
Bethesda, MD 20892-3665
Toll-Free: 877-946-4627
Phone: 202-828-1025
Fax: 202-828-1028
Website: www.niddk.nih.gov/
health-information/health-
communication-programs/win/
win-health-topics/media-kit/
Documents/WIN_MediaKit.pdf
E-mail: win@info.niddk.nih.gov

Allergies and Asthma

American College of Rheumatology (ACR)
2200 Lake Blvd. N.E.
Atlanta, GA 30319
Phone: 404-633-3777
Fax: 404-633-1870
Website: www.rheumatology.org/
Contact
E-mail: website@rheumatology.
org

Arthritis Foundation
National Office
1355 Peachtree St. N.E.
Ste. 600
Atlanta, GA 30309
Toll-Free: 800-283-7800
Phone: 404-872-7100
Website: www.arthritis.org/
about-us/contact-us.php

Asthma and Allergy Foundation of America (AAFA)
8201 Corporate Dr.
Ste. 1000
Landover, MD 20785
Toll-Free: 800-7-ASTHMA
(800-727-8462)
Website: www.aafa.org
E-mail: info@aafa.org

National Institute of Arthritis and Musculoskeletal and Skin Diseases (NIAMS)
Information Clearinghouse
1 AMS Cir.
Bethesda, MD 20892-3675
Toll-Free: 877-22-NIAMS
(877-226-4267)
Phone: 301-495-4484
TYY: 301-565-2966
Fax: 312-718-6366
Website: www.niams.nih.gov/
About_Us/Contact_Us/default.
asp
E-mail: NIAMSinfo@mail.nih.
gov

National Osteoporosis Foundation (NOF)
1150 17th St. N.W.
Ste. 850
Washington, DC 20036
Toll-Free: 800-231-4222
Phone: 202-223-2226
Fax: 202-223-2237
Website: www.nof.org/
privacy-policy
E-mail: info@nof.org

Cancer

American Cancer Society (ACS)
250 Williams St. N.W.
Atlanta, GA 30303
Toll-Free: 800-227-2345
Website: www.cancer.org/
about-us/online-help/contact-us.
html

Foundation for Women's Cancer (FWC)
230 W. Monroe St.
Ste. 710
Chicago, IL 60606-4902
Toll-Free: 800-444-4441 (hotline)
Phone: 312-578-1439
Fax: 312-235-4059
Website: www.
foundationforwomenscancer.org/
contact-us
E-mail: FWCinfo@sgo.org

National Cancer Institute (NCI)
9609 Medical Center Dr.
BG 9609 MSC 9760
Bethesda, MD 20892-9760
Toll-Free: 800-4-CANCER
(800-422-6237)
Toll-Free TTY: 800-332-8615
Website: www.cancer.gov/
contact

National Ovarian Cancer Coalition (NOCC)
2501 Oak Lawn Ave.
Ste. 435
Dallas, TX 75219
Toll-Free: 888-OVARIAN
(888-682-7426)
Phone: 214-273-4200
Fax: 214-273-4201
Website: www.ovarian.org
E-mail: nocc@ovarian.org

The Skin Cancer Foundation (SCF)
149 Madison Ave.
Ste. 901
New York, NY 10016
Phone: 212-725-5176
Website: www.skincancer.org/
contact-us

Susan G. Komen for the Cure
5005 LBJ Fwy
Ste. 250
Dallas, TX 75244
Toll-Free: 877-GO-KOMEN
(877-465-6636)
Website: ww5.komen.org/
Contact.aspx
E-mail: Helpline@komen.org

Children and Young Adults

Eunice Kennedy Shriver
National Institute of
Child Health and Human
Development (NICHD)
Information Resource Center
P.O. Box 3006
Rockville, MD 20847
Toll-Free: 800-370-2943
Toll-Free TTY: 888-320-6942
Toll-Free Fax: 866-760-5947
Website: www.nichd.nih.gov/
Pages/Contact.aspx
E-mail: NICHDInformation
ResourceCenter@mail.nih.gov

GirlsHealth.gov
200 Independence Ave. S.W.
Rm. 712E
Washington, DC 2020
Toll-Free: 800-994-9662
Website: www.girlshealth.gov/
contact

Diabetes

American Diabetes
Association (ADA)
Center for Information
2451 Crystal Dr.
Ste. 900
Arlington, VA 22202
Toll-Free: 800-DIABETES
(800-342-2383)
Website: www.diabetes.org/
about-us/contact-us/center-for-
information.html
E-mail: askada@diabetes.org

National Diabetes Education
Program (NDEP)
1 Diabetes Way
Bethesda, MD 20814-9692
Toll-Free: 888-693-NDEP
(888-693-6337)
TTY: 866-569-1162
Fax: 703-738-4929
Website: www.ndep.nih.gov
E-mail: ndep@mail.nih.gov

National Diabetes
Information Clearinghouse
(NDIC)
1 Information Way
Bethesda, MD 20892-3560
Toll-Free: 800-860-8747
TTY: 866-569-1162
Fax: 703-738-4929
Website: www.diabetes.niddk.
nih.gov
E-mail: ndic@info.niddk.nih.gov

Eating Disorders

National Association of
Anorexia Nervosa and
Associated Disorders (ANAD)
220 N. Green St.
Chicago, IL 60607
Toll-Free Helpline: 630-577-
1330 (9 a.m. to 5 p.m. CST,
Monday–Friday)
Phone: 630-577-1333
Website: www.anad.org/
get-information/about-anad
E-mail: hello@anad.org

National Eating Disorders Association (NEDA)
200 W. 41st St.
Ste. 1203
New York, NY 10036
Toll-Free Hotline: 800-931-2237
Phone: 212-575-6200
Fax: 212-575-1650
Website: www.
nationaleatingdisorders.org/
contact-us
E-mail: info@
NationalEatingDisorders.org

Gastrointestinal and Digestive Disorders

Academy of Nutrition and Dietetics
120 S. Riverside Plaza
Ste. 2190
Chicago, IL 60606-6995
Toll-Free: 800-877-1600
Phone: 312-899-0040
Website: www.eatrightpro.org/
resource/about-us/academy-
vision-and-mission/who-we-are/
contact-us
E-mail: knowledge@eatright.org

American Celiac Disease Alliance (ACDA)
2504 Duxbury Pl.
Alexandria, VA 22308
Phone: 703-622-3331
Website: www.americanceliac.
org
E-mail: info@americanceliac.org

American College of Gastroenterology (ACG)
6400 Goldsboro Rd.
Ste. 200
Bethesda, MD 20817
Phone: 301-263-9000
Website: www.gi.org
E-mail: info@gi.org

American Gastroenterological Association (AGA)
4930 Del Ray Ave.
Bethesda, MD 20814
Phone: 301-654-2055
Fax: 301-654-5920
Website: www.gastro.org/
contact/contact-aga
E-mail: member@gastro.org

Celiac Disease Foundation (CDF)
20350 Ventura Blvd.
Ste. 240
Woodland Hills, CA 91364
Phone: 818-716-1513
Toll-Free Fax: 818-267-5577
Website: www.celiac.org
E-mail: cdf@celiac.org

Crohn's and Colitis Foundation of America (CCFA)
733 3rd Ave., Ste. 510
New York, NY 10017
Toll-Free: 800-932-2423
Phone: 212-685-3440
Fax: 212-779-4098
Website: www.ccfa.org
E-mail: info@
crohnscolitisfoundation.org

National Digestive Diseases Information Clearinghouse (NDDIC)
2 Information Way
Bethesda, MD 20892-3570
Toll-Free: 800-891-5389
TTY: 866-569-1162
Fax: 703-738-4929
Website: www.digestive.niddk.nih.gov
E-mail: nddic@info.niddk.nih.go

Immunizations

Immunization Action Coalition (IAC)
2550 University Ave. W.
Ste. 415 N.
Saint Paul, MN 55114
Phone: 651-647-9009
Fax: 651-647-9131
Website: www.immunize.org/aboutus/contactus.asp
E-mail: admin@immunize.org

National Center for Immunization and Respiratory Diseases (NCIRD)
1600 Clifton Rd.
Atlanta, GA 30329-4027
Toll-Free: 800-CDC-INFO
(800-232-4636)
Toll-Free TTY: 888-232-6348
Website: www.cdc.gov/ncird/contact.html
E-mail: ncirddvdinquiry@cdc.gov

Heart and Lung Health

American Heart Association (AHA)
7272 Greenville Ave.
Dallas, TX 75231
Toll-Free: 800-AHA-USA-1
(800-242-8721)
Website: www.americanheart.org/HEARTORG

American Lung Association
1301 Pennsylvania Ave. N.W.
Ste. 800
Washington, DC 20004
Toll-Free: 800-LUNGUSA
(800-548-8252)
Phone: 212-315-8700
Fax: 202-452-1805
Website: www.lungusa.org
E-mail: info@lung.org

National Heart, Lung, and Blood Institute (NHLBI)
NHLBI Health Information Center
P.O. Box 30105
Bethesda, MD 20824-0105
Phone: 301-592-8573
TTY: 240-629-3255
Fax: 301-592-8563
Website: www.nhlbi.nih.gov/about/contact
E-mail: nhlbiinfo@nhlbi.nih.gov

WomenHeart: The National Coalition for Women with Heart Disease
1100 17th St. N.W.
Ste. 500
Washington, DC 20036
Phone: 202-728-7199
Fax: 202-728-7238
Website: www.womenheart.
org/?page=ContactUs
E-mail: mail@womenheart.org

Mental Health

National Institute of Mental Health (NIMH)
6001 Executive Blvd.
Rm. 6200 MSC 9663
Bethesda, MD 20892-9663
Toll-Free: 866-615-6464
Phone: 301-443-4513
Toll-Free TTY: 866-415-8051
TTY: 301-443-8431
Fax: 301-443-4279
Website: www.nimh.nih.gov/site-info/contact-nimh.shtml
E-mail: nimhinfo@nih.gov

Substance Abuse and Mental Health Services Administration (SAMHSA)
SAMHSA's Health Information Network
P.O. Box 2345
Rockville, MD 20847-2345
Toll-Free: 877-SAMHSA-7
(877-726-4727)

Neurological Disorders

National Institute of Neurological Disorders and Stroke (NINDS)
P.O. Box 5801
Bethesda, MD 20824
Toll-Free: 800-352-9424
Phone: 301-496-5751
Website: www.ninds.nih.gov/
Contact-Us

Reproductive Health

American Pregnancy Association
3007 Skyway Cir. N., Ste. 800
Irving, TX 75038
Toll-Free: 800-672-2296
Phone: 972-550-0140
Website: www.
americanpregnancy.org/contact
E-mail: info@
americanpregnancy.org

March of Dimes
1275 Mamaroneck Ave.
White Plains, NY 10605
Phone: 914-997-4488
Website: www.marchofdimes.
org/contact-us.aspx

Planned Parenthood Federation of America
123 William St.
10th Fl.
New York, NY 10038
Toll-Free: 800-230-PLAN
(800-230-7526)
Phone: 212-541-7800
Fax: 212-245-1845
Website: www.
plannedparenthood.org/
about-us/contact-us

Urologic Health

National Kidney and Urologic Diseases Information Clearinghouse (NKUDIC)

3 Information Way
Bethesda, MD 20892-3580
Toll-Free: 800-891-5390
Toll-Free TTY: 866-569-1162
Fax: 703-738-4929
Website: www.kidney.niddk.nih.
gov
E-mail: nkudic@info.niddk.nih.
gov

Urology Care Foundation

1000 Corporate Blvd.
Linthicum, MD 21090
Toll-Free: 800-828-7866
Phone: 410-689-3700
Fax: 410-689-3998
Website: www.urologyhealth.org
E-mail: info@
UrologyCareFoundation.org

Index

Index

Page numbers followed by 'n' indicate a footnote. Page numbers in *italics* indicate a table or illustration.